Wound Healing

METHODS IN MOLECULAR MEDICINE™

John M. Walker, SERIES EDITOR

85. **Novel Anticancer Drug Protocols,** edited by *John K. Buolamwini and Alex A. Adjei,* 2003

84. **Opioid Research:** *Methods and Protocols,* edited by *Sabire Özcan,* 2003

83. **Diabetes Mellitus:** *Methods and Protocols,* edited by *Zhizhong Z. Pan,* 2003

82. **Hemoglobin Disorders:** *Molecular Methods and Protocols,* edited by *Ronald L. Nagel,* 2003

81. **Prostate Cancer Methods and Protocols,** edited by *Pamela J. Russell, Paul Jackson, and Elizabeth A. Kingsley,* 2003

80. **Bone Research Protocols,** edited by *Stuart H. Ralston and Miep H. Helfrich,* 2003

79. **Drugs of Abuse:** *Neurological Reviews and Protocols,* edited by *John Q. Wang,* 2003

78. **Wound Healing:** *Methods and Protocols,* edited by *Luisa A. DiPietro and Aime L. Burns,* 2003

77. **Psychiatric Genetics:** *Methods and Reviews,* edited by *Marion Leboyer and Frank Bellivier,* 2003

76. **Viral Vectors for Gene Therapy:** *Methods and Protocols,* edited by *Curtis A. Machida,* 2003

75. **Lung Cancer:** *Volume 2, Diagnostic and Therapeutic Methods and Reviews,* edited by *Barbara Driscoll,* 2003

74. **Lung Cancer:** *Volume 1, Molecular Pathology Methods and Reviews,* edited by *Barbara Driscoll,* 2003

73. **E. coli:** *Shiga Toxin Methods and Protocols,* edited by *Dana Philpott and Frank Ebel,* 2003

72. **Malaria Methods and Protocols,** edited by *Denise L. Doolan,* 2002

71. *Hemophilus influenzae* **Protocols,** edited by *Mark A. Herbert, Derek W. Hood, and E. Richard Moxon,* 2002

70. **Cystic Fibrosis Methods and Protocols,** edited by *William R. Skach,* 2002

69. **Gene Therapy Protocols,** *2nd ed.,* edited by *Jeffrey R. Morgan,* 2002

68. **Molecular Analysis of Cancer,** edited by *Jacqueline Boultwood and Carrie Fidler,* 2002

67. **Meningococcal Disease:** *Methods and Protocols,* edited by *Andrew J. Pollard and Martin C. J. Maiden,* 2001

66. **Meningococcal Vaccines:** *Methods and Protocols,* edited by *Andrew J. Pollard and Martin C. J. Maiden,* 2001

65. **Nonviral Vectors for Gene Therapy:** *Methods and Protocols,* edited by *Mark A. Findeis,* 2001

64. **Dendritic Cell Protocols,** edited by *Stephen P. Robinson and Andrew J. Stagg,* 2001

63. **Hematopoietic Stem Cell Protocols,** edited by *Christopher A. Klug and Craig T. Jordan,* 2001

62. **Parkinson's Disease:** *Methods and Protocols,* edited by *M. Maral Mouradian,* 2001

61. **Melanoma:** *Methods and Protocols,* edited by *Brian J. Nickoloff,* 2001

60. **Interleukin Protocols,** edited by *Luke A. J. O'Neill and Andrew Bowie,* 2001

59. **Molecular Pathology of the Prions,** edited by *Harry F. Baker,* 2001

58. **Metastasis Research Protocols:** *Volume 2, Cell Behavior In Vitro and In Vivo,* edited by *Susan A. Brooks and Udo Schumacher,* 2001

57. **Metastasis Research Protocols:** *Volume 1, Analysis of Cells and Tissues,* edited by *Susan A. Brooks and Udo Schumacher,* 2001

56. **Human Airway Inflammation:** *Sampling Techniques and Analytical Protocols,* edited by *Duncan F. Rogers and Louise E. Donnelly,* 2001

METHODS IN MOLECULAR MEDICINE™

Wound Healing

Methods and Protocols

Edited by

Luisa A. DiPietro

*Department of Surgery, Burn and Shock Trauma Institute,
Loyola University Medical Center, Maywood, IL*

and

Aime L. Burns

*Department of Surgery, Burn and Shock Trauma Institute,
Loyola University Medical Center, Maywood, IL*

Humana Press Totowa, New Jersey

BS

Production Editor: Tracy Catanese
Cover design by Patricia F. Cleary.

Cover illustration: Figures 3E and F from Chapter 13/Growth of Human Blood Vessels in Severe Combined Immunodeficient Mice: A New In Vivo Model System of Angiogenesis by Peter J. Poverini, Jacques E. Nör, Martin C. Peters, and David J. Mooney.

Printed in the United States of America. 10 9 8 7 6 5 4 3 2 1

Library of Congress Cataloging in Publication Data

Wound healing : methods and protocols / edited by Luisa A. DiPietro and Aime L. Burns.
       p. cm. -- (Methods in molecular medicine ; 78)
    Includes bibliographical references and index.
       ISBN 0-89603-999-4 (alk. paper);1-59259-332-1 (e-book)
       1. Wound healing--Research. 2. Wound healing--Animal models. I. DiPietro, Luisa A.
II. Burns, Aime L. III. Series.

RD94.W695 2003
617.1'4027--dc21   2002027304

8/27/04

Preface

During the past decade, significant progress in molecular and cellular techniques has greatly advanced our understanding of the wound healing process. Many of these new techniques have been utilized in the context of more classic models of wound healing. The combination of new and classic approaches has allowed scientists to make exciting discoveries in the field of tissue repair, resulting in an explosion of information about the healing process. Importantly, these new findings have great relevance beyond wound healing itself. The injury repair process cuts across many disciplines, extending to such broad fields as cancer, inflammation, and atherosclerosis. The relevance of the field to these many disciplines has generated great interest in models and methods for the study of wound healing. The goal of *Wound Healing: Methods and Protocols* is to provide scientists from many disciplines with a compendium of classic and contemporary protocols from recognized experts in the field of wound healing. We hope this volume will be useful not only to those working within the field itself, but also to scientists from other disciplines who wish to adapt wound healing models to their own experimental needs.

The process of wound healing encompasses many different biologic processes, including epithelial growth and differentiation, fibrous tissue production and function, angiogenesis, and inflammation. For this reason, the choice of model systems is broad, and includes a large array of both in vivo and in vitro models. We could not, of course, include all of the many available experimental models of wound healing. Instead, we have attempted to assemble a cross section of practical techniques, many of which are widely used.

This volume is organized into two broad sections. Part I presents model systems for the study of wound healing, whereas Part II describes methods for the analysis and manipulation of the healing wound. Part I includes thirteen separate in vivo models and four in vitro models of wound healing, as well as several reviews of specific model systems in which underlying systemic and genetic conditions influence the healing process. Part II provides multiple methods for the analysis of the individual biologic processes observed in the healing wound. In many cases, several different approaches to a single process are provided in order to allow the scientist to select the approach most applicable to the problem at hand. We hope this text will become a valuable reference source for both basic and clinical scientists interested in initiating or expanding their efforts in the study of wound healing.

We are very grateful to our large group of contributors who gave so willingly of their expertise and provided the chapters within this volume. We wish to thank the series editor, Dr. John Walker, for his guidance during the development and realization of this book, and the president of Humana Press, Mr. Thomas Lanigan, for the opportunity to prepare this volume. We also thank Mr. Craig Adams at Humana Press and Mr. Benjamin Levi for their valuable editorial assistance. Finally, our sincere thanks to our families for their patience and encouragement during the completion of this book.

Luisa A. DiPietro
Aime L. Burns

Contents

Preface v

Contributors xi

PART I. EXPERIMENTAL MODELS OF WOUND HEALING

A. In Vivo Animal Models

1 Excisional Wound Healing:
   An Experimental Approach
   Stefan Frank and Heiko Kämpfer 3

2 Methods in Reepithelialization:
   A Porcine Model of Partial-Thickness Wounds
   Heather N. Paddock, Gregory S. Schultz, and Bruce A. Mast 17

3 Incisional Wound Healing:
   Model and Analysis of Wound Breaking Strength
   Richard L. Gamelli and Li-Ke He 37

4 Animal Models of Ischemic Wound Healing:
   *Toward an Approximation of Human Chronic
   Cutaneous Ulcers in Rabbit and Rat*
   Mark Sisco and Thomas A. Mustoe 55

5 Corneal Injury:
   *A Relatively Pure Model of Stromal-Epithelial Interactions
   in Wound Healing*
   **Steven E. Wilson, Rahul R. Mohan, Renato Ambrosio,
   and Rajiv R. Mohan** 67

6 Subcutaneous Sponge Models
   David T. Efron and Adrian Barbul 83

7 A Mouse Model of Burn Wounding and Sepsis
   Julia M. Stevenson, Richard L. Gamelli, and Ravi Shankar 95

8 A Porcine Burn Model
   Adam J. Singer and Steve A. McClain 107

9 Wound Healing in Airways In Vivo
   Steven R. White 121

10 Murine Models of Intestinal Anastomoses
    David L. Williams and I. William Browder 133

11 Murine Model of Peritoneal Adhesion Formation
    **Andrew E. Jahoda, Mary Kay Olson,
    and Elizabeth J. Kovacs** 141

vii

12 Methods for Investigating Fetal Tissue Repair
    **Ziv M. Peled, Stephen M. Warren, Pierre J. Bouletreau,
    and Michael T. Longaker** *149*

13 Growth of Human Blood Vessels in Severe Combined
    Immunodeficient Mice:
    A New in Vivo Model System of Angiogenesis
    **Peter J. Polverini, Jacques E. Nör, Martin C. Peters,
    and David J. Mooney** *161*

B. Reviews of Specific Model Systems

14 Tissue Repair in Models of Diabetes Mellitus: *A Review*
    David G. Greenhalgh *181*

15 Wound Healing Studies in Transgenic and Knockout Mice:
    A Review
    Richard Grose and Sabine Werner *191*

16 Wound Repair in Aging: *A Review*
    May J. Reed, Teruhiko Koike, and Pauli Puolakkainen *217*

C. Human Wound Healing Models

17 Specimen Collection and Analysis: *Burn Wounds*
    Areta Kowal-Vern and Barbara A. Latenser *241*

18 Suction Blister Model of Wound Healing
    Vesa Koivukangas and Aarne Oikarinen *255*

19 Implantable Wound Healing Models and the Determination
    of Subcutaneous Collagen Deposition in Expanded
    Polytetrafluoroethylene Implants
    **Lars Nannestad Jorgensen, Søren Munk Madsen,
    and Finn Gottrup** *263*

D. In Vitro Models

20 The Fibroblast Populated Collagen Lattice:
    A Model of Fibroblast Collagen Interactions in Repair
    H. Paul Ehrlich *277*

21 A Quantifiable In Vitro Model to Assess Effects
    of PAI-1 Gene Targeting on Epithelial Cell Motility
    **Kirwin M. Providence, Lisa Staiano-Coico,
    and Paul J. Higgins** *293*

22 Human Skin Organ Culture
    Ingrid Moll *305*

23 In Vitro Matrigel Angiogenesis Model
    Anna M. Szpaderska and Luisa A. DiPietro *311*

Part II. Analysis and Manipulation of Wound Healing

24 Quantification of Wound Angiogenesis
    Quentin E. H. Low and Luisa A. DiPietro 319

25 In Vivo Matrigel Migration and Angiogenesis Assays
    Katherine M. Malinda 329

26 Endothelial Cell Migration Assay:
    A Quantitative Assay for Prediction of In Vivo Biology
    Mark W. Lingen 337

27 Analysis of Collagen Synthesis
    Robert F. Diegelmann 349

28 Method for Detection and Quantitation of Leukocytes
    During Wound Healing
    Iulia Drugea and Aime L. Burns 359

29 Detection of Reactive Oxygen Intermediate Production
    by Macrophages
    Jorge E. Albina and Jonathan S. Reichner 369

30 Measurement of Chemokines at the Protein Level in Tissue
    **Robert M. Strieter, Marie D. Burdick, John A. Belperio,
    and Michael P. Keane** 377

31 Methods of Measuring Oxygen in Wounds
    **Harriet W. Hopf, Thomas K. Hunt, Heinz Scheuenstuhl,
    Judith M. West, Lisa M. Humphrey, and Mark D. Rollins** 389

32 Isolation, Culture, and Characterization of Human Intestinal
    Smooth Muscle Cells
    Martin Graham and Amy Willey 417

33 Use of High-Throughput Microarray Membranes
    for cDNA Analysis of Cutaneous Wound Repair
    Nicole S. Gibran and F. Frank Isik 425

34 Particle-Mediated Gene Therapy of Wounds
    **Jeffrey M. Davidson, Sabine A. Eming,
    and Jayasri Dasgupta** 433

Index 453

Contributors

JORGE E. ALBINA • *Division of Surgical Research, Department of Surgery, Rhode Island Hospital and Brown Medical School, Providence, RI*

RENATO AMBROSIO • *Department of Ophthalmology, University of Washington School of Medicine, Seattle, WA, and Department of Ophthalmology, University of Sao Paulo, Sao Paulo, Brazil*

ADRIAN BARBUL • *Department of Surgery, Sinai Hospital, and Johns Hopkins Medical Institution, Baltimore, MD*

JOHN A. BELPERIO • *The Division of Pulmonary and Critical Care Medicine, Department of Medicine, UCLA School of Medicine, Los Angeles, CA*

PIERRE J. BOULETREAU • *Children's Surgical Research Program, Stanford University School of Medicine, Stanford, CA, and Department of Maxillofacial Surgery, Centre Hospitalier Lyon-Sud, Pierre-Benite, France*

I. WILLIAM BROWDER • *Department of Surgery, James H. Quillen College of Medicine, East Tennessee State University, Johnson City, TN, and James H. Quillen Veterans Affairs Medical Center, Mountain Home, TN*

MARIE D. BURDICK • *The Division of Pulmonary and Critical Care Medicine, Department of Medicine, UCLA School of Medicine, Los Angeles, CA*

AIME L. BURNS • *Department of Surgery, Burn and Shock Trauma Institute, Loyola University Medical Center, Maywood, IL*

JAYASRI DASGUPTA • *Department of Pathology, Vanderbilt University School of Medicine, Nashville, TN*

JEFFREY M. DAVIDSON • *Department of Pathology, Vanderbilt University School of Medicine, Nashville, TN, and Department of Veterans Affairs Medical Center, Nashville, TN*

ROBERT F. DIEGELMANN • *Department of Biochemistry, Medical College of Virginia, Virginia Commonwealth University, Richmond, VA*

LUISA A. DIPIETRO • *Department of Surgery, Burn and Shock Trauma Institute, Loyola University Medical Center, Maywood, IL*

IULIA DRUGEA • *Department of Surgery, Burn and Shock Trauma Institute, Loyola University Medical Center, Maywood, IL*

DAVID T. EFRON • *Department of Surgery, Sinai Hospital, and Johns Hopkins Medical Institution, Baltimore, MD*

H. PAUL EHRLICH • *Division of Plastic Surgery, Hershey Medical Center, Hershey, PA*

SABINE A. EMING • *Department of Dermatology, Cologne University, Cologne, Germany*

STEFAN FRANK • *Pharmazentrum Frankfurt, Klinikum der Johann Wolfgang Goethe-Universität, Frankfurt am Main, Germany*

RICHARD L. GAMELLI • *Department of Surgery, Burn and Shock Trauma Institute, Loyola University Medical Center, Maywood, IL*

NICOLE S. GIBRAN • *Department of Surgery, University of Washington, Seattle, WA*

FINN GOTTRUP • *Copenhagen Wound Healing Center, Bispebjerg University Hospital, Copenhagen, Denmark*

MARTIN GRAHAM • *Laboratory of Tissue Repair, Department of Pediatrics, Virginia Commonwealth University, Medical College of Virginia, Richmond, VA*

DAVID G. GREENHALGH • *Department of Surgery, University of California, Davis, and Shriners Hospitals for Children Northern California, Sacramento, CA*

RICHARD GROSE • *Cancer Research UK, London Research Institute, Viral Carcinogenesis, London, UK*

LI-KE HE • *Department of Surgery, Burn and Shock Trauma Institute, Loyola University Medical Center, Maywood, IL*

PAUL J. HIGGINS • *Center for Cell Biology and Cancer Research, Albany Medical College, Albany, NY*

HARRIET W. HOPF • *Department of Anesthesia and Perioperative Care, and Department of Surgery, University of California, San Francisco, CA*

LISA M. HUMPHREY • *Department of Anesthesia and Perioperative Care, University of California, San Francisco, CA*

THOMAS K. HUNT • *Department of Surgery, University of California, San Francisco, CA*

F. FRANK ISIK • *Department of Surgery, University of Washington, Seattle, WA*

ANDREW E. JAHODA • *Department of Urology, Burn and Shock Trauma Institute, Loyola University Chicago, Maywood, IL*

LARS NANNESTAD JORGENSEN • *Department of Surgical Gastroenterology K, Bispebjerg University Hospital, Copenhagen, Denmark*

HEIKO KÄMPFER • *Pharmazentrum Frankfurt, Klinikum der Johann Wolfgang Goethe-Universität, Frankfurt am Main, Germany*

MICHAEL P. KEANE • *Division of Pulmonary and Critical Care Medicine, Department of Medicine, UCLA School of Medicine, Los Angeles, CA*

TERUHIKO KOIKE • *Department of Medicine, Nagoya University Graduate School of Medicine, Nagoya, Japan*

VESA KOIVUKANGAS • *Departments of Dermatology and Surgery, University of Oulu, Finland*

ELIZABETH J. KOVACS • *Department of Surgery, Department of Cell Biology, Neurobiology, and Anatomy, Burn and Shock Trauma Institute, Loyola University Chicago, Maywood, IL*

ARETA KOWAL-VERN • *Sumner L. Koch Burn Center, Cook County Hospital, Chicago, IL*

BARBARA A. LATENSER • *Sumner L. Koch Burn Center, Cook County Hospital, Chicago, IL*

MARK W. LINGEN • *Department of Pathology, The University of Chicago, Chicago, IL*

MICHAEL T. LONGAKER • *Children's Surgical Research Program, Stanford University School of Medicine, Stanford, CA*

QUENTIN E. H. LOW • *Burn and Shock Trauma Institute, Loyola University Medical Center, Maywood, IL*

SØREN MUNK MADSEN • *Parker Institute, Frederiksberg Hospital, Copenhagen, Denmark*

KATHERINE M. MALINDA • *EntreMed, Inc., Rockville, MD*

BRUCE A. MAST • *Department of Surgery, University of Florida College of Medicine, Gainesville, FL*

STEVE A. MCCLAIN • *Department of Emergency Medicine, University Hospital and Medical Center, State University of New York, Stony Brook, NY*

RAHUL R. MOHAN • *Department of Ophthalmology, University of Washington School of Medicine, Seattle, WA*

RAJIV R. MOHAN • *Department of Ophthalmology, University of Washington School of Medicine, Seattle, WA*

INGRID MOLL • *Universitätsklinikum Hamburg-Eppendorf, Klinik und Poliklinik für Dermatologie und Venerologie, Hamburg, Germany*

DAVID J. MOONEY • *Department of Biologic and Materials Sciences, School of Dentistry, and Department of Biomedical Engineering, School of Engineering, University of Michigan, Ann Arbor, MI*

THOMAS A. MUSTOE • *Division of Plastic and Reconstructive Surgery, Wound Healing Research Laboratory, Northwestern University Medical School, Chicago, IL*

JACQUES E. NÖR • *Department of Cariology, Restorative Sciences, and Endodontics, School of Dentistry, University of Michigan, Ann Arbor, MI*

AARNE OIKARINEN • *Department of Dermatology, University of Oulu, Finland*

MARY KAY OLSON • *Department of Cell Biology, Neurobiology, and Anatomy, Loyola University Chicago, Maywood, IL*

HEATHER N. PADDOCK • *Department of Surgery, University of Florida College of Medicine, Gainesville, FL*

ZIV M. PELED • *Children's Surgical Research Program, Stanford University School of Medicine, Stanford, CA, and University of Connecticut School of Medicine, Farmington, CT*

MARTIN C. PETERS • *Department of Biomedical Engineering, School of Engineering, University of Michigan, Ann Arbor, MI*

PETER J. POLVERINI • *Department of Oral Sciences, University of Minnesota School of Dentistry, Minneapolis, MN*

KIRWIN M. PROVIDENCE • *Center for Cell Biology and Cancer Research, Albany Medical College, Albany, NY*

PAULI PUOLAKKAINEN • *Department of Surgery, Helsinki University Central Hospital, Helsinki, Finland*

MAY J. REED • *Division of Geriatric Medicine, Department of Medicine, University of Washington, Seattle, WA*

JONATHAN S. REICHNER • *Division of Surgical Research, Department of Surgery, Rhode Island Hospital and Brown Medical School, Providence, RI*

MARK D. ROLLINS • *Department of Anesthesia and Perioperative Care, University of California, San Francisco*

HEINZ SCHEUENSTUHL • *Department of Surgery, University of California, San Francisco, CA*

GREGORY S. SCHULTZ • *Department of Obstetrics and Gynecology, University of Florida College of Medicine, Gainesville, FL*

RAVI SHANKAR • *Department of Surgery, Burn and Shock Trauma Institute, Loyola University Medical Center, Maywood, IL*

ADAM J. SINGER • *Department of Emergency Medicine, University Hospital and Medical Center, State University of New York, Stony Brook, NY*

MARK SISCO • *Division of Plastic and Reconstructive Surgery, Wound Healing Research Laboratory, Northwestern University Medical School, Chicago, IL*

LISA STAIANO-COICO • *Department of Surgery, Weill Medical College of Cornell University, New York, NY*

JULIA M. STEVENSON • *Department of Surgery, Burn and Shock Trauma Institute, Loyola University Medical Center, Maywood, IL*

ROBERT M. STRIETER • *The Division of Pulmonary and Critical Care Medicine, Department of Medicine, UCLA School of Medicine, Los Angeles, CA*

ANNA M. SZPADERSKA • *Department of Surgery, Burn and Shock Trauma Institute, Loyola University Medical Center, Maywood, IL*

STEPHEN M. WARREN • *Children's Surgical Research Program, Stanford University School of Medicine, Stanford, CA, and Oregon Health Sciences University, Portland, OR*

SABINE WERNER • *Insitute of Cell Biology, ETH Hönggerberg, Zürich, Switzerland*

JUDITH M. WEST • *Department of Surgery, University of California, San Francisco, CA*

STEVEN R. WHITE • *Section of Pulmonary and Critical Care Medicine, Department of Medicine, University of Chicago, Chicago, IL*

AMY WILLEY • *Laboratory of Tissue Repair, Department of Pediatrics, Virginia Commonwealth University, Medical College of Virginia, Richmond, VA*

DAVID L. WILLIAMS • *Department of Surgery, James H. Quillen College of Medicine, East Tennessee State University, Johnson City, TN, and James H. Quillen Veterans Affairs Medical Center, Mountain Home, TN*

STEVEN E. WILSON • *Department of Ophthalmology, University of Washington School of Medicine, Seattle, WA*

I

EXPERIMENTAL MODELS OF WOUND HEALING

A. IN VIVO ANIMAL MODELS

1

Excisional Wound Healing

An Experimental Approach

Stefan Frank and Heiko Kämpfer

1. Introduction

Wound healing disorders present a serious clinical problem and are likely to increase since they are associated with diseases such as diabetes, hypertension, and obesity. Additionally, increasing life expectancies will cause more people to face such disorders and further aggravate this medical problem. Thus, several animal models have been established to serve as an experimental basis to determine molecular and cellular mechanisms underlying and controlling an undisturbed healing process. Here we describe a model of excisional skin wounding in mice that can be used to assess molecular, cellular, and tissue movements in healthy mice as well as in mouse models characterized by impaired or altered healing conditions such as genetically deficient or transgenic animals. Moreover, we point out that the presented model of excisional skin wounding can be easily adapted from a basic experimental model to a model that deals with more detailed questions of interest.

The presented method represents an animal model that provides access to investigate complex tissue movements associated with repair such as hemorrhage, granulation tissue formation, reepithelialization, and angiogenic processes *(1–3)*. These processes are initiated by the complete removal of the skin including epidermis, dermis, sc fat and the underlying panniculus carnosus smooth muscle layer by excising skin areas (about 5 mm in diameter) from the backs of the animals. Accordingly, repair of injured skin areas now requires coordinated cellular movements to restore epidermal, dermal, and sc tissue

From: *Methods in Molecular Medicine, vol. 78: Wound Healing: Methods and Protocols*
Edited by: Luisa A. DiPietro and Aime L. Burns © Humana Press Inc., Totowa, NJ

structures. These processes can be analyzed by different techniques, namely gene expression studies, immunoblot, and histological analyses.

Mice of comparable age and weight should be used for each single experimental setup to guarantee the comparability and reproducibility of independent animal experiments. Wounding experiments are started by anesthetizing the animals. The fur of the whole back skin area is removed from the anesthetized mice using an electric razor. This step is important to subsequently allow precise removal of skin areas from the backs of the mice and, moreover, easy handling of skin wound biopsy specimens. The wounding is done with fine scissors, and the cut removes the epidermal, dermal, and sc layer including the panniculus carnosus. Thus, because wounding is severe, this excisional model provides the possibility of investigating central tissue movements associated with repair, starting with hemorrhage followed by reepithelialization, granulation tissue formation, and angiogenesis *(1–3)*. Experience shows that wounded mice will cope well with the injuries; mice start to climb, clean, and feed soon after the end of anesthesia. A few hours after wounding, the wounded area will first be closed by a thin scab, which becomes stronger within the first 2 d of repair. After wounding, mice are kept in a 12-h light/12-h dark regimen, usually four animals per cage, and are fed ad libitum.

Mice are sacrificed at the desired experimental time points. Usually, mice should be killed at day 1, 3, 5, 7, and 13 postwounding to remove the wounded tissues, as these time points reflect central time points of repair including inflammation, keratinocyte migration and proliferation, and the formation of new stroma (d 1–7) *(1–3)* as well as the end point of the acute healing process (d 13). Thus, the abovementioned experimental time points provide access to characterize representative expressional kinetics for genes of interest during the whole process of acute wound repair.

For analysis, wounds are removed from sacrificed animals using scissors. First, it is important to remove the wound biopsy specimens including a sufficient but constant amount of the surrounding wound margin skin tissue. Second, cutting of wound tissue must be performed deep into the underlying tissue, because only this procedure ensures that the complete granulation tissue is isolated and not lost, at least partially, on the backs of the animals. Both points are crucial for further analysis of wound-derived gene expression or histological analysis, since the wound margins as well as the granulation tissue are central to the repair process. Excised wound tissue should be immediately snap-frozen in liquid nitrogen, or directly embedded into tissue-freezing medium for histology. Snap-frozen or embedded wound tissue should be stored at –80°C until used for isolation of total cellular RNA and protein, or sectioning.

Finally, we point out that the model of excisional wounding described in this chapter can be easily adapted to investigate more detailed aspects of skin repair. To this end, mice that are characterized by wound-healing disorders *(4)*, or transgenic animals *(5)*, can be used. Moreover, the presented model provides access to investigate the impact of pharmacological substances (e.g., enzymatic inhibitors) or recombinant growth factors on normal and disturbed wound-healing conditions, because it allows an accompanying treatment of wounded animals by systemic or topical application of these substances during repair *(6,7)*.

2. Materials

2.1. Excisional Wounding

1. Anesthesia solution: Ketavet® (2-[2-chlorphenyl]-2-methylaminocyclohexanon-hydrochloride) (ketamine hydrochloride), 100 mg/mL solution, stable to date as given by the manufacturer (Pharmacia & Upjohn GmbH, Erlangen, Germany); and Rompun® (5,6-dihydro-2-[2,6-xylidino]-4H-1,3-thiazinhydrochloride) (xylazine-hydrochloride), 20 mg/mL solution, stable to date as given by the manufacturer (Bayer, Leverkusen, Germany). Immediately prior to use, add 800 µL of Ketavet and 500 µL of Rompun to 25 mL of sterile Dulbecco's phosphate-buffered saline (PBS) using a sterile 50-mL polypropylene conical tube. Mix carefully by inverting the tube (*see* **Note 1**).
2. Dulbecco's PBS without sodium bicarbonate (Life Technologies, Karlsruhe, Germany).
3. EtOH (70% [v/v] solution in H_2O).
4. Single-use, sterile, nontoxic, nonpyrogenic syringes (3 mL) (*see* **Fig. 1**).
5. Single-use, sterile, nontoxic, nonpyrogenic needles (0.5 × 25 mm) (*see* **Fig. 1**).
6. Paper towels, examination gloves, 50-mL polypropylene conical tubes (Falcon, Becton Dickinson, Franklin Lakes, NJ).
7. Electric razor (*see* **Fig. 1**).
8. Scissors and forceps (*see* **Fig. 1**).

2.2. Isolation of Wound Biopsy Specimens

1. Scissors and forceps (*see* **Fig. 1).**
2. Paper towels, examination gloves, polypropylene conical tubes (50 mL).
3. Liquid nitrogen.

2.3. Preparation of Total Cellular RNA from Isolated Wound Tissue

1. Paper towels, examination gloves, polypropylene conical tubes (50 mL).
2. Ultra Turrax®, electric tissue homogenizer.
3. GSCN solution (components from Sigma, Deisenhofen, Germany): 50% (w/v) guanidinium thiocyanate, 0.5% (w/v) sodium laurylsarcosyl, 15 mM sodium citrate, 0.7% (v/v) β-mercaptoethanol; must be stored at 4°C, stable for 6 wk.

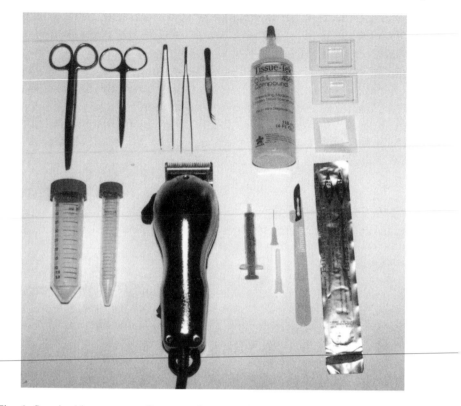

Fig. 1. Surgical instruments for wound preparation. Clockwise from upper left-hand corner: scissors, forceps, embedding media, cryomolds, single-use scalpel, syringes, electric razor, conical tubes.

4. 2 M Sodium acetate (NaOAc), pH 4.0.
5. 3 M NaOAc, pH 5.2.
6. Acidic, nonbuffered phenol (H_2O saturated).
7. Chloroform.
8. EtOH.
9. Diethylpyrocarbonate (DEPC)-treated H_2O: Dissolve DEPC (Sigma) at a final concentration of 0.1% (v/v) in distilled H_2O by stirring overnight. Inactivate DEPC by autoclaving.
10. Buffered phenol/chloroform solution: Dissolve 22.5 mL of phenol in 22.5 mL of chloroform. Adjust phenol/chloroform solution to pH 8.0 by adding 5 mL of Tris-HCl (1 M, pH 9.5). Mix vigorously and store overnight to separate organic and aqueous phases.

2.4. Preparation of Total Cellular Protein from Isolated Wound Tissue

1. Paper towels, examination gloves, polypropylene conical tubes (50 mL).
2. Ultra Turrax, electric tissue homogenizer.
3. Proteinase inhibitor phenylmethylsulfonyl fluoride (PMSF) (Sigma): 100 mM in 70% EtOH. Store in the dark at 4°C.
4. Proteinase inhibitor leupeptin (Sigma): 1 mg/mL in H$_2$O. Store in aliquots at –20°C.
5. Protein homogenization buffer (stable when stored at 4°C): 137 mM NaCl, 20 mM Tris-HCl, 5 mM EDTA, pH 8.0, 10% (v/v) glycerol, 1% (v/v) Triton X-100. Immediately before use, add to a final concentration 1 mM PMSF, 1 µg/mL of leupeptin.

2.5. Embedding Isolated Wound Tissue for Histology

1. Tissue Tek® cryomold® intermediate, disposable vinyl specimen molds (15 × 15 × 5 mm). (Miles, Diagnostic Division, Elkhart, IN) (*see* **Fig. 1**).
2. Tissue Tek®, O.C.T. compound, embedding medium for frozen tissue specimens (Sakura Finetek, Torrance, CA) (*see* **Fig. 1**).
3. Polyvinyl difluoride (PVDF) membrane (Immobilon-P). (Millipore, Bedford, MA) (*see* **Fig. 1**).
4. Single-use, disposable scalpel (*see* **Fig. 1**).
5. Forceps.
6. Dry ice.

2.6. Standard Laboratory Equipment Needed

1. Centrifuge for use with 50-mL polypropylene conical tubes: Heraeus Megafuge 1.0, rotor 7570F (Heraeus, Hanau, Germany).

3. Methods
3.1. Excisional Wounding

1. Freshly prepare Ketavet (ketamine)/Rompun (xylazine) solution for anesthesia. Prepare the single-use syringe for injection.
2. For ip injection, hold the mouse at its neck directly behind the ears and grasp the tail (*see* **Fig. 2A**) while holding the mouse with its head down.
3. Inject as 0.5 mL of anesthetizing solution shown in **Fig. 2B** (*see* **Note 2**).
4. Put the mouse back in a cage, so that the mouse will not become agitated. Anesthesia should take effect after 5–10 min.
5. Shave the back of the anesthetized mouse using the electric razor. Carefully remove the hair from the complete back of the animal (*see* **Fig. 2C**).

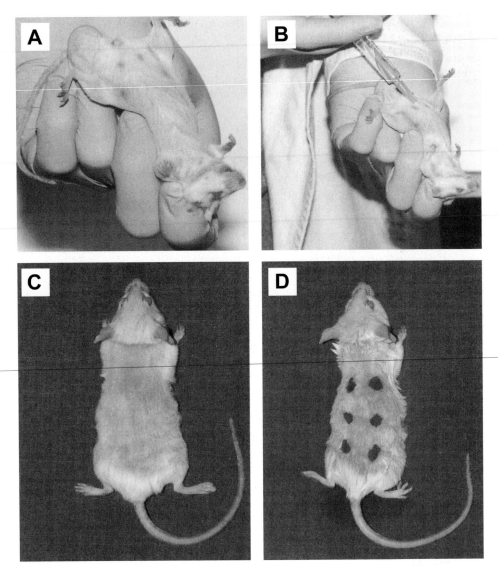

Fig. 2. Steps in excisional wound preparation. (**A**) For ip injection, hold the mouse at its neck directly behind the ears and grasp the tail holding the mouse with its head down. (**B**) Inject anesthetizing solution as shown. (**C**) Remove the hair from the complete back of the animal. (**D**) Place a total of six wounds on the back of each mouse.

6. Place the anesthetized and shaved mouse on a paper towel.
7. Wipe the shaved back of the animal with a sufficient amount of 70% EtOH.
8. Use **Fig. 2D** as a guide for the final localization of all six wounds before you start to excise the skin areas (*see* **Note 3**).

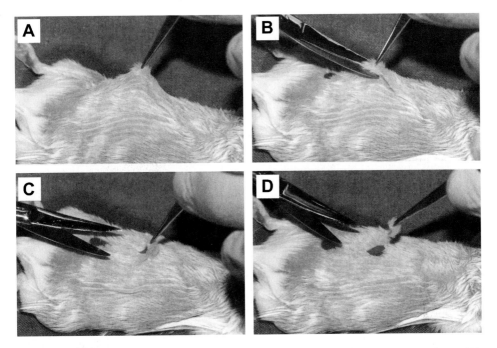

Fig. 3. Preparation of excisional wounds. (**A**) Lift the back skin using forceps. (**B**) Incise the skin with a first and careful cut using scissors. (**C**) Following the first cut, hold the partially removed skin area using scissors. (**D**) Complete the excision with two to three additional cuts.

9. Lift back the skin using forceps (*see* **Figure 3A**).
10. Incise the skin with a first and careful cut using the scissors (*see* **Fig. 3B**). Lifting up the skin will ensure that the incision will move through the panniculus carnosus.
11. Following the first cut, hold the partially removed skin area using forceps (*see* **Fig. 3C**).
12. Complete the excision with two to three additional cuts (*see* **Fig. 3D**) (*see* **Note 4**).
13. Repeat **steps 9–12** to create a total of six wounds on the back of each mouse (*see* **Fig. 2D**).
14. After completion of excisional wounding, transfer the animals into cages that are covered with two to three layers of paper towels (*see* **Note 5**).

3.2. Isolation of Wound Biopsy Specimens

1. Choose the experimental time point of interest (*see* **Notes 6** and **7**).
2. Prior to isolation of wound biopsy specimens, sacrifice mice painlessly using a carbon dioxide (CO_2) chamber followed by cervical dislocation. Cervical

dislocation must be carried out carefully to avoid disruption of the weak wound tissue (*see* **Note 7**). A mouse that has been sacrificed at day 3 postwounding is shown in **Fig. 4A** to demonstrate wound contraction during healing.

3. Hold the sacrificed mouse in one hand and begin to remove wound tissue using scissors (*see* **Fig. 4B–E**). It is important to include about 2 mm of the directly adjacent skin, which represents the wound margin tissue (*see* **Fig. 4B,C** and **Note 9**) when cutting out the wound from the dorsal skin surface.
4. Complete your cut, which now includes the whole wound (*see* **Fig. 4C**).
5. Lift the skin tissue with forceps (*see* **Fig. 4D**).
6. Remove the wound tissue from the body (*see* **Fig. 4D,E**).
7. Immediately snap-freeze the wounds in liquid nitrogen.
8. Repeat **steps 4–8** to remove all wounds from the back of the animal.
9. Remove the same amount of normal skin from the backs of nonwounded animals for use as a control, or from the same animal to analyze for systemic effects of the wounding procedure.

3.3. Preparation of Total Cellular RNA from Isolated Wound Tissue

This method has been adapted from the acid guanidinium thiocyanate–phenol–chloroform extraction protocol by Chomczynski and Sacchi (*8*).

1. Prepare a 50-mL polypropylene conical tube with 5 mL of GSCN solution at room temperature.
2. Add 16 wounds to the tube (**Note 7**).
3. Immediately homogenize the tissue for 30–45 s using the Ultra Turrax homogenizer.
4. Clear the solution of hair and insoluble debris by centrifuging at 3000*g* for 10 min.
5. Transfer the supernatant to a fresh 50-mL polypropylene conical tube (*see* **Note 8**).
6. Add 400 µL of 2 *M* NaOAc (pH 4.0) to the remaining 4 mL of GSCN wound lysate supernatant.
7. Add 4 mL of acidic phenol (H_2O saturated).
8. Add 1.2 mL of chloroform.
9. Mix vigorously for 30 s by vortexing.
10. Incubate on ice for 15 min.
11. Separate the aqueous and organic phases by centrifuging at 3000*g* for 10 min.
12. Transfer the supernatant (aqueous phase) to a fresh 50-mL tube (*see* **Note 9**).
13. Precipitate total cellular RNA by adding 10 mL of EtOH.
14. Incubate for at least 1 h at –20°C.
15. Pellet the RNA (Heraeus Megafuge 1.0, 3000*g* for 30 min).
16. Discard the supernatant, and let the RNA pellet dry for 5 min.
17. Dissolve the RNA pellet in 4 mL of DEPC-treated H_2O.
18. Add 4 mL of buffered phenol/chloroform (pH 8.0) and mix vigorously by vortexing (1 min).

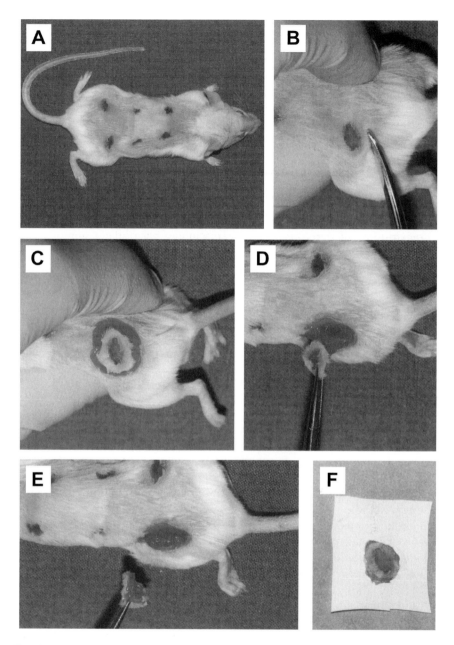

Fig. 4. Harvesting of excisional wounds. (**A**) A mouse that has been sacrificed at d 3 postwounding demonstrates wound contraction during healing. (**B**) To harvest the wound, hold the sacrificed mouse in one hand and begin to remove wound tissue using scissors. (**C**) Include about 2 mm of the directly adjacent skin, which represents the wound margin tissue. (**D**) Lift the skin tissue with forceps. (**E**) Remove the wound tissue from the body. (**F**) For embedding, place freshly isolated wound tissue scab side up directly onto a piece of PVDF membrane.

19. Separate the aqueous and organic phases by centrifuging at 3000g for 10 min.
20. Transfer the supernatant (aqueous phase) to a fresh 50-mL tube (*see* **Note 12**).
21. Add 400 µL of 3 M NaOAc (pH 5.2) and 10 mL of EtOH.
22. Precipitate the RNA by incubating at –20°C for at least 1 h.
23. Pellet the RNA by centrifuging at 3000g for 30 min.
24. Discard the supernatant, and let the RNA pellet dry for 5 min.
25. Dissolve the RNA pellet in 0.5 mL of DEPC-treated H_2O (aqueous RNA solution remains stable when stored at –80°C).

3.4. Preparation of Total Cellular Protein from Isolated Wound Tissue

1. Prepare a 50-mL polypropylene conical tube with 4 mL of homogenization buffer at room temperature.
2. Add eight wounds to the tube (**Note 7**).
3. Immediately homogenize the tissue for 30–45 s using the Ultra Turrax homogenizer.
4. Clear the solution of hair and insoluble debris by centrifuging at 3000g for 10 min.
5. Transfer the supernatant to a fresh 50-mL polypropylene conical tube (*see* **Note 8**).
6. Determine protein concentration using standard techniques.

3.5. Embedding Isolated Wound Tissue for Histology

1. Place freshly isolated wound tissue (*see* **Subheading 3.2.**, item 6) scab side up directly onto a piece of PVDF membrane (*see* **Fig. 4F** and **Note 11**).
2. Bisect the wound using a new single-use scalpel. The cut should also pass through the membrane.
3. Add a small droplet of Tissue Tek O.C.T. compound to the middle of a Tissue Tek cryomold.
4. Place the cryomold on a piece of dry ice.
5. When the O.C.T. compound starts freezing, put one half of the bisectioned wound with the sectioned side down directly into the droplet (using small forceps).
6. Hold the bisectioned biopsy until the droplet of O.C.T. compound is frozen.
7. Carefully fill up the Tissue Tek cryomold with Tissue Tek O.C.T. compound. Avoid air bubbles.
8. Wait until the embedding medium is completely frozen.
9. Store embedded wounds at –80°C until use.

4. Notes

1. Injecting 0.5 mL of this solution per animal provides a final dose of 80 mg/kg of ketamine and 10 mg/kg of xylazine, which represents the ideal dose for a 20-g mouse.
2. Avoid entering too deeply into the peritoneum and try to insert the injection needle in an obtuse angle.

3. Wound localization is important, because the wounds should be separated by a sufficient amount of nonwounded skin. Most important, the uppermost two wounds must not be localized too close to the neck for two practical reasons (*see* **Fig. 2D**). First, the animal will be sacrificed using a CO_2 chamber followed by cervical dislocation. To this end, one must leave enough space between the neck of the mouse and the uppermost wounds if one intends to avoid a rupture of the wound areas when killing the animal. Second, in the case that the mouse must be handled throughout the experiment (e.g., further injections during the healing period), one must be able to hold the animal at its neck without disturbing the uppermost wound areas.

4. The excised skin area (the skin area that one now holds between the forceps; *see* **Fig. 3D**) should be approx 5 mm in diameter. The diameters of all six wounds should be constant; this provides the basis for comparable data among different animals, or even different experimental setups. Sometimes injury is associated with rupture of a small artery located where the two uppermost wounds are created. In our experience, hemorrhage is not severe and will stop within minutes.

5. It is important to avoid standard animal litter as long as the wounds are not covered by a stable and dry scab. In our experience, paper towels should not be replaced by litter within the first 24 h after wounding. This avoids the possibility that litter particles will become enclosed within the drying wound. Mice will wake up from anesthesia within 2 to 3 h after the initial injection. Within 4–6 h after surgery, the animals will feed, clean themselves, and climb around.

6. In general, to obtain useful and clear kinetics (e.g., for RNA or protein expression) representing important phases of the repair process, we suggest the following experimental time points to isolate wound tissue: d 1, 3, 5, 7, and 13 postwounding. In our experience, most of the extensive gene expression events occur during the first 7 d of healing, which are characterized by inflammatory, reepithelialization and granulation tissue formation processes. In most cases, the d 13 postwounding time point represents the end of acute repair. Thus, we recommend starting with the suggested time points of analysis and then to use additional time points depending on specific questions of interest.

7. In our experience, a minimum of four animals is needed for each experimental time point. From these animals ($n = 4$ mice), a total of 16 wounds (4 wounds from each mouse of the corresponding group) for RNA and a total of 8 wounds (2 wounds from each mouse of the corresponding group) for protein isolation as a standard procedure can be isolated. These wounds are pooled prior to isolation of total cellular RNA ($n = 16$ wounds) and protein ($n = 8$ wounds). More wounds are needed for RNA preparation than protein preparation, since the amounts of total RNA isolated from wound tissue always represent the limiting factor of the described experimental setup. By contrast, the total amount of protein that is isolated from the eight wounds removed for protein preparation will not be limiting in any case. We strongly recommend pooling the wounds prior to analysis rather than isolating RNA or protein from single wounds. RNA or protein isolated from single wounds would have the advantage that one can

compare expression levels for the genes of interest among each wound, thus estimating the deviations among individual wounds. However, this procedure has a major disadvantage: the low yield of RNA isolated from a single wound will limit the number of genes analyzed per animal experiment. Accordingly, pooling wounds ($n = 16$ for RNA and $n = 8$ for protein analysis) for each experimental time point will balance out the intra- (among different wounds from the same animal) and interindividual (among wounds of different animals) expressional differences among the wound tissues. This will allow a direct comparison of independent animal experiments from which differential gene expression is easily reproducible using the presented method.

8. The dorsal skin wound tissue is fragile until d 5–7 postwounding. Keep in mind not to disrupt the wound tissue during the procedure of cervical dislocation (when the mouse becomes stretched), since rupture of the wounds will lead to mechanical destruction of newly formed tissue structures; ruptured wounds are not suitable for a histological analysis.

9. The correct and precise excision and, most important, the removal of wound tissue with constant proportions are central for analysis and reproducibility of the animal experiments. Thus, one must guarantee that constant amounts of wound margin and granulation tissue are removed from the backs of the mice with each single wound when the wounds are excised (*see* **Fig. 4C,D**). Most of the wound-derived gene expression occurs within the epithelial wound margins and the granulation tissue. Thus, we strongly recommend including a consistent amount of the wound margins (about 2 mm) when excising the wounds from the back skin. Moreover, do not hesitate to cut deep into the muscle tissue underlying the wounds when finally removing the wound tissue from the animals' backs, in order to guarantee that the granulation tissue is not partially lost.

10. Be careful not to transfer parts of the solid pellet that consist of insoluble cellular debris and hair.

11. It is important not to disturb the large interphase.

12. It is important not to disturb the traces of the small interphase that will form.

13. Press the wound tissue onto the membrane carefully (*see* **Fig. 4F**). The wound should remain completely flat on the membrane. This is important because the wound margins tend to roll inside.

References

1. Clark, R. A. F. (1996) Wound repair: overview and general considerations, in *The Molecular and Cellular Biology of Wound Repair* (Clark, R. A. F., ed.), Plenum, New York, pp. 3–50.
2. Singer, A. J. and Clark, R. A. F. (1999) Cutaneous wound healing. *N. Engl. J. Med.* **341,** 738–746.
3. Martin, P. (1997) Wound healing—aiming for perfect skin regeneration. *Science* **276,** 75–81.
4. Wetzler, C., Kämpfer, H., Stallmeyer, B., Pfeilschifter, J., and Frank, S. (2000) Large and sustained induction of chemokines during impaired wound healing in the

genetically diabetic mouse: prolonged persistence of neutrophils and macrophages during the late phase of repair. *J. Invest. Dermatol.* **115,** 245–253.

5. Yamasaki, K., Edington, H. D. J., McClosky, C., Tzeng, E., Lizonova, A., Kovesdi, I., Steed, D. L., and Billiar, T. R. (1998) Reversal of impaired wound repair in iNOS-deficient mice by topical adenoviral-mediated iNOS gene transfer. *J. Clin. Invest.* **101,** 967–971.

6. Stallmeyer, B., Kämpfer, H., Kolb, N., Pfeilschifter, J., and Frank, S. (1999) The function of nitric oxide in wound repair: inhibition of inducible nitric oxide-synthase severely impairs wound reepithelialization. *J. Invest. Dermatol.* **113,** 1090–1098.

7. Frank, S., Stallmeyer, B., Kämpfer, H., Kolb, N., and Pfeilschifter, J. (2000) Leptin enhances wound re-epithelialization and constitutes a direct function of leptin in skin repair. *J. Clin. Invest.* **106,** 501–509.

8. Chomczynski, P. and Sacchi, N. (1987) Single-step method of RNA isolation by acid guanidinium thiocyanate-phenol-chloroform extraction. *Anal. Biochem.* **162,** 156–159.

2

Methods in Reepithelialization

A Porcine Model of Partial-Thickness Wounds

Heather N. Paddock, Gregory S. Schultz, and Bruce A. Mast

1. Introduction

1.1. General Aspects of Wound Healing

The healing of skin wounds progresses through sequential and overlapping phases of inflammation, repair, and remodeling (**Fig. 1A**). Each phase of healing is directed by the complex coordination and interaction of several cell types contained within the wound, including inflammatory cells such as neutrophils, macrophages, lymphocytes, and platelets. Native skin cells such as fibroblasts, keratinocytes, and vascular endothelial cells are also intricately involved in these processes. Although these processes are well described at the macroscopic cell biology level, until recently they were poorly understood at the molecular level.

Studies of wound fluid and biopsies collected during the phases of wound healing have begun to elucidate the molecular interactions that regulate wound healing. In the early phases of wound healing, chemokines and cytokines regulate chemotaxis and activation of inflammatory cells, as well as synthesis of proteases and protease inhibitors. Growth factors play dominant roles in regulating cell proliferation, differentiation, and synthesis of extracellular matrix. The analysis of fluids and biopsies collected from nonhealing wounds has also provided insight into the molecular differences between healing and nonhealing wounds. Compared with nonhealing wounds, healing wounds characteristically have lower levels of inflammatory cytokines and proteases and higher levels of growth factor activity. Furthermore, as nonhealing wounds

From: *Methods in Molecular Medicine, vol. 78: Wound Healing: Methods and Protocols*
Edited by: Luisa A. DiPietro and Aime L. Burns © Humana Press Inc., Totowa, NJ

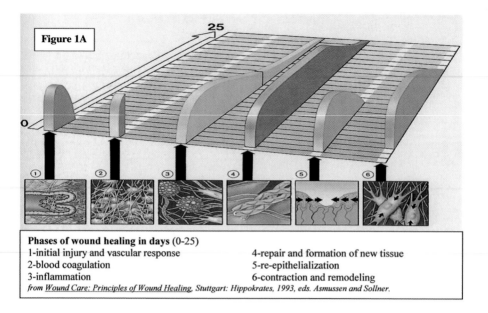

Figure 1A

25

0

① ② ③ ④ ⑤ ⑥

Phases of wound healing in days (0-25)
1-initial injury and vascular response
2-blood coagulation
3-inflammation
4-repair and formation of new tissue
5-re-epithelialization
6-contraction and remodeling

from Wound Care: Principles of Wound Healing, Stuttgart: Hippokrates, 1993, eds. Asmussen and Sollner.

Figure 1B

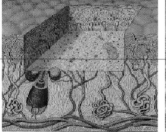

A. Partial thickness wound

B. Re-epithelialization via dermal appendages

C. Early scar

Figure 1C

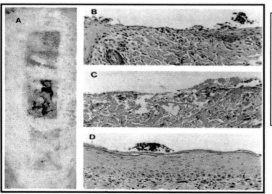

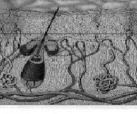

Effects of different treatments on thermal partial thickness wounds in the same animal 7 days after wounding:
A- Gross appearance
B- Histology Silvadine treated wound (top)
C- Histology untreated wound (middle)
D- Histology EGF treated wound (bottom)
Reprinted from Brown et al., 1986

Fig. 1.

begin to heal, these molecular abnormalities begin to reverse, resulting in a molecular milieu similar to healing wounds *(1–5)*.

As the molecular and cellular regulation of wound healing becomes better understood, new approaches to enhancing wound healing will become possible. Animal models of wound healing that closely mimic human wound healing are needed to evaluate new treatments. Several different animal models have been developed to study healing of partial-thickness skin wounds, and these models have played key roles in developing wound treatments such as early debridement and moist healing. More recently, animal models of partial-thickness skin wound healing have been vital in helping to develop new treatments that utilize growth factors to accelerate the healing of burn wounds *(6)*. In addition, many of the general principles that have been learned from growth factor treatment of partial-thickness skin injuries have found direct application in development of growth factors for treatment of nonhealing full-thickness skin wounds *(7)*.

1.2. Aspects of Epidermal Regeneration

A partial-thickness skin injury can be simply defined as a wound that extends completely through the epidermal layer and only partially through the dermal layer. Epithelial cells that line hair follicles, sweat glands, or sebaceous glands extending into the deep dermis remain viable after a partial-thickness injury. In large partial-thickness injuries, these epithelial cells proliferate and migrate onto the surface of the wound, where they differentiate into epidermal keratinocytes (**Fig. 1B**). Because of the large number of epithelial cell–lined appendages within the dermis, the epidermal cells migrating from these structures account for a majority of the new epidermal cells following a partial-thickness skin injury. However, reepithelialization is also necessary for other types of skin wounds, including surgical incisions, skin grafts for burns or venous stasis ulcers, and other open wounds. Thus, studies that increased the understanding of the cellular and molecular regulation of epidermal regeneration have led to improvements in healing of most types of skin wounds.

As described previously, the healing of skin wounds involves a complex system of integrated molecular signals and interactions among many different types of cells within a wound. For some types of experimental questions, it is desirable to simplify the experimental system and isolate the single variable of interest. Frequently, this is best approached using an in vitro cell culture system. With a single type of cultured cell, the number of experimental variables can be dramatically reduced compared to a similar experiment performed in an animal. For example, if one hypothesized that hypertrophic scars developed because of an increased sensitivity to a growth factor, an important in vitro experiment would be to compare the mitogenic response of cultures of fibroblasts established from normal skin or from hypertrophic scar tissue to the growth factor. However, simplified in vitro cell culture systems inherently lack other components that may influence the responses of cells in vivo. For example, study of the response of pure cultures of fibroblasts to a scrape injury (as a model of an incision wound) does not include the contribution of paracrine growth factors and cytokines that may be secreted by epidermal keratinocytes or inflammatory cells. Although constraints exist, both in vitro and in vivo model systems provide important information about aspects of skin wound healing.

During the development of new therapeutic strategies to augment wound healing, experiments utilizing animal models of wound healing have played important roles by helping to define concentrations of factors, dosing regimens, and vehicles. Several substances have been successfully developed and are now in clinical development and use. Examples include topical epidermal growth factor (EGF) or Gentel® *(8)*; recombinant human platelet-derived growth factor or Regranex®; fibroblast growth factor (FGF) *(6)*; and keratinocyte growth factor or Repifermin *(9)*. Recently, several novel gene therapies have been tested in animal models of skin wound healing *(10)*.

1.3. Animal Models of Epidermal Healing

In vivo animal models of epidermal wound healing have been developed in several different species including rats, mice, rabbits, and pigs. We have utilized several of these different animal models, and each has unique advantages and disadvantages. The investigator will need to assess which model provides the best balance for his or her experimental objectives.

1.3.1. Tape Abrasion

Tape abrasion is perhaps the simplest method of creating an epithelial injury. Once hair is depilated (*see* **Subheading 3.2.**) and the skin is disinfected, adherent tape is applied to the skin and then quickly removed with a quick stripping motion moving nearly parallel to the skin, thereby removing the top layers of skin cells. This can be repeated several times until the desired depth of injury is attained. The advantage of this method is that it is inexpensive and very simple to perform. However, the injury is limited to the epidermis, and most often basal cells will be left intact. The depth of the epidermal injury varies depending on the number of repetitive strippings performed, the adhesiveness of the tape, and the pressure used to apply the tape. This model is not used frequently probably because the wound is superficial and not precisely reproducible.

1.3.2. Partial-Thickness Excisions

A method that is frequently used to study epidermal wound healing in animal models involves excising a partial-thickness layer of skin with a tissue planer, called an electrokeratome or dermatome. The procedure and injury created are essentially the same as those used clinically to harvest skin for split-thickness skin grafts. The technique of creating partial-thickness excision wounds is extremely effective when performed correctly, but it is very operator dependent. The dermatome is basically a razor blade that is rapidly oscillated by a high-speed electric motor. The depth of the excision can be varied and is generally set at a depth of 0.005 in (0.013 cm) to remove just the top epithelial layer of the skin. Oil may be applied to the clean skin to assist in lubricating the area to be "shaved." The skin must be pulled taught in the direction of the blade and constant downward pressure applied to ensure an even depth of skin removal. If the dermatome is not operated correctly, the depth of excision will vary and small "islands" of epidermis will be left within the excised wound. The probability of uneven skin removal using this technique is moderate, even in experienced hands. Furthermore, the bleeding induced by the epithelial shaving is significant owing to the dermal arterioles that supply nutrients to the epithelial layer. Cutaneous blood supply is similar in swine and humans. Once a wound is created, the area usually needs to be treated with topical epinephrine and manual pressure until all bleeding stops and the arterial myoepithelial cells react to the bleeding from the arterioles. Once bleeding is stopped, the experimental treatment may be applied; one must be sure to remove as much of the remaining blood clot from the wound area as possible prior to the application. Maintaining a constant depth of excisions among different wounds is challenging. This is not especially problematic in humans when harvesting skin for grafting because most often the donor skin is meshed prior to being placed onto the graft site. However, this would become problematic in an experimental study in which the rate of epidermal wound healing is being studied since deeper excision wounds tend to heal more slowly than shallow excision wounds.

1.3.3. Suction Blisters

Dry suction has been used to create skin blisters for more than 100 yr. In 1950, this technique was used experimentally for the first time to separate epidermis from dermis *(11)*. In recent years, this technique has been used successfully to study healing of epidermal injuries in several animal species including rat, guinea pigs, and swine *(12–14)*. Briefly, this technique involves the application of vacuum suction to skin for a period of time ranging from several minutes to an hour or more. This induces slow separation of the epidermis and dermis at their interface followed by fluid filling the intradermal space. Time to create a blister can be decreased by increasing the amount of suction or by warming the skin 3 to 4°C. Several devices have been developed to deliver continuous and uniform suction to skin that effectively creates a blister *(15–17)*. One advantage of this technique is that it causes minimal damage to the underlying dermis and separation of the epidermis from the dermis in a defined tissue plane (i.e., at the level of the basement membrane separating the epidermis and dermis).

1.3.4. Water Scald Burns

Constant temperature water scald burn models have been created in several species including mice *(18)* and pigs *(19)*. Typically, the skin is shaved, and in the case of mice or rats, the animal is placed in a tubelike structure that contains a cutout area that exposes only a fixed area of the dorsal skin. The unit is then partially submerged in a constant temperature water bath for a fixed time period. To create a uniform depth of scald injury, it is important in this technique to halt the burn process, which is usually accomplished by applying ice-cold water to the scald. In approx 1 to 2 h a blister will form over the burn, which can be deroofed to expose the wound. One difficulty in utilizing this technique is creating watertight structures that hold the rodent and prevent scalding of tissue past the intended site. In addition, creating a partial-thickness burn to the desired depth may require several trials at different temperatures and times of exposure to calibrate the exposure conditions.

1.3.5. Partial-Thickness Thermal Injury

We have found the partial-thickness thermal burn model in pigs or piglets to provide a good balance of accuracy, reproducibility, cost, and ease of use. Test agents usually are applied topically to the injury rather than systemically because of the large size of the animals. Some of the investigations that we have performed using this model are topical recombinant EGF stimulation of reepithelialization *(8)*, topical transforming growth factor-β stimulation of reepithelialization *(20)*, and topical EGF on keratinocyte collagenase-1 expression *(21)*.

The key to creating consistent partial-thickness thermal skin injuries is to reproducibly apply an amount of thermal energy to the skin that kills all the epithelial cells in the epidermal layer, and cells in the dermis to a defined depth. The thermal energy will also denature most of the proteins in the dermal matrix to a consistent depth. The cell death and protein denaturation will rapidly induce an inflammatory response owing to the release of chemokines. These chemokines increase local vascular permeability, which causes edema in the wound and subsequently produces a blister that usually forms within an hour of the burn injury. The blister roof (bollous) can be removed to expose the dermis, and the experimental treatment can be applied. One major difference between partial-thickness thermal injuries and partial-thickness excision injuries caused by a dermatome is that thermal injuries cause extensive denaturation of dermal collagen that remains in the wound bed. Excisional wounds produce much less denatured collagen. Because denatured extracellular matrix proteins (primarily collagen and proteoglycans) must be removed and replaced by new matrix proteins that are necessary for epithelialization (mainly through the actions of proteases released from inflammatory cells), burn wounds typically have higher levels of inflammation for a longer period of time than partial-thickness excisional wounds.

Several techniques can be used to create a partial-thickness thermal injury. The shape and size of the wound can be varied, according to the experimental design. In previous studies, we have created 3 × 3 cm square wounds or 2 × 3 cm rectangular wounds. However, other researchers have advocated the use of circular wounds because they have a larger ratio of total wound area to migrating wound edge and the wound edge is symmetrical to the wound center *(22)*. The depth of the burn wound can be varied by adjusting the temperature, the time of exposure of the skin to the heated template, or the weight of the template.

1.3.5.1. ADVANTAGES OF A PORCINE PARTIAL-THICKNESS THERMAL INJURY MODEL

One advantage of using the porcine model of partial-thickness skin wound healing is that porcine skin is more similar histologically to human skin than is rodent skin. Human epidermis comprises five layers: stratum corneum, stratum lucidum, stratum granulosum, stratum spinosum, and stratum basale. Pigs have a similar epithelial structure. Swine, like humans, have "fixed skin," which adheres tightly to subdermal structures and has similar deposition of subdermal fat. Rodents have a subdermal muscle layer called the panniculus carnosus, which is not present in human or swine skin. The interaction between the panniculus carnosus and the overlying dermal and epidermal layers is not fully understood and, therefore, may confound extrapolation of data obtained from rodents to humans.

Swine are relatively hairless compared with rodents, and their dorsal hair undergoes sporadic hair growth and replacement or "mosaic pattern" similar to humans. Rodent dorsal hair grows in a denser pattern and is replaced in what is termed *Mexican waves* starting at the head and progressing to the tail *(23,24)*. Because the epithelial cells lining hair follicles contribute substantially to the healing of partial-thickness wounds, the density and pattern of hair growth can influence healing of partial-thickness wounds.

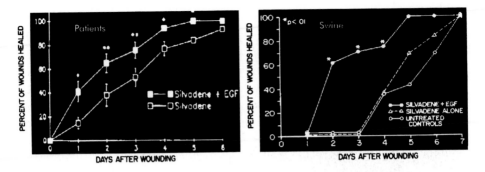

Fig. 2. Similar healing patterns in human patients (**A**) and swine (**B**) treated with and without EGF.

Pigs also have a larger dorsal surface area than rodents. This facilitates performing experiments with multiple test agents and controls on the same animal, which reduces interanimal variation and allows maximal information to be collected with fewer animals. Most important, results from studies of experimental treatments in the porcine model of partial-thickness wound healing have correlated well the results of clinical studies. For example, results of a study on the effects of topical EGF on healing of partial-thickness excision wounds in pigs (*8*) correlated well with the results reported for a clinical study of paired skin graft donor sites in patients undergoing skin grafting (*25*). Therefore, the porcine model of partial-thickness skin wound healing has been validated and appears to predict effectively the effects of novel treatments in humans (**Figs. 1C and 2**).

1.3.5.2. DISADVANTAGES OF A PORCINE PARTIAL-THICKNESS THERMAL INJURY MODEL

Although the pig model of partial-thickness skin wound healing has many advantages and correlates well with results of clinical studies in patients, it is not a perfect model. For example, porcine skin does not contain apocrine sweat glands, which are glandular structures in the dermis of humans that contain cells that participate in regeneration of the epidermis following partial-thickness injuries. Both pigs and humans have hair and sebaceous glands in similar number and distribution. However, the absence of apocrine sweat glands in porcine skin does not appear to appreciably alter healing of pig wounds compared with human wounds.

Migration of epithelial cells depends on the recognition of nondenatured extracellular matrix proteins by integrin receptors in the plasma membrane of epidermal cells. Thus, in a partial-thickness thermal wound, epithelial cells migrate underneath the denatured dermal collagen. By contrast, epithelial cells migrate more across the surface of an excised partial-thickness wound. This

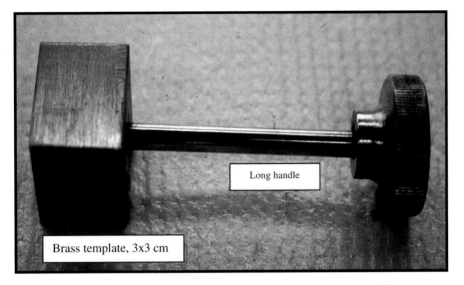

Fig. 3. Solid brass template block with long handle.

migration pattern may alter planimetric analysis but will not affect results as long as the wound technique is consistent.

Size, expense, and difficulty handling pigs are also disadvantages of this model of partial-thickness wound healing. However, as pointed out previously, fewer animals can be used and each animal can function as its own control because many wounds can be made on the swine dorsum without difficulty. The ability to perform paired wound healing measurements reduces the effect of interanimal variability on healing and permits the use of the more robust paired analysis statistical tests.

2. Materials

1. Hampshire or Yorkshire adult pigs (20–30 kg), Yorkshire piglets, or adult Yucatan miniature pigs (available from many vendors, such as Vita-Vet Laboratories, Marion, ID, as well as local farms) (*see* **Note 1**).
2. Template or metal block made of solid brass weighing approx 1 kg with a 3 × 4 cm square surface or circular rod 12 to 19 mm in diameter (**Fig. 3**) (*see* **Note 2**).
3. A constant temperature water bath heated to 70°C.
4. A bioocclusive dressing such as Op-site™ or Steri-Drape™ (*see* **Note 3**).
5. Test material optimally formulated in an ointment or cream with a viscosity and rheology that permits easy application and persistence in the applied area (*see* **Note 4**).
6. Vet-wrap™, a self-adhesive elastic tape.

7. Anesthestic agents (*see* **Note 5**).
8. A long-acting analgesic such as buprenorphine.
9. Penicillin G.
10. Electric clippers.
11. Nair™.
12. Gauze.
13. Stopwatch.
14. Tweezers.
15. Cotton swabs.
16. 35-mm Slide film camera or digital camera.
17. Sigma Scan™.

3. Methods

3.1. Anesthesia

1. Weigh the pig or piglet directly or by subtraction method (weight of pig and researcher minus researcher's weight).
2. Initially anesthetize the pig or piglet by im injection of ketamine and xylazine (20 mg/kg of ketamine + 2 mg/kg of xylazine) mixed in one injection.
3. After the animal is manageable, transfer it to an operating table.
4. Maintain anesthesia with inhalation of 1.5% isoflurane at a flow rate of 1 L O_2/min (*see* **Notes 6** and **7**).
5. Give a prophylactic im injection of penicillin G (4000 IU/kg) at least 30 min prior to placing the first burn wound.

3.2. Creation of Burn Injury

1. Trim dorsal skin hair with an electric clipper. Remove hair shafts using a commercially available hair depilatory. We use Nair applied in a thick layer evenly covering the hair stubble (*see* **Note 8**).
2. After 30 min, completely remove the depilatory agent from the skin by several washings and scrubbing with coarse gauze (*see* **Notes 9** and **10**).
3. Dry the skin thoroughly with gauze.
4. While the depilatory is working, prepare the template block by heating to 70°C in a constant temperature water bath (this takes 20–30 min).
5. Remove the template block from the water bath, and quickly wipe with a towel to remove any water droplets.
6. Apply the heated template to prearranged sites on the dorsum evenly. Avoid bony prominences and ribs. Do not press down on the template (*see* **Notes 11–13**).
7. Hold the block in place for 10 s measured by an accurate stopwatch. Maintain deep inhalation anesthesia throughout this process.
8. Remove the template and place it back into the constant temperature water bath for 5 min to reheat.
9. Repeat this process for each burn site, leaving at least 1 cm between each burn (*see* **Note 14**). On removal of the heated block from the skin you should note a

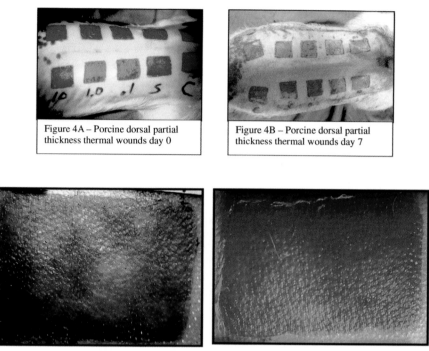

Figure 4A – Porcine dorsal partial thickness thermal wounds day 0

Figure 4B – Porcine dorsal partial thickness thermal wounds day 7

Figure 4C – Blister formation

Figure 4D – After blister roof

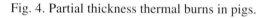

Fig. 4. Partial thickness thermal burns in pigs.

distinct bright red or pink appearance to the epithelium (**Fig. 4A,B**). A thin blister should develop at the injury site over the next 60 min (**Fig. 4C**).

10. Gently tease off the blister covering from the center of the blister to the edges using tweezers and cotton-tipped swabs (*see* **Note 15**).

11. At the edge of the burn, cut sharply and discard the separated epithelium, leaving the viable unburned skin at the wound edges intact (**Fig. 4D**).

3.3. Treatment and Dressing of Burn Injury

1. Once the burned epithelium is removed, apply a test cream to completely cover the burn surface. If desired, a precise volume of the test material can be applied per square centimeter of surface area (*see* **Note 16**).

2. Place a secure biooclusive dressing on the burn area. We use one large sheet of Steri-Drape, which has the ability to adhere to the interwound spaces of normal skin and prevent cross-contamination of topical treatments.

3. Apply the adhesive occlusive dressing in the following manner: Have one person uncover the adhesive surface, and beginning at the rostral end, attach

the dressing to the skin with about 5-cm of border to the most anterior burn. Have a second person expose more of the adhesive dressing surface and elevate the dressing, while the first person gently presses the adhesive dressing surface around the burns, ensuring that the topical creams do not migrate between burns (*see* **Note 17**).

4. Apply the dressing laterally with about a 5-cm border extending past the lateral edges of the burns.
5. Secure the occlusive adhesive dressing to the animal using an elastic self-adhesive tape such as Vet-wrap. This should be wrapped around the torso of the animal using a figure eight crossed about the shoulders then continued in a spiral wrap down the torso. This should secure the dressing fully for at least 24 h.
6. Recover the animal on its side under a warming light or on a warming blanket.

3.4. Monitoring of Wounds and Analgesia

1. Assess wounds during treatment and dressing changes for signs of infection, including erythema around the wound, purulent discharge, or foul odor. The rate of infection is very low (<1%) in this model. If an infection does develop, treat the wound aggressively with topical antibiotics and exclude it from data analysis.
2. Second-degree partial-thickness burns can cause significant pain during the first few hours after injury, but this usually subsides within 12–24 h. The animal will, however, be anesthetized during the most painful portion of the procedure. Administer a long-acting analgesic such as buprenorphine (5–10 µg/kg every 12 h) during anesthesia recovery and for the first 12–24 h to provide postburn pain relief.
3. Monitor animals for any other changes in behavior that may indicate excessive pain or distress such as decreased eating, decreased locomotion, or weight loss.

3.5. Measurements of Epidermal Healing

Measurements of healing can generally be performed in one of two ways: a noninvasive, repeated measurement of epidermal healing of each wound over the entire course of the experiment; or an invasive, onetime measurement of each wound at a selected time point during the experiment. A 9-cm^2 partial-thickness burn (3 × 3 cm) will consistently reepithelialize within 14 d with good wound care.

3.5.1. Noninvasive Measurement: Planimetric Wound-Healing Analysis

1. Typical noninvasive, repeated measurement of epidermal healing utilizes photography of the burn. Photograph the wound with a 35-mm slide film camera using a circular (or ring) flash with a close-up lens.
2. Project each slide onto white paper at a constant distance, and trace the area of nonhealed wound or healed wound (*see* **Note 18**).

3. Integrate the areas of healed epidermis using a digitizing tablet and program from Sigma Scan.
4. Calibrate the size of the original wound and set to a known area. The program will calculate the percentage of the wound surface that is healed or not healed based on area. This can be repeated at many different time points during healing. We previously photographed wounds at each daily dressing change while the pig was under general anesthesia. Digital cameras can also be used and the projected digital images traced and processed as for the slide images.

3.5.2. Invasive Measurement: Strip Biopsy

One invasive method used to measure epidermal healing uses a biopsy specimen that is collected at a single time point. A strip biopsy can be taken across the diagonal of a rectangular or square burn, or taken through the center of a circular burn. The biopsy is fixed in formalin, processed for paraffin sectioning, and representative tissue sections stained with hematoxylin and eosin (H&E) are examined microscopically *(26)*. The entire length of the biopsy can be examined and the length of the epithelialized surface can be measured very accurately with a micrometer and compared to the full length of the wound (*see* **Note 19**).

3.5.3. Invasive Measurement: Wound Excision

Another invasive technique that is used to measure epidermal healing of partial-thickness wounds takes advantage of the ability of dispase, an enzyme that digests the desmosome proteins, to separate the epidermal layer of cells from the dermis. In this technique, a partial thickness wound is completely excised and incubated overnight in the dispase enzyme, and then the epidermal layer is carefully dissected from the dermis *(27)*. If the epidermis is fully healed, the epidermal layer will form an intact sheet of tissue. If the epidermis is not fully healed, there will be a central hole in the epidermal sheet where the epidermal cells have not regenerated an intact layer of cells. Wounds are graded as completely healed or not completely healed. Separating the epidermis from the dermis is an effective way to determine the percentage of fully healed wounds (**Fig. 5**).

3.5.4. Noninvasive: Evaporimeter

A second noninvasive technique that has been used in other laboratories is to measure water vapor pressure gradients above a wound *(28–30)*. This technique measures late wound healing because a substantial layer of keratinized cells must be present to affect the vapor pressure above a wound.

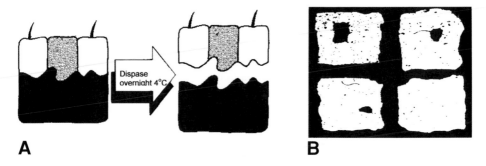

Fig. 5. Assessment of wound healing by dispase digestion. Full thickness excisions of wounds are digested overnight in dispase solution and the epidermal layer is separated from the dermis (**A**). Wounds that are fully epithelialized produce an intact sheet of epidermis while partially healed wounds produce a sheet with holes (**B**).

This procedure must be conducted in a temperature-controlled room with minimal air drafts. An open cylinder detection probe is placed onto the skin about the healing wound and is allowed to equilibrate. The detection probe has two sets of thermistors and humidity sensors at fixed points above the wound. The difference in temperature and partial pressure of water at the different locations is calculated to give the water vapor transmission rate.

3.6. Data Analysis

If noninvasive, repeated measurements are made of wounds, data may be graphed as the average percentage of the surface area of the burns that has reepithelialized for each of the treatment groups vs the time after injury. The appropriate statistical test to determine whether there is a difference in the amount of healing among any of the groups at a specific time point (e.g., 7 d after injury) is the repeated measures analysis of variance followed by a post-hoc multiple comparison test such as the Tukey test to determine where differences exist. The data also can be analyzed for the time to achieve 25, 50, 75, and 100% healing by interpolating values from the best-fit curves of healing vs time graphs (*see* **Note 20**).

In addition, the data can be analyzed using multiple regression analysis to determine whether healing rates differ among treatments over time, even if the overall time to complete healing may be similar among different treatments. In this way, early and late healing stages may be examined under different treatment conditions. For example, it was found that growth factors such as basic FGF are more important in the early stages of wound healing (decreases time to initiation of wound healing) but may not affect overall healing time using multiple regression analysis *(31)*. If measurements of healing such as the enzymatic separation of epidermis and dermis are used, data may be analyzed using nonparametric frequency tables such as χ^2 analysis that evaluate categorical data (healed vs nonhealed).

4. Notes

1. Epithelial wounds will heal quickly in nutritionally replete swine, but healing rates appear to be faster in Yorkshire piglets than in mature Yucatan miniature pigs.
2. The template block that we use is solid brass and weighs 714 g with a square heated surface measuring 3 × 3 cm. It has a long handle attached to the middle of the block to facilitate handling. We have found this type of template to be best in this partial-thickness thermal injury technique.
3. We have found Op-site or Steri-Drape, which are adherent to normal skin but not to injured skin, to be particularly suitable bioocclusive dressings. These dressings provide optimal coverage of the wounds to prevent contamination.
4. The test material and vehicle should be available in amounts that permit repeat applications (usually once a day) for up to 2 wk.
5. Optimal anesthesia is crucial for the smooth completion of the experiment. It is important to ensure deep anesthesia during the application of the heated template, which is best attained by inhalation anesthesia (especially isofluorane). Ketamine and xylazine injection can be used for initial anesthesia followed by isofluorane inhalation anesthesia.
6. The animals will undergo repeated anesthesia for repeated application of test materials or repeat measurements of healing at multiple time points. Therefore, it is necessary to utilize an anesthetic regimen that permits rapid recovery and minimizes the need to fast (withhold nutrition) the animals prior to anesthesia.
7. Inhalation anesthesia can be given by a nose cone that can be purchased from a veterinary supply or fashioned from a large funnel with a latex glove stretched over the opening.
8. Skin preparation is very important in this model. Porcine hair tends to be coarse and should be trimmed with an electric trimmer and then removed by a depilatory agent. The depilatory agent should be evenly applied and remain on the skin for at least as long as the directions indicate (usually 20–30 min).
9. Once the depilatory agent has been applied for the required amount of time, the skin must be washed thoroughly with water to completely remove the depilatory agent. This may require multiple washings to remove residual depilatory agent from hair follicles and gland structures in the dermis. This is an important step because any depilatory agent that remains in the epidermal skin appendages (such as hair follicles) will cause a chemical burn to the epithelial cells when heat is applied in the next step and extend the burn more deeply than intended, affecting the reepithelialization rate.
10. Once the skin has been thoroughly washed, it should be dried with rough gauze to further remove any remaining depilatory agent.
11. It is important *not to press down* on the heated block template during application to the dorsal skin. Rather, the operator should only stabilize the brass block to

ensure that the entire surface of the block remains in contact with the skin. The weight of the block provides constant pressure of the block on the skin.

12. The depth of the thermal burn is dependent on three major factors: the temperature of the block, the time the block is exposed to the skin, and how much force is applied to the block. These three factors are easily controlled using a good water bath that maintains a constant temperature, using an accurate stopwatch, and using only the weight of the brass block or rod to apply force to the skin. Prior to initiating the experimental protocol, histological analysis of test burns must be made to establish the depth and consistency of the burning technique. Representative tissue sections should be stained by H&E and be examined by a pathologist. All epidermal cells should be killed, and the depth of the thermal denaturation of the extracellular matrix will be revealed by a difference in staining, with the denatured matrix staining a lighter and brighter shade of pink.

13. When applying the heated block, it is important to avoid bony prominences and ribs because the pressure will be increased at these sites, resulting in deeper wounds. This is more easily accomplished if one chooses pigs with significant sc fat.

14. Depending on the size of the burn wound, multiple burns can be created. We usually create a total of eight 3 × 3 cm burns on a 25 kg pig. If smaller square burns or circular burns are created, as many as 20 burns can be created on a pig. We recommend no more than three burns per (experimental) treatment.

15. Prior to applying the test treatments, the burn blister must be deroofed completely to permit penetration of the test materials into the dermis. The keratinized epidermis and blister fluid may be barriers to some test agents.

16. Typically, the treatments tested include no treatment (desiccating wound), vehicle, vehicle with drug dose no. 1, and vehicle with drug dose no. 2, for a total of four treatments per subject. For example, the dorsum of the pig could be divided into four quadrants (e.g., A, B, C, and D) using the spine and navel as references. We usually place up to six (though we recommend no more than three) 3 × 3 cm square or 3-cm-diameter circular burn wounds in each quadrant, approx 1 cm apart. Each treatment (e.g., 1, 2, 3, and 4) should be randomly assigned to each quadrant of the first subject, making sure to vary the positions of the treatments by quadrant on each subsequent subject. In this manner, each treatment will occur at least once in each location (e.g., treatment no. 1 will occur in each of quadrants A, B, C, and D). This variation in treatment placement will control for any variability in healing among quadrants; it is possible that the right hind quadrant may have a slightly different blood supply than the left upper quadrant and affect healing rates.

17. Multiple thermal burns can be made on the pig dorsum on either side of the spine but there should be at least 1 cm of normal skin between each burn. This will permit the occlusive dressing to be applied to intact skin between burn sites and prevent migration of test agents between burn sites.

18. It is important when using planimetric analysis to photograph burns at a constant magnification and to project the images at a constant enlargement to ensure accurate measurement among wounds.

19. Some investigators believe this is a more accurate method to assess the percentage of the burn surface that has epithelialized. Although this morphometric histological technique very accurately determines the percentage of epithelial healing in the biopsy, it only examines the region of the burn where the biopsy was taken and does not assess the entire burn surface.

20. We recommend a repeated-measures design for the reasons stated in **Subheading 3.6.** We also suggest consulting a statistician prior to starting a study to conduct a POWER analysis, which will provide an appropriate number of subjects and wounds per treatment necessary to reach the study's goals. This analysis made *a priori* may reduce the numbers of animals and wounds per animal before beginning the study. The number of subjects necessary for the study is dependent on the number of levels of treatments to be tested and the study design (e.g., parallel arm vs repeated-measures design). One advantage of using swine is that their large dorsal area allows several treatments to be compared in one animal, which permits more robust statistical analysis of effects using paired tests. However, it is important that the positions of different treatments on the pigs be randomized to avoid the possibility of artifacts owing to slight differences in skin thickness, hair density, skin pigmentation, and so forth. For example, if four treatment levels are to be tested (e.g., desiccation, vehicle, vehicle with 0.1-mg drug dose, and vehicle with 1.0-mg drug dose), each treatment should be placed in a separate dorsal quadrant. The location of the treatments in each quadrant of the other pigs should vary. Therefore, each treatment should be located in each quadrant at least once. More information can be gained by increasing the number of pigs instead of increasing the number of wounds per pig.

References

1. Trengove, N. J., Bielefeldt-Ohmann, H., and Stacey, M. C. (2000) Mitogenic activity and cytokine levels in non-healing and healing chronic leg ulcers. *Wound Repair Regen.* **8,** 13–25.
2. Trengove, N. J., Stacey, M. C., MacAuley, S., Bennett, N., Gibson, J., Burslem, F., Murphy, G., and Schultz, G. (1999) Analysis of the acute and chronic wound environments: the role of proteases and their inhibitors. *Wound Repair Regen.* **7,** 442–452.
3. Wysocki, A. B., KKusakabe, A. O., Chang, S., and Tuan, T. L. (1999) Temporal expression of urokinase plasminogen activator, plasminogen activator inhibitor and gelatinase-B in chronic wound fluid switches from a chronic to acute wound profile with progression to healing. *Wound Repair Regen.* **7,** 154–165.
4. Wysocki, A. B. (1992) Fibronectin in acute and chronic wounds. *J. ET. Nurs.* **19,** 166–170.

5. Wysocki, A. B. and Grinnell, F. (1990) Fibronectin profiles in normal and chronic wound fluid. *Lab. Invest.* **63,** 825–831.

6. Fu, X., Shen, Z., Chen, Y., Xie, J., Guo, Z., Zhang, M., and Sheng, Z. (1998) Randomised placebo-controlled trial of use of topical recombinant bovine basic fibroblast growth factor for second-degree burns. *Lancet* **352,** 1661–1664.

7. Rees, R. S., Robson, M. C., Smiell, J. M., and Perry, B. H. (1999) Becaplermin gel in the treatment of pressure ulcers: a phase II randomized, double-blind, placebo-controlled study. *Wound Repair Regen.* **7,** 141–147.

8. Brown, G. L., Nanney, L. B., Griffen, J., Cramer, A. B., Yancey, J. M., Curtsinger, L. J., Holtzin, L., Schultz, G. S., Jurkiewicz, M. J., and Lynch, J. B. (1989) Enhancement of wound healing by topical treatment with epidermal growth factor. *N. Engl. J. Med.* **321,** 76–79.

9. Han, D. S., Li, F., Holt, L., Connolly, K., Hubert, M., Miceli, R., Okoye, Z., Santiago, G., Windle, K., Wong, E., and Sartor, R. B. (2000) Keratinocyte growth factor-2 (FGF-10) promotes healing of experimental small intestinal ulceration in rats. *Am. J. Physiol. Gastrointest. Liver Physiol.* **279,** G1011–G1022.

10. Nanney, L. B., Paulsen, S., Davidson, M. K., Cardwell, N. L., Whitsitt, J. S., and Davidson, J. M. (2000) Boosting epidermal growth factor receptor expression by gene gun transfection stimulates epidermal growth in vivo. *Wound Repair Regen.* **8,** 117–127.

11. Falabella, R. (2000) Suction blistering as a research and therapeutic tool in dermatology. *Int. J. Dermatol.* **39,** 670–671.

12. Rommain, M., Brossard, C., Piron, M. A., and Smets, P. (1991) A skin suction blister model in hairless rats: application to the study of anti-inflammatory and immunomodulatory drugs. *Int. J. Immunopharmacol.* **13,** 379–384.

13. Mousa, S. A., Brown, R., Chan, Y., Hsieh, J., and Smith, R. D. (1990) Evaluation of the effect of azapropazone on neutrophil migration in anaesthetized swine using a multichamber blister suction technique. *Br. J. Pharmacol.* **99,** 233–236.

14. Nanchahal, J. and Riches, D. J. (1982) The healing of suction blisters in pig skin. *J. Cutan. Pathol.* **9,** 303–315.

15. Kiistala, U. (1968) Suction blister device for separation of viable epidermis from dermis. *J. Invest. Dermatol.* **50,** 129–137.

16. Dittmar, H. C., Weiss, J. M., Termeer, C. C., Denfeld, R. W., Wanner, M. B., Skov, L., Barker, J. N., Schopf, E., Baadsgaard, O., and Simon, J. C. (1999) In vivo UVA-1 and UVB irradiation differentially perturbs the antigen-presenting function of human epidermal Langerhans cells. *J. Invest. Dermatol.* **112,** 322–325.

17. Feliciani, C., Di Muzio, M., Mohammad Pour, S., Allegretti, T., Amerio, P., Toto, P., Coscione, G., Proietto, G., and Amerio, P. (1998) Suction split as a routine method to differentiate epidermolysis bullosa acquisita from bullous pemphigoid. *J. Eur. Acad. Dermatol. Venereol.* **10,** 243–247.

18. Cribbs, R. K., Luquette, M. H., and Besner, G. E. (1998) A standardized model of partial thickness scald burns in mice. *J. Surg. Res.* **80,** 69–74.

19. Brans, T. A., Dutrieux, R. P., Hoekstra, M. J., Kreis, R. W., and du Pont, J. S. (1994) Histopathological evaluation of scalds and contact burns in the pig model. *Burns* **20(Suppl. 1),** S48–S51.
20. Jones, S. C., Curtsinger, L. J., Whalen, J. D., Pietsch, J. D., Ackerman, D., Brown, G. L., and Schultz, G. S. (1991) Effect of topical recombinant TGF-beta on healing of partial thickness injuries. *J. Surg. Res.* **51,** 344–352.
21. Pilcher, B. K., Dumin, J., Schwartz, M. J., Mast, B. A., Schultz, G. S., Parks, W. C., and Welgus, H. G. (1999) Keratinocyte collagenase-1 expression requires an epidermal growth factor receptor autocrine mechanism. *J. Biol. Chem.* **274,** 10,372–10,381.
22. Brahmatewari, J., Serafini, A., Serralta, V., Mertz, P. M., and Eaglstein, W. H. (2000) The effects of topical transforming growth factor-beta2 and anti-transforming growth factor-beta2,3 on scarring in pigs. *J. Cutan. Med. Surg.* **4,** 126–131.
23. Hansen, L. S., Coggle, J. E., Wells, J., and Charles, M. W. (1984) The influence of the hair cycle on the thickness of mouse skin. *Anat. Rec.* **210,** 569–573.
24. Saitoh, M., Uzuka, M., and Sakamoto, M. (1970) Human hair cycle. *J. Invest. Dermatol.* **54,** 65–81.
25. Brown, G. L., Nanney, L. B., Griffen, J., Cramer, A. B., Yancey, J. M., Curtsinger, L. J., Holtzin, L., Schultz, G. S., Jurkiewicz, M. J., and Lynch, J. B. (1989) Enhancement of wound healing by topical treatment with epidermal growth factor. *N. Engl. J. Med.* **321,** 76–79.
26. Benn, S. I., Whitsitt, J. S., Broadley, K. N., Nanney, L. B., Perkins, D., He, L., Patel, M., Morgan, J. R., Swain, W. F., and Davidson, J. M. (1996) Particle-mediated gene transfer with transforming growth factor-beta1 cDNAs enhances wound repair in rat skin. *J. Clin. Invest.* **98,** 2894–2902.
27. Davis, S. C., Mertz, P. M., Bilevich, E. D., Cazzaniga, A. L., and Eaglstein, W. H. (1996) Early debridement of second-degree burn wounds enhances the rate of epithelization—an animal model to evaluate burn wound therapies. *J. Burn Care Rehabil.* **17,** 558–561.
28. Wu, P., Nelson, E. A., Reid, W. H., Ruckley, C. V., and Gaylor, J. D. (1996) Water vapour transmission rates in burns and chronic leg ulcers: influence of wound dressings and comparison with in vitro evaluation. *Biomaterials* **17,** 1373–1377.
29. Barel, A. O. and Clarys, P. (1995) Study of the stratum corneum barrier function by transepidermal water loss measurements: comparison between two commercial instruments: Evaporimeter and Tewameter. *Skin Pharmacol.* **8,** 186–195.
30. Pirone, L. A., Bolton, L. L., Monte, K. A., and Shannon, R. J. (1992) Effect of calcium alginate dressings on partial-thickness wounds in swine. *J. Invest. Surg.* **5,** 149–153.
31. Hebda, P. A., Klingbeil, C. K., Abraham, J. A., and Fiddes, J. C. (1990) Basic fibroblast growth factor stimulation of epidermal wound healing in pigs. *J. Invest. Dermatol.* **95,** 626–631.

32. Asmussen, P. D. and Sollner, B. (1993) Wound Care: Principles of Wound Healing. Biersdorf Medical Bibliothek, Hamburg, Germany.
33. Brown, G. B., Curtsinger, L., Brightwell, J. R., Ackerman, D. M., Tobin, G. R., Polk, H. C., Jr., George-Nascimento, C., Valenzuela, P., and Schultz, G. S. (1986) Enhancement of epidermal regeneration by biosynthetic epidermal growth factor. *J. Exp. Med.* **163,** 1319–1324.

3

Incisional Wound Healing

Model and Analysis of Wound Breaking Strength

Richard L. Gamelli and Li-Ke He

1. Introduction

The nature and mechanism of incisional wound healing has been and continues to be of interest to clinicians and wound biologists. More than 46 million operations are performed in the United States alone each year *(1)*. To shorten the time required for incisional wound healing is not only relevant to reducing postoperative pain and impairment as well as convalescence but is also cost-effective. It is very important to understand the nature, the mechanism, and the process of incisional wound healing before designing an experiment.

1.1. Incisional Wound Healing

A clean, uninfected incision, surgically reapproximated, causes the least amount of epithelial and connective tissue cell death and limits the extent of epithelial basement membrane disruption. As does any type of injury, incisional wounds alter the homeostatic state of the organism and trigger a sequence of events that constitutes three typical pathological phases. In the acute inflammatory phase, infiltrating phagocytes protect the wounded tissue from infection and remove necrotic debris. Chemical mediators are formed and play a crucial role in the development of inflammation. The proliferative phase is characterized by the formation of granulation tissue, which is mainly composed of fibroblasts and newly formed blood vessels. Intracellular synthesis and extracellular deposition of collagen and matrix molecules are also active during this phase. The maturation phase, also called the remodeling phase, is characterized by fibroplasia and progressive alignment of collagen bundles.

From: *Methods in Molecular Medicine, vol. 78: Wound Healing: Methods and Protocols*
Edited by: Luisa A. DiPietro and Aime L. Burns © Humana Press Inc., Totowa, NJ

Scar modification during this phase adds further to the restoration of wound tensile strength. Although the process involves intense and complex cell-cell, cell-matrix, and cell-environment interactions, the phases of wound healing are closely merged one into another without clear boundaries. The overall course of wound healing is typically orderly, precise, and well timed.

Within 24 h of wounding, the first inflammatory cells, neutrophils, appear at the margins of the incision and move toward the fibrin clot, which fills the narrow incisional space immediately after wounding. On d 2, the basal cells of the epidermis demonstrate mitotic activity, migrate, and grow along the cut margins. By d 3, granulation tissue progressively grows into the wound cleft. Collagen fibers also appear at the wound margins. Neutrophils are largely replaced by macrophages during this time. At about d 5, neovascularization is maximal in the granulation tissue, and abundant collagen fibrils begin to bridge the incision. Meanwhile, the epidermis recovers its normal thickness with progressive keratinization. During the second week, the inflammatory infiltrates have largely disappeared. Clinically the wound's appearance changes from pink to pale, suggesting continued collagen accumulation and fibroblast proliferation, as well as the regression of vascular channels. This process lasts for 3 to 4 wk, after which the biosynthesis and degradation of collagen is nearly in a state of dynamic equilibrium. Further increases in wound strength are no longer related to collagen deposition. The ultimate scar comprises acellular connective tissue devoid of inflammatory infiltrates and covered by intact epidermis. After 2 to 3 mo, wound strength plateaus at 70–90% of unwounded skin strength values.

The discussed process of incisional wound healing is referred to as healing by primary (first) intention. When tissue loss is extensive, an exuberant inflammatory response ensues in association with extensive granulation tissue formation. Such wounds heal by secondary intention, which involves a more complex series of events and may include significant degrees of wound contraction. Most surgical incisions are created to affect healing by primary intention. Systemic and local factors, as well as certain therapeutic agents, may affect the adequacy of the inflammatory-reparative response, resulting in delayed or dysfunctional healing.

1.2. Impaired Wound Healing

Malnutrition has long been observed to profoundly influence wound healing at multiple points in the phases of wound repair. Protein malnutrition or vitamin C deficiency directly inhibits collagen synthesis and deposition, leading to a retardation of the healing process (*2–5*). Patients with malignancies frequently have impaired nutrient intake and potentially tumor-induced altered substrate utilization. Various antitumor treatments such as chemotherapy and radiation therapy, beyond direct effects at the site of wounding, may add further to impaired nutritional status *(6)*. In such patients subjected to surgery, there is an increased risk of wound-healing complications *(7)*. Diabetes is often associated with poor wound healing, which is related in part to alteration in granulocyte function, altered microvasculature, and frequently coexistent atherosclerotic vascular disease *(8,9)*. Local infection is one of the single most important causes of defective wound repair *(10,11)*. The development of a major wound infection in a surgical incision can lead to a complete failure of healing by primary intention. When ultimately healed by secondary intention, such wounds experience impaired wound strength and often contain excessive scarring. Additional, well-recognized factors that can lead to impairments in repair include aging *(7,12,13)*; anemia and hypoxia *(14)*; jaundice *(15)*; uremia *(16)*; use of steroids *(17,18)*; and local factors including irradiation treatment *(19,20)*; retained foreign bodies *(21)*; and nonviable tissue *(22)*.

1.3. Determination of Wound Breaking Strength

A critical outcome of the wound repair process is restoration of the mechanical properties of tissue strength. Measurement of wound strength provides highly quantifiable estimates of the efficacy of the aggregate healing process. Determination of various individual components of the phases of healing can provide important insights about events operative during repair. However, if sufficient wound strength is not attained, the net effect may be wound failure. Factors that modulate wound repair can be evaluated according to their influence on the development of wound strength.

Various methods have been used to estimate the strength of healing wounds. Harvey *(23)* developed a technique of estimating the tensile strength of wounds in hollow viscera by removing them from the body, tying one end, and pumping air into the other until the wound burst. The pressure at which bursting occurred was recorded on a revolving drum attached to a sphygmomanometer *(23)*. The method for testing hollow viscera was modified by Lanman and Ingalls *(24)*, who used a lumbar-puncture needle attached by rubber tubing to a sphygmomanometer. The needle could be inserted into the peritoneal cavity or any hollow viscus to measure the wound bursting pressure *(24)*. Howes and Harvey *(25)* also tested the breaking strength of excised wounds by attaching them to a standard thread-testing machine. Tension was sequentially increased and wound strength determined at the load value of wound disruption *(25)*. Testing equipment for incisional wounds was also developed by Hartzell and Stone *(26)* and Jones et al. *(27)*. In 1944, the apparatus used for testing tensile strengths of incisional wounds by Bourne *(5)* was a simple gallows device. Excised pieces of skin bearing the wound were hung onto the top of a rack by one end and weights were attached to the free end until the wound disrupted *(5)*.

During the past several decades, manufactured materials testing instrumentation have improved in both sophistication and availability. Instron brought one of the first commercially available material tensile testers to the market in 1946. The Instron model series 5540 single-column tester combines a broad range of testing capabilities with a computerized operating system *(28)*. The materials tester used in our own laboratory was designed and built locally by the Department of Surgery and Instrument Models Facility at the University of Vermont *(29)*. The degree of elongation and load applied to a tissue specimen is determined via Wheatstone bridges, which are coupled to a differential transformer and load transducer (Entran Devices, Fairfield, NJ). The load deformation curves are obtained by a continuous recording on an X-Y plotter, and the maximum load or wound breaking strength (in grams) is displayed via a digital readout. This particular design has proven to be accurate, stable, and simple to use; to provide reliable results; and to be economically feasible to fabricate (**Fig. 1**).

1.4. Studies with Lower Mammals

Experimental studies of wound breaking strength have commonly utilized guinea pigs, rats, and mice. These animal models of healing do not totally replicate healing in humans. Animals are not as susceptible to wound infections as are humans. Scar formation is significantly less in these animals and is for all practical purposes not problematic.

Histologically, a thin sheet of skeletal muscle in the dermis at its boundary with the subcutis, known as panniculus carnosus, is extensively distributed in the head, neck, and trunk regions of lower mammals but not in humans. The presence of this layer of muscle within the underlying loose areolar tissue allows the voluntary motions of the local skin and facilitates contraction of an excised skin wound. Anatomically, the skin in these animals moves easily over the underlying fascia because of a prominent layer of loose areolar tissue underlying the panniculus carnosus muscle. In humans, however, dermal mobility is reduced because of the development of more skin attachments to underlying structures. These factors must be borne in mind in experimental studies examining the rate of wound closure of excisional wounds and their implications for the healing of wounds in humans.

1.5. Breaking Strength and Tensile Strength

Breaking strength and *tensile strength* are the two most commonly used terms to describe the wound strength in nonhollow structures such as skin. For decades, a diversity of opinion has existed over the issue of which one of these parameters best reflects the nature of a wound's strength *(30)*. *Tensile strength*

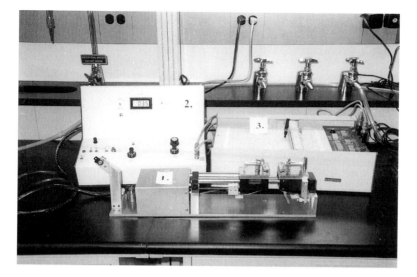

Fig. 1. Material tester (1), digital readout (2), and X-Y plotter (3) used in our laboratory.

is defined as the load per unit of cross-sectional area at rupture. *Breaking strength* is simply the load required to break a wound and does not account for wound geometry. The proponents of tensile strength determinations stress the point that a greater breaking strength would not necessarily reflect enhanced healing in those circumstances of a wound specimen that was thicker. We, the authors, appreciate this consideration but prefer to use breaking strength. Tensile strength is of more benefit when one is comparing homogeneous structure, because it eliminates a physical variable, i.e., thickness, and emphasizes the nature of the material and its tensile property. However, in the clinical situation, the surgeon is interested more in the force required to break a wound, regardless of thickness. For example, a pathological situation may impair wound healing by inhibiting collagen formation, thus thinning the tissue. The treatment would seek to increase the synthesis and accumulation of collagen, thereby thickening the wound. Study results if analyzed via tensile strength may well be uninformative whereas determination of the breaking strength would support the assessment of a favorable response. Furthermore, estimating cross-sectional areas of fresh, newly healed wounded tissues is often difficult and alters the wound. The accuracy of such determinations precisely at the wound cleft in biological specimens adds the very real potential for significant measurement error, which would confound the assessment of the strength properties of the wound.

1.6. Formalin Fixation in Wound-Healing Studies

Formalin-fixed specimens are often tested as a component of a wound study, to evaluate the status of collagen biosynthesis. Collagen is the ultimate product of fibroblast and contributes to wound strength as early as d 3 postinjury. Collagen accounts for approx 70% of the dry weight of skin. The biosynthesis and modifications of collagen involves both intracellular and extracellular processing. Following synthesis on the ribosome, the α-chains are subjected to a number of enzymatic modifications, including hydroxylation of proline—hence, the characteristically high hydroxyproline content of collagen. The hydroxylation of collagen, which is dependent on the availability of vitamin C, is necessary for triple helix formation. The procollagen molecule is soluble at this stage of formation. After the excretion from the cell and enzymatic modifications, procollagen molecules are converted to tropocollagen units and then assemble spontaneously into fibrils within the extracellular space. The immature fibrils give strength to connective tissue mainly by hydrogen bonds, which are relatively weak. The ultimate tensile strength of the collagen fibrils is provided by the formation of covalent crosslinkages. The first step in the formation of crosslinkages is lysyl oxidase–induced deamination of certain lysine and hydroxylysine residues, which results in highly reactive aldehyde groups. The free aldehyde groups then react spontaneously to form intramolecular and intermolecular covalent crosslink bonds. Crosslinking, in addition to being a major contributor to the tensile strength of collagen, is also the basis of collagen's structural stability. Mediated through methylene bridges formed between amino groups, formalin (40% formaldehyde) fixation maximally increases the formation of the covalent crosslinkages and results in a significant increase in wound breaking strength (31,32). Studies have revealed that as collagen maturation occurs, the effect of formalin fixation plateaus. Thus, the effect of formalin treatment is proportionately much greater with immature, early, less dense, and finer collagen fibrils as compared with late, more compact, and coarser fibrils (33,34). When the relative increases in breaking strength are compared between formalin-fixed and fresh wound specimens, the seemingly increased strength of the fixed specimens reflects not a greater collagen content but, rather, the status of collagen crosslinkage. Such data provide additional insights into the status of the healing process, particularly in studies of impaired wound healing.

2. Materials

The materials and methods presented in this chapter are based on the use of mice as the experimental animal (**Fig. 2**).

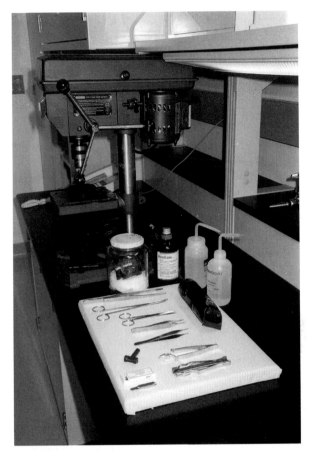

Fig. 2. Materials required for procedure.

1. Inhalation anesthesia administration:
   a. Metofane (Schering-Plough Animal Health, Union, NJ), or halothane (Halo-carbon, River Edge, NJ).
2. Dissecting forceps:
   a. One 8-in. serrated forceps.
   b. Two 5-in. single/double-toothed forceps.
3. Operating scissors:
   a. One 6-in. straight, sharp-blunt scissor.
   b. One 5-in. straight, sharp-sharp scissor.
4. Wound closure system:
   a. One autoclip applier (for 9-mm clips).
   b. Autoclips (9-mm) (about three clips per wound).
   c. Autoclip-removing forceps (Roboz, Rockville, MD).

5. Wound-harvesting system:
   a. Specially designed dumbbell-shaped wound cutters.
   b. Punch press for wound cutters (a simple drill press with a standard chuck holder works quite well).
6. Material tester and recording system (Instron, Canton, MA).
7. Hair clipper with size 40 blades.
8. Rubber hockey pucks (several).
9. Operating board (corkboard).
10. See-through jar with lid and gauze bedding.
11. 75% Alcohol in squirt bottle.
12. Normal saline in squirt bottle.
13. 10% Formalin in sealable container.
14. Tissue cassettes (one per wound).
15. Pushpins.

3. Methods

3.1. Wounding

1. The initial animal body weight as well as weight changes throughout the course of an experiment may be an important parameter in wound-healing studies. The breaking strength of unwounded skin increases almost linearly with animal weight but correlates poorly with the thickness or weight of skin *(33)*. Therefore, it is important to control for animal weights in such studies so that perceived differences in wound strength are not an artifact of the study design. A significant loss of animal body weight should also be considered in evaluating the breaking strength of test wound because the experimental conditions may have had the unintended consequences of introducing nutritional status into the study outcome *(11)*. Weigh and record animal weights; exclude animals with weights that vary by more than 3 g from the group mean. Stratify animal groupings according to weights, so that the average weights of all groups are comparable (*see* **Note 1**).
2. Lightly anesthetize a mouse in a see-through chamber (jar) bedded with gauze containing 15 mL of metofane (sufficient for 30 animals) (*see* **Note 2**).
3. Quickly remove the mouse from the anesthesia chamber with the long forceps and clip the hair from the entire trunk. All mice to be studied should first be shaved before proceeding with the wounding protocol (*see* **Note 3**).
4. Following the hide prepping of all animals, the wounding protocol can begin. After the induction of surgical anesthesia, quickly move each animal onto the operating board, which has been covered with a sterile surgical sheet. Position animals prostrate and pointed in a caudal direction toward the operator (*see* **Note 2**).
5. Apply 75% alcohol for skin preparation (*see* **Note 4**).
6. Use the tooth forceps to elevate the starting point of the incision at the lower left posterior flank, about 1 cm lateral to the spine (*see* **Note 5**).

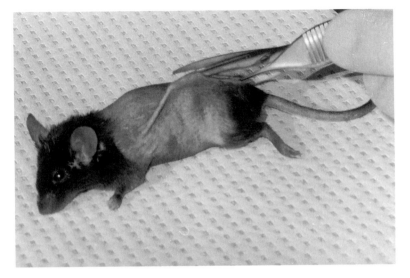

Fig. 3. Creation of incisional wound with scissors.

7. Use the sharp-blunt scissors to make a small cut through the whole thickness of the skin. Insert the blunt tip of the scissors through the cut and into the loose areolar tissue (*see* **Notes 6** and **7**).

8. Reposition the forceps to hold the tissue at the incision site and "push cut" the skin with the scissors along the paraspinous longitudinal line until a 4-cm incision is made (**Fig. 3**).

9. Position the animal's head to the left of the operator. Grasp both ends of the wound with forceps to create a wound pocket and apply test materials if this to be done per the experimental plan (*see* **Note 8**).

10. With one end of the wound under tension applied to the grasped wound, approximate the wound margins with three evenly spaced autoclips (**Fig. 4**) (*see* **Notes 9–11**).

3.2. Removal of Clips

Wound clips typically can be removed on d 5 after wounding.

1. After induction of light anesthesia, quickly move the animal from the jar to the operating board (*see* **Note 2**).

2. With one hand holding the clip, remove the clips one by one with the removing forceps (*see* **Notes 12** and **13**).

3. Weigh and record animal weights (*see* **Note 1**).

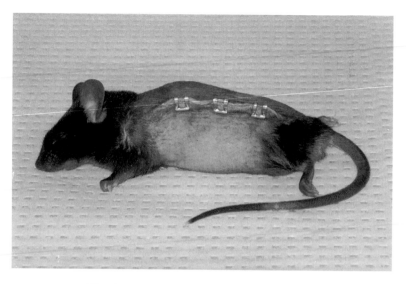

Fig. 4. Wound closed with three autoclips.

3.3. Determination of Wound Disruption Strength

1. Weigh the animal and then euthanize.
2. Place the animal on its back oriented in a caudal direction to the operator.
3. Elevate the skin at the lowest point in the midline with the toothed forceps. Using scissor dissection, harvest the animal's pelt by incising the whole thickness of the skin along the ventral midline to the neck, rotate the corpse onto its side, then cut around the body passing through both axillae, and complete the incision over both hind legs from the midline to the paws (**Fig. 5**).
4. Separate the pelt from one side of the corpse with blunt finger dissection, attach the pelt to a corkboard with two pushpins, and then repeat the process on the contralateral side. After the four corners of the pelt are transfixed, apply cervical traction while elevating the animal's torso, free the pelt with sharp dissection from its underlying attachments, and transect it at the level of the rear paws. A square of the pelt is now spread on the corkboard (**Fig. 6**) (*see* **Note 14**).
5. Coat the pelt with saline, and then place a rubber cutting block (a hockey puck is ideal) on the pelt between the four push pins. Remove the pins and flip the block over. The pelt will be on the top of the block, ready to be sampled (*see* **Note 15**).
6. Cut the wound sample strips with the dumbbell-shaped wound mount in the punch press perpendicular to the long axis of the incision (scar) avoiding the clip closure application sites (**Fig. 7**) (*see* **Notes 16** and **17**).
7. Load the sample strip on the materials tester. Tightly secure the ends of the strip and set the tester elongation rate at 3 cm/min, until the disruption of the healed wound occurs. The results will be recorded in grams (*see* **Notes 18–21**).

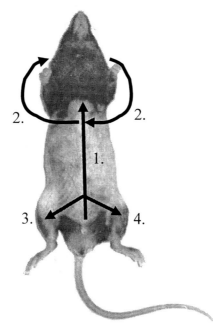

Fig. 5. Incisions for pelt harvest with scissors.

8. At least two strips per wound should be tested. If a formalin-fixed sample is to be tested, place the strip in a marked tissue cassette and then fix in 10% formalin for 24 h. To avoid twisting of the wound strips after fixation, a piece of sponge for support may be needed in the cassette. Appropriate materials should be prepared for special needs, such as cryogenic vials and liquid nitrogen for frozen sections.

4. Notes

1. Since total body weight is closely relevant to the wound disruption strength, organizing experimental groups by weights is a prerequisite to achieve valid test data. The animal weights should be recorded at least three times during the experiment: immediately before the operation, at the time of clip removal, and on the day of wound harvest. Under the stress induced by wounding and closure, normal animals typically experience some weight loss during the first 5 d postwounding, then regain the weight thereafter.
2. Anesthetic management is critical to the success of the study because it is performed on four occasions. The final occasion should not be a particular problem since it is designed to euthanize the animal. The first anesthetic allows shaving of the animals and requires only a brief period of anesthesia and not a deep plane of anesthesia. The second anesthetic requires a somewhat deeper plane to achieve surgical anesthesia for the creation of the wound, application

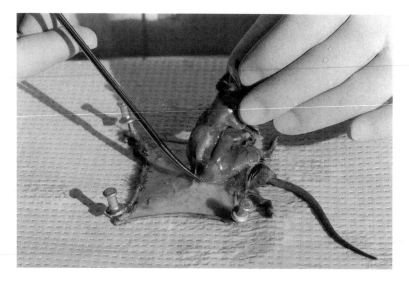

Fig. 6. Pelt transfixion to corkboard and removal from animal torso.

of any test materials, and proper wound closure of a fully anesthetized animal. The animals should be placed prone during their postanesthetic period for recovery and be warmed until fully recovered. The third anesthetic is again a light anesthesia for clip removal, which must be done in an atraumatic fashion to prevent any inadvertent injury to the healing wound. An alternative approach to this procedure is the use of ip sodium pentobarbital (0.8 mg/10 g of body wt per mouse), which provides a greater duration of anesthesia but is not as readily reversible as the inhalation technique. In general, the various wounding protocols require only brief periods of anesthesia; thus, inhalation anesthesia is the preferred method. Metofane, if available, is the first choice because it is very safe and quickly reversed by simply removing the animal from the anesthesia chamber. Alternatively, halothane anesthesia requires careful attention to the depth and rate of the animal's breathing; it is not as readily reversed as is metofane, and an anesthetic overdose is a distinct possibility. If an extended period of anesthesia is required during a procedure, supplemental dosing can be accomplished by placing a small flask (50 mL) containing a piece of gauze moistened with the anesthetic agent over the animal's nose.

3. The anesthetic chamber should be opened only briefly during animal handling to preserve the life of the anesthetic agent and prevent exposure to the operator. Anesthetic agents should be used in an area with a scavenge-type ventilation system.

4. The wounding procedure should be performed with an aseptic technique, and debris such as hair fragments should not be allowed to contaminate the wound site. Wound infection is a relatively uncommon occurrence in lower mammals if these basis principles are followed.

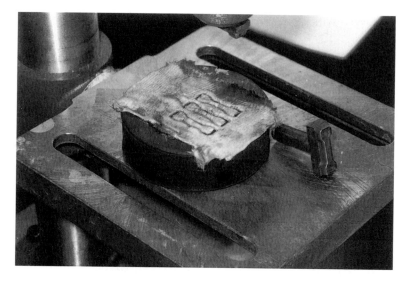

Fig. 7. Pelt mounted at hockey puck with three sample strips cut to long axis of incision (scar).

5. If both left and right paraspinous incisions are desired, the two sites should be alternated to avoid bias. Based on our experience, right paraspinous incisions seem to induce more bleeding than left.
6. The rationale for using scissors but not a scalpel to make the incision is (1) that mouse skin is highly mobile and can be easily distorted when attempting a scalpel incision and (2) that it is difficult to achieve a consistent and uniform depth of cut with a scalpel. The use of scissors results in a proper depth of incision, a sharply demarcated wound margin, avoidance of injury to adjacent structures, and is quickly performed.
7. The "tricks" for making the incisions with scissors are as follows:
   a. The long axis of the small cut should be parallel to the spine.
   b. The blunt tip should be slightly elevated when the scissor is advanced to avoid injuring deeper tissues.
   c. The cut should be made in a single plane and continuously to avoid an uneven wound edge.
   d. The incision is actually made more easily by pushing the scissors when they are maintained sharp than by cutting.
   e. Using the toothed forceps to apply tension at the starting point for the incision will assist in making a precise cut.
   f. Marking out the dimensions (length) of the wound to avoid the creation of an overly extended incision may be advisable.
8. The local administration of test compounds into a wound cleft is a standard approach in studies seeking to determine the ability of a drug to alter incisional healing. Unfortunately, the vehicle carrier may prove to be problematic and not

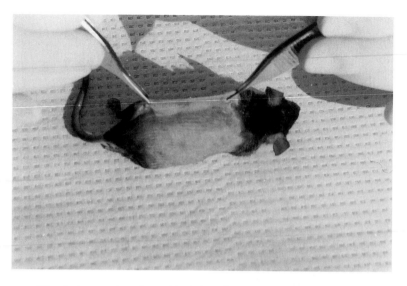

Fig. 8. Approximation of incisional wound with two forceps.

represent a valid delivery system. Liquid delivery systems often leak from the wound and the administered dose is not retained. More viscous vehicles may have limited absorbability. The vehicle may persist intact at the wound site and serve as a foreign body, which may well impair or totally inhibit healing. Studies such as this are then compromised by design and cannot answer the question, Is the test compound of value? Additionally, if cross-species reactions occur to foreign proteins, an immune reaction may further confuse the observations. Attention to these aspects of the experimental design are critical to the conduct of valid wound treatment studies.

9. Wound occlusion is facilitated by holding both ends of the wound with forceps and slightly lifting and pulling the wound. This is also the easiest and fastest way to approximate the two edges of the wound during the application of test materials (**Fig. 8**).

10. Wound closure is performed by pinching together one end of the incision with forceps under tension and applying a wound clip. Grasp the clip just applied with one hand and raise the skin slightly off of the mouse. With your free hand, pinch the two sides of the wound together while advancing the forceps along the incision to the next clip application site (approx 0.75 cm). Apply the second wound clip. This sequence is continued along the wound until it is closed with clips; most wounds require three clips. The clips should be evenly spaced over the wound. Poorly approximated wounds will have delayed and altered healing.

11. The clips must be applied in a secure fashion, since the mice, on recovering from anesthesia, will attempt to remove them. All animals should be checked during the experiment. Animals with clip loss may need to be removed from the study.

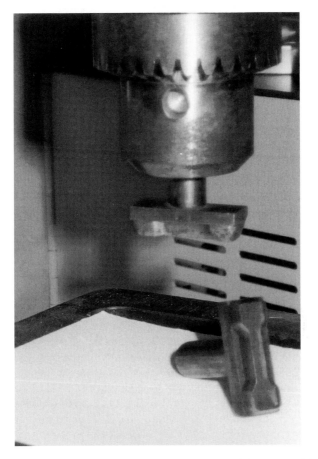

Fig. 9. Dumbbell-shaped cutter mounted in chuck of drill press with rod end.

12. The use of the autoclip remover is awkward. The trick is to hold the clip and let the tips of the remover fit in completely, and then squeeze the remover. One must avoid traumatizing the wound during this procedure.
13. The wound will demonstrate a ridge of healing induration at clip removal on d 5. Within 24 h after clip removal, considerable flattening will have occurred.
14. Leaving the dorsal skin attached to the body at the time of pelt harvest when blunt finger dissection is being performed will protect the wound from the mechanical trauma of the dissection.
15. Moistening the pelt with saline will prevent adhesion to the rubber block (hockey puck). Do not use alcohol; it will fix the tissue.
16. Since mice have minimal scarring, the wound may not be visible from the external surface after 3 wk. Maintaining the orientation of the pelt during

harvesting and mounting on the cutting block is important. One can check the deeper side (flip the pelt over) if it is necessary, to see the exact position of the wound on the pelt.

17. The specially designed cutter that we use is dumbbell shaped with the narrow portion measuring 4 mm wide and 12 mm long, which contains the test incision. The wider portion is 7 mm wide and 7 mm long at either end and is the site for attachment to the jaws of the materials tester (**Fig. 9**).

18. To avoid postmortem autolysis, harvested wound strips should be tested immediately after the pelt is prepared. This is particularly true for tests performed in the early phases of wound healing.

19. Not only the force applied to the wound but the rates of elongation are important. We have found that the rate of 3 cm/min is optimal.

20. Studies that require wound strength determination within the first week postwounding must be carefully performed, because many such wounds are relatively fragile and can be damaged with less than proper surgical technique.

21. As a testing time point, the first wk (d 5–7) postwounding is a window to check on the epidermal healing, since collagen deposition is not significant yet. The second and third weeks (d 10–21) may be the best time points to determine the effect of collagen deposition on wound-breaking strength. The increased breaking strength in the first three to five wk (d 21–35) after wounding is no longer related to collagen deposition but reflects the phase of wound remodeling. This period may also be the time point to check on wound tensile strength since tensile strength is gained during this phase. The rate of breaking strength may reach a plateau after 8 wk of wounding (d 56–90).

References

1. Owings, M. F. and Kozak, L. J. (1998) Ambulatory and inpatient procedures in the United States, 1996. *Vital Health Stat.—Ser. 13* **139,** 1–119.
2. Rhoads, S. L., Fliegelman, M. T., and Paner, L. M. (1942) The mechanism of delayed wound healing in the presence of hypoproteinemia. *JAMA* **118,** 21–23.
3. Pollack, S. V. (1979) Wound healing: a review. III. Nutritional factors affecting wound healing. *J. Dermatol. Surg. Oncol.* **5,** 615–619.
4. Modolin, M., Bevilacqua, R. G., Margarido, N. F., and Lima-Goncalves, E. (1984) The effects of protein malnutrition on wound contraction: an experimental study. *Ann. Plast. Surg.* **12,** 428–430.
5. Bourne, G. H. (1944) Effect of vitamin-C deficiency on experimental wounds. *Lancet* **27,** 688–692.
6. Greenhalgh, D. G. and Gamelli, R. L. (1988) Do nutritional alterations contribute to adriamycin-induced impaired wound healing? *J. Surg. Res.* **45,** 261–265.
7. Reitamo, J. and Moller, C. (1972) Abdominal wound dehiscence. *Acta Chir. Scand.* **138,** 170–175.
8. Mowat, A. G. and Baum, J. (1971) Chemotaxis of polymorphonuclear leukocytes from patients with diabetes mellitus. *N. Engl. J. Med.* **284,** 621–627.

9. Bybee, J. D. and Rogers, D. E. (1964) The phagocytic activity of polymorpho-nuclear leukocytes obtained from patients with diabetes mellitus. *J. Lab. Clin. Med.* **64,** 1–13.

10. Robson, M. C., Stenberg, B. D., and Heggers, J. P. (1990) Wound healing altera-tions caused by infection. *Clin. Plast. Surg.* **17,** 485–492.

11. Greenhalgh, D. G. and Gamelli, R. L. (1987) Is impaired wound healing caused by infection or nutritional depletion? *Surgery* **102,** 306–312.

12. Mendoza, C. B., Postlethwait, R. W., and Johnson, W. D. (1970) Incidence of wound disruption following operation. *Arch. Surg.* **101,** 396–398.

13. Boynton, P. R., Jaworski, D., and Paustian, C. (1999) Meeting the challenges of healing chronic wounds in older adults. *Nurs. Clin. North Am.* **34,** 921–932.

14. Heughan, C., Grislis, G., and Hunt, T. K. (1974) The effect of anemia on wound healing. *Ann. Surg.* **179,** 163–167.

15. Armstrong, C. P., Dixon, J. M., Duffy, S. W. Elton, R. A., and Davies, G. C. (1984) Wound healing in obstructive jaundice. *Br. J. Surg.* **71,** 267–270.

16. Goodson, W. H., Lindenfeld, S. M., Omachi, R. S., and Hunt, T. K. (1982) Chronic uremia causes poor healing. *Surg Forum* **33,** 54–56.

17. Furst, M. B., Stromberg, B. V., Blatchford, G. J., Christensen, M. A., and Thorson, A. G. (1994) Colonic anastomoses: bursting strength after corticosteroid treatment. *Dis. Colon Rectum* **37,** 12–15.

18. Eubanks, T. R., Greenberg, J. J., Dobrin, P. B., Harford, F. J., and Gamelli, R. L. (1997) The effects of different corticosteroids on the healing colon anastomosis and cecum in a rat model. *Am. Surg.* **63,** 266–269.

19. Moore, M. J. (1984) The effect of radiation on connective tissue. *Otolaryngol. Clin. North Am.* **17,** 389–399.

20. Joseph, D. L. and Shumrick, D. L. (1973) Risks of head and neck surgery in previously irradiated patients. *Arch. Otolaryngol.* **97,** 381–384.

21. Whelan, D. M., van Beusekom, H. M., and van der Giessen, W. J. (1997) Foreign body contamination during stent implantation. *Cathet. Cardiovasc. Diagn.* **40,** 328–332.

22. Troyer-Caudle, J. (1993) Debridement: removal of non-viable tissue. *Ostomy Wound Manage.* **39,** 24–32.

23. Harvey, S. C. (1929) The velocity of the growth of fibroblasts in the healing wound. *Arch. Surg.* **18,** 1227–1240.

24. Lanman, L. H. and Ingalls, T. H. (1937) Vitamin C deficiency and wound healing. *Ann. Surg.* **105,** 616–646.

25. Howes, E. L. and Harvey, S. C. (1929) The strength of the healing wound in relation to the holding strength of the catgut suture. *N. Engl. J. Med.* **200,** 1285–1291.

26. Hartzell, J. B. and Stone, W. E. (1942) The relationship of the concentration of ascorbic acid of the blood to the tensile strength of wounds in animals. *Surg. Gynecol. Obstet.* **75,** 1–7.

27. Jones, C. M., Bartlett, M. K., Ryan, A. E., and Drummey, G. D. (1943) The effect of sulfanilamide powder on the healing of sterile and infected wounds. *N. Engl. J. Med.* **229,** 642–646.

28. Berger, A. C., Feldman, A. L., Gnant, M. F. X., Kruger, E. A., Sim, B. K. L., Hewitt, S., Figg, W. D., Alexander, H. R., and Libutti, S. K. (2000) The angiogenesis inhibitor, endostatin, does not affect murine cutaneous wound healing. *J. Surg. Res.* **91,** 26–31.

29. Greenhalgh, D. G., Gamelli, R. L., Foster, R. S., and Chester, A. (1985) Inhibition of wound healing by corynebacterium parvum. *J. Surg. Res.* **41,** 209–214.

30. Levenson, S. M., Crowley, L. V., Geever, E. F., Rosen, H., and Berard, C. W. (1964) Some studies of wound healing: experimental methods, effect of ascorbic acid and effect of deuterium oxide. *J. Trauma* **4,** 543–566.

31. Dexter, F. and Edsall, J. T. (1945) The reactions of formaldehyde with amino acids and proteins. *Adv. Protein Chem.* **2,** 277–335.

32. Hopwood, B. (1969) Fixatives and fixation: a review. *Histochem. J.* **1,** 322–360.

33. Levenson, S. M., Geever, E. F., Crowley, L. V., Oates, J. F., Berard, C. W., and Rosen, H. (1965) The healing of rat skin wounds. *Ann. Surg.* **161,** 293–308.

34. Miles, R. H., Paxton, T. P., Zacheis, D., Dries, D. J., and Gamelli, R. L. (1994) Systemic administration of interferon-γ impairs wound healing. *J. Surg. Res.* **56,** 288–294.

4

Animal Models of Ischemic Wound Healing

Toward an Approximation of Human Chronic Cutaneous Ulcers in Rabbit and Rat

Mark Sisco and Thomas A. Mustoe

1. Introduction

Chronic wounds are defined as wounds that heal with a significant delay, usually over a period of more than 2 mo. The morbidity associated with delayed wound healing imposes an enormous social and financial burden on the health care system. Clinical observations suggest that persistent tissue ischemia in the vicinity of the wound is an important underlying feature of chronic wounds that severely impairs the healing process. Prolonged ischemia subjects wounds to infection, inflammation, and necrosis and is a significant contributor to delayed healing in the settings of diabetes, pressure sores, peripheral vascular disease, and venous stasis. In addition, research shows that the physiological response to wounding is deranged in the elderly. This cumulative effect has been demonstrated when topical agents that improve wound healing in the young failed to work in the aged *(1–3)*.

Currently, there is no ideal animal model of the chronic wound. Several models have been developed to study the effects of ischemia on wound healing, most of which are based on cutaneous flaps. Quirina and colleagues *(4,5)* developed an H-shaped random pattern flap in the rat dorsum, in which the horizontal line of the *H* is the ischemic incision and the vertical arms of the *H* are control wounds. Perfusion to the flap is immediately reduced by 93% and increases in a linear fashion until control levels are reached at d 16. This model is easy to create and is elegantly designed. However, such models have limitations. The rapidity with which the tissue returns to normal levels of

From: *Methods in Molecular Medicine, vol. 78: Wound Healing: Methods and Protocols*
Edited by: Luisa A. DiPietro and Aime L. Burns © Humana Press Inc., Totowa, NJ

perfusion precludes extended testing of potential vulnerary agents. Meanwhile, it is difficult to assess wound healing in incisional wounds, since breaking strength measurements reflect only one aspect of healing.

The model described in **Subheading 3.2.** *(6)*, in which the left ear of a rabbit is made ischemic, was designed to approximate three important characteristics of human chronic cutaneous ulcers. First, ischemia is significant and prolonged *(7)*, allowing repeated or continuous testing of therapeutic agents. In the ischemic ear, we have found pO_2 to be significantly decreased at d 14 postwounding, with a trend still apparent at d 28 *(8)*. Using this model, ischemia has been confirmed using dermofluorometry, tissue PO_2 measurements, venous pO_2 and pH sampling, and tissue temperature measurements. Second, wound contraction is minimal since the dermis is tightly adherent to the underlying cartilage, which essentially splints the wound as it heals *(9,10)*. Third, the model is well tolerated by aged animals, which are more sensitive to anesthesia and surgery.

The rabbit model has additional benefits. Since healing takes place only from the periphery of the wound, the healing time is extended even in the nonischemic wounds. This allows relative ease in detecting a statistically significant difference between control wounds and treatment wounds, even after modest stimulation or inhibition of healing. In addition, the end points of this model are reproducible and quantifiable. Histology can provide discrete quantitative data on epithelialization and deposition of granulation tissue. Immunohistochemistry and *in situ* hybridization can provide additional information. Finally, creating control wounds in each animal increases the statistical power of the data and reduces the number of animals required.

We have successfully performed this model in the rat with minor modifications (*see* **Note 1**) *(11)*. Although the size of the rat allows for the creation of only one wound per ear, the rat model has several advantages. More genomic sequence data and molecular reagents are available, aged animals are more easily obtained, and the cost per animal for procurement and maintenance is lower.

2. Materials

2.1. Preparation of Animals

1. New Zealand white rabbit, about 3 kg (*see* **Note 2**).
2. Ketamine (Ketaset™) and xylazine (X-ject™).
3. 3-cc Syringe with 25-gage needle.
4. Electric shaver.
5. Depilatory agent (Nair™).
6. Sterile gauze.
7. Povidone-iodine solution (Betadine™).
8. Sterile drape.

2.2. Pedicle Dissection

1. Scalpel handle with no. 15 blade.
2. Sterile gauze.
3. Blunt tissue-dissecting scissors.
4. Microscissors and forceps.
5. Operating microscope (loupes can be substituted; we suggest using ×2.5 or greater magnification).
6. Monofilament nylon suture (5-0) on a cutting needle (Ethilon™).
7. Needle driver and Adson forceps with teeth.

2.3. Wounding

1. Disposable skin biopsy punch, 6 mm.
2. Sterile gauze.
3. Microscissors and forceps.
4. Operating microscope (loupes can be substituted).
5. Freer double-ended periosteal elevator, 3 mm wide.
6. Cotton swabs.
7. Skin adhesive (Mastisol™).
8. Polyurethane occlusive dressing (Tegaderm™), cut into 1.5-cm squares.

2.4. Harvesting of Wounds

1. Ketamine and xylazine.
2. 3-cc Syringe with 25-gage needle.
3. Scalpel with no. 10 blade or razor blade.
4. Histological cassettes.
5. Plastic specimen container with lid.
6. Fixative (*see* **Note 3**).
7. Liquid nitrogen (optional).

2.5. Microscopic Analysis

1. Light microscope (capable of ×200 magnification) with reticle.

3. Methods

3.1. Preparation of Animals

1. Weigh rabbit and anesthetize using 60 mg/kg of ketamine, and 5 mg/kg of xylazine intramuscularly. Ketamine and xylazine can be mixed in one syringe prior to injection.
2. Shave the inside and outside of each ear. Shave the base of the left ear circumferentially. Apply the depilatory agent generously to the inside of both ears and allow 5 min for it to take effect. The hair and depilatory agent can then be removed with moist gauze.
3. Prep each ear with surgical scrub and allow it to dry.
4. Drape the rabbit such that the entire left ear is exposed.

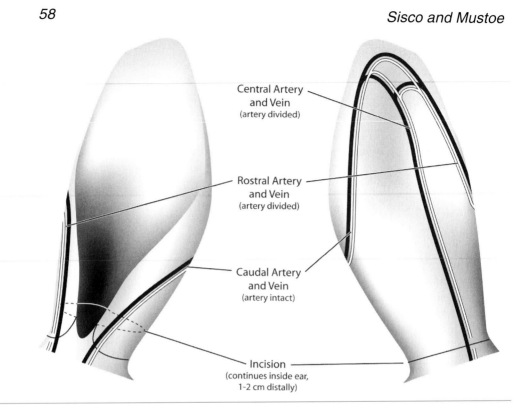

Central Artery
and Vein
(artery divided)

Rostral Artery
and Vein
(artery divided)

Caudal Artery
and Vein
(artery intact)

Incision
(continues inside ear,
1-2 cm distally)

Fig. 1. Vascular anatomy of left rabbit ear.

3.2. Pedicle Dissection

In this model, the left ear is rendered ischemic. The right ear serves as a paired control.

1. The rabbit ear is supplied by three major vascular pedicles: the rostral, central, and caudal (*see* **Figs. 1** and **2**). These are easily visible on the dorsum of the ear. Note their locations before starting. Using a no. 15 blade, circumferentially incise the dermis on the outside of the ear 1 cm distal to the base of the left ear. Do not incise more deeply at this time.
2. Identify each pedicle underneath the dermis. Under the microscope, dissect each pedicle from the surrounding tissue using blunt dissecting scissors. This can be best accomplished by gently spreading the scissors in the direction of the vessels, perpendicular to the incision (*see* **Note 4**).
3. Taking care to protect each pedicle, deepen the circumferential incision to the level of the cartilage. This incision will interrupt the subcutaneous microvasculature. Control bleeding with bipolar electrocautery.
4. Under the microscope, divide the rostral and central arteries after cauterizing them. Preserve all veins and the caudal artery.

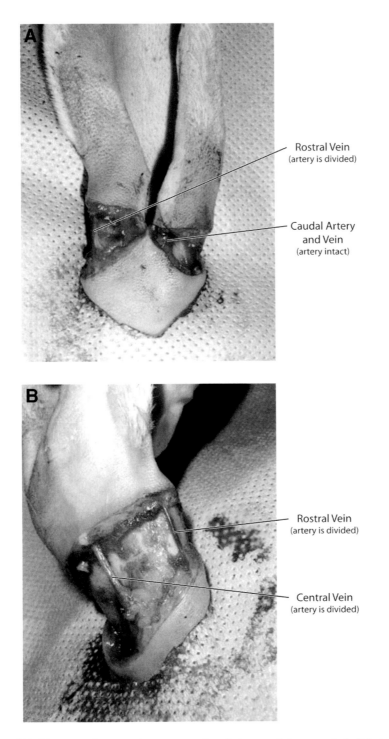

Fig. 2. **(A)** The rostral artery is transected and the caudal artery is left intact. **(B)** The rostral and central arteries are transected.

5. Extend the dermal incision (from **Step 2**) across the inside of the ear (*see* **Fig. 2**). This may be done 1 to 2 cm distal to the incision on the outside of the ear.
6. Reapproximate the dermis using 5–0 nylon. On the inside of the ear, sutures may not be necessary if the dermal incision has not spread open.

3.3. Wounding

In this model, four circular full-thickness ulcers are created on each ear. The base on which granulation and epithelization take place is the avascular cartilage.

1. Redrape the rabbit such that both ears are exposed.
2. Using a 6-mm-diameter biopsy punch, create four circular wounds through the skin to the level of the cartilage on the ventral aspect of each ear (*see* **Note 5** and **Fig. 3**).
3. Using forceps and a periosteal elevator, raise the skin inside the punch wound from the cartilage. Remove the perichondrium from the cartilage as well. This may come up with the skin or may have to be removed separately (*see* **Note 6**).
4. When the wounds on both ears are completed, wipe each ear with sterile gauze and swab adhesive around each wound site.
5. Apply an occlusive dressing to each wound site (*see* **Note 7**).

3.4. Treatment

The dermis should be injected subcutaneously within 1 mm of the wound, since most wound-healing activity is thought to take place in this area *(12)*. Topical agents may be applied using a sterile cotton swab or syringe.

3.5. Harvesting of Wounds

In the control wounds, 50% of wounds will be fully epithelialized by d 7. In ischemic wounds, no wounds will be epithelialized by d 7. By d 7, 39% of ischemic wounds are completely covered by granulation tissue. Sixty-three percent of control wounds are completely covered by granulation tissue at the same time point.

1. Heavily anesthetize the rabbit as described in **Subheading 3., step 1** prior to harvest (*see* **Note 8**).
2. Shave the backs of the ears and remove the occlusive dressings.
3. Note any wounds that appear dried out or infected; these factors will affect results.
4. Amputate the ears with a razor blade or scalpel.
5. Cut the wounds out, one at a time, in a rectangular shape, 2–5 mm outside the circle.
6. Bisect the wounds slightly off center (*see* **Fig. 4**).

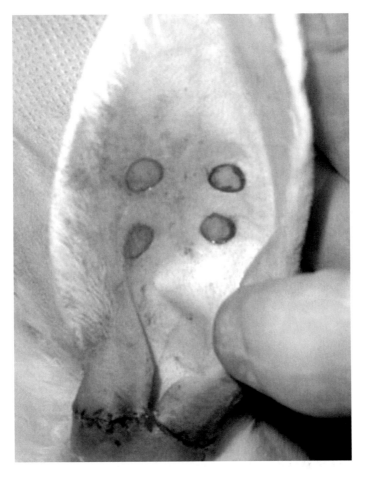

Fig. 3. After closure of the incision, four partial-thickness wounds are made on the inside of the ear.

7. Place the larger half of the wound into a cassette for fixation and processing (*see* **Note 9**). The other half of the bisected wound may be flash-frozen in liquid nitrogen for molecular biological assays (*see* **Note 10**).
8. Euthanize the rabbit.

3.6. Microscopic Analysis (see Note 11 and Fig. 5)

Conventional histology can be analyzed using a standard light microscope.

1. Verify that you are looking at a section cut near the middle of the punch wound by locating the nicks in the cartilage made by the biopsy punch. These nicks

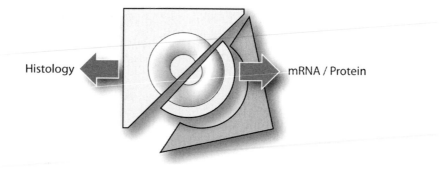

Fig. 4. One half of each wound can be used for histology. The other half can be used for molecular assays. Note that the wound is transected slightly off center so that tissue can be wasted during cutting before the center of the wound is reached.

     should be about 6 mm apart. If they are absent, the location of the original wound margin can be estimated by finding the interface between granulation tissue and the preexisting dermis. On a trichrome-stained section, this interface will appear as a shift from mostly blue (mature collagen) to mostly pink (granulation tissue).

2. Using the reticle, measure and record the cross-sectional area of the granulation tissue (*see* **Note 12** and **Figure 5B**) on either side of the wound.
3. Measure and record the granulation tissue gap (*see* **Fig. 5A**).
4. Measure and record the epithelial gap (*see* **Fig. 5A**).

4. Notes

1. This model can be achieved in the rat with the following modifications:
   a. When prepping the rat, shaving and applying the depilatory agent to the inside of the ear is not necessary.
   b. When rendering the ear ischemic, the rostral and central arteries *and veins* are divided. We cauterize the entire dermis circumferentially as well.
   c. When wounding the ear, use a 5-mm biopsy punch. Make one wound per ear. Since the cartilage in the rat ear is only three to four cells thick, it is easy to transect it when using the biopsy punch. Furthermore, scoring the cartilage (*see* **Note 4**) is nearly impossible. We use the biopsy punch to score the skin and a microsurgical scalpel to incise the edge of the wound.
2. Paired wounds generally allow reproducible results when 8–10 animals are used.
3. For routine histology, we use 10% formalin overnight. Other applications such as immunohistochemistry may require other methods of fixation.
4. Do not fully dissect the caudal pedicle. Leaving a 1-mm cuff of tissue around it will prevent damage or spasm of the arterial supply to the ear.

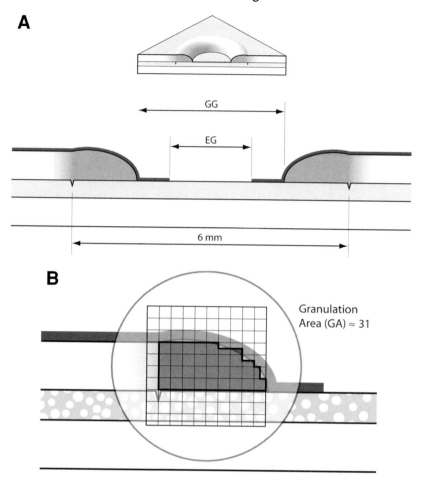

Fig. 5. (**A**) Schematic of histologic analysis. EG, epithelial gap; GG, granulation gap. (**B**) The reticle can be used to calculate the area of new granulation tissue.

5. Take care not to perforate the cartilage. Scoring the cartilage is acceptable and indeed will facilitate histological analysis by marking the initial wound margin.
6. The perichondrium appears as a fibrous, transparent layer over the cartilage. Remove this layer using sterile gauze of the periosteal elevator. The cartilage should appear clean and shiny.
7. The use of occlusive dressings to maintain a moist wound environment is critical to this model. Desiccation of the cartilage will result in necrosis, which will significantly impair healing of the wound. Animals should be checked daily

to ensure integrity of the dressings. The use of one dressing for each wound makes it less likely that all of the wounds will go uncovered for any period of time.

8. If RNA is to be extracted from the tissues, it is better to harvest the wounds from the animal while it is alive since RNA starts to degrade within minutes of death. It is important to heavily anesthetize the animal when doing so since rabbits are extremely sensitive to amputation of the ear. If routine histology is all that is needed, we recommend euthanizing the rabbit immediately prior to harvest.

9. When cutting tissue for histology, attempt to take sections from the first millimeter or so. As deeper sections approach the wound edge, analysis of wound-healing parameters, such as granulation tissue area, becomes difficult.

10. The amount of cartilage present in these samples may make disruption and homogenization of the tissue difficult when extracting RNA. We use a motorized rotor-stator homogenizer on our samples. The amount of collagen in the samples has prompted us to use a Proteinase K step in our RNA extractions. These steps have improved our yields greatly.

11. For routine histology, we use hematoxylin and eosin (H&E) and trichrome stains. Granulation tissue can be best measured using a trichrome stain while epithelialization can be best assessed using H&E.

12. We have found that the area of granulation tissue, in cross section, correlates best with conventional wound-healing parameters. The granulation tissue gap is an important corroborating value, since inflammation at the wound site (owing to infection or necrosis of the cartilage) may spuriously increase the granulation tissue area. Therefore, elevated granulation tissue values in the setting of a large granulation gap should be interpreted with caution.

References

1. Wu, L., Xia, Y. P., Roth, S. I., Gruskin, E., and Mustoe, T. A. (1999) Transforming growth factor-beta1 fails to stimulate wound healing and impairs its signal transduction in an aged ischemic ulcer model: importance of oxygen and age. *Am. J. Pathol.* **154,** 301–309.

2. Mustoe, T. A., Cutler, N. R., Allman, R. M., Goode, P. S., Deuel, T. F., Prause, J. A., Bear, M., Serdar, C. M., and Pierce, G. F. (1994) A phase II study to evaluate recombinant platelet-derived growth factor-BB in the treatment of stage 3 and 4 pressure ulcers. *Arch. Surg.* **129,** 213–219.

3. Richard, J. L., Parer-Richard C., Daures, J. P., Clouet, S., Vannereau, D., Bringer, J., Rodier, M., Jacob, C., and Comte-Bardonnet, M. (1995) Effect of topical basic fibroblast growth factor on the healing of chronic diabetic neuropathic ulcer of the foot. A pilot, randomized, double-blind, placebo-controlled study. *Diabetes Care* **18,** 64–69.

4. Quirinia, A., Taagehoj, F., and Viidik, A. (1992) Ischemia in wound healing I: design of a flap model-changes in blood flow. *Scand. J. Plast. Reconstr. Hand Surg.* **26,** 21–28.

5. Quirinia, A. and Viidik, A. (1992) Ischemia in wound healing II: design of a flap model-biomechanical properties. *Scand. J. Plast. Reconstr. Hand Surg.* **26,** 133–139.
6. Ahn, S. T. and Mustoe, T. A. (1990) Effects of ischemia on ulcer wound healing: a new model in the rabbit ear. *Ann. Plast. Surg.* **24,** 17–23.
7. Bonomo, S. R., Davidson, J. D., Tyrone, J. W., Lin, X., and Mustoe, T. A. (2000) Enhancement of wound healing by hyperbaric oxygen and transforming growth factor beta3 in a new chronic wound model in aged rabbits. *Arch Surg.* **135,** 1148–1153.
8. Wu, L. and Mustoe, T. A. (1994) Effect of ischemia on growth factor enhancement of wound healing. *Surgery* **117(5),** 570–576.
9. Joseph, J. and Townsend, F. J. (1961) The healing of defects in immobile skin in rabbits. *Br. J. Surg.* **48,** 557–564.
10. Zahir, M. (1964) Contraction of wounds. *Br. J. Surg.* **31,** 456–461.
11. Zhao, L., Sisco, M., Mogford, J. E., and Mustoe, T. A. (2000) Effects of ischemia on a model of non-contractile cutaneous wound healing in the rat. *Wound Healing Soc.* (Abstract).
12. Bevin, A. and Madden, J. (1969) The localization of collagen synthesis in healing wounds. *Surg. Forum* **20,** 65–66.

5

Corneal Injury

A Relatively Pure Model of Stromal-Epithelial Interactions in Wound Healing

Steven E. Wilson, Rahul R. Mohan, Renato Ambrosio, and Rajiv R. Mohan

1. Introduction

Wound healing is a complex cascade that varies depending on the organ being studied. However, many components of the response are similar in different organs. Stromal-epithelial interactions are critical to wound healing in tissues in which epithelium and stroma are conjoined. The cornea provides a relatively pure model of stromal-epithelial interactions since there are no blood vessels, sebaceous glands, hair follicles, or other structures involved in the response (**Fig. 1**). There are Langerhan's cells distributed within the epithelium, and sensory nerve endings innervate the basal epithelium, but otherwise the system is pure. Another advantage of the cornea is unambiguous localization of epithelial and stromal (keratocyte) cells. This is convenient when monitoring the expression of mRNAs and proteins by these cells during the wound-healing response. The tissue is also tough and stands up well to cryofixation and cryosectioning. This facilitates the use of antibodies in immunocytochemistry that cannot be used with formalin-fixed tissues. Terminal deoxyribonucleotidyl transferase–mediated dUTP-digoxigenin nick end labeling (TUNEL) assay to detect apoptosis can be performed on either cryofixed or formalin-fixed corneal sections. Finally, the cornea is amenable to a variety of manipulations, such as epithelial scrape, lamellar flap formation, microinjection of cytokines, exposure to toxic chemicals, and infection with microorganisms, that facilitate study of the wound-healing response. The most

From: *Methods in Molecular Medicine, vol. 78: Wound Healing: Methods and Protocols*
Edited by: Luisa A. DiPietro and Aime L. Burns © Humana Press Inc., Totowa, NJ

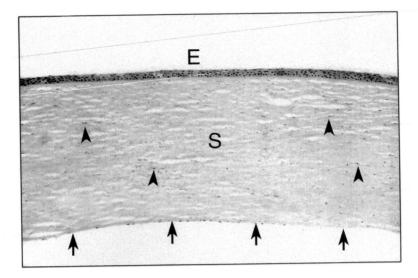

Fig. 1. The cornea has epithelial (E), stromal (S), and endothelial (arrows) layers that are well delineated and unambiguous. Keratocytes (arrowheads) are the cells that are embedded in the stroma composed of collagen, glycosaminoglycans, and other connective-tissue components. Special stains are required to identify occasional Langerhan's cells in the epithelium or sensory nerve trunks that run through the stroma and terminate adjacent to the basal epithelium. These cannot be detected in this H&E-stained section. This particular specimen is from human and has an approximate central thickness of 500 μm. Magnification: ×100.

common animal models used in corneal wound-healing studies are the mouse and rabbit. This chapter details methods for initiating the healing response in the cornea and some of the manipulations that can be applied to investigate stromal-epithelial interactions in this organ.

2. Materials

2.1. Animals

Six- to 8-wk-old Balb/c mice and 8-wk-old New Zealand white rabbits are most commonly used for corneal wound-healing studies *(1,2)*. Other strains of mice and rabbits are acceptable. Rats are less commonly used and the methods for studying this species are not covered here. The principles, however, are similar to those used in mice. The effects of gene knockout of growth factors, receptors, matrix components, and other factors on corneal wound healing are also commonly tested in mice.

2.2. Anesthesia and Euthanasia

1. Xylazine hydrochloride and ketamine hydrochloride, for injected anesthesia.
2. Topical Ophthaine, Tetracaine (1%), or Proparacaine (1%) drops, for local anesthesia.
3. Pentobarbitol, for euthanasia.
4. Topical Ocuflox drops (Allergan, Irvine, CA), to inhibit microbial infection.
5. Sterile syringes (5 cc) with 25-gage 1.5-in. needles (Fisher, Pittsburgh, PA), for ip and iv injections.

2.3. Wounding Methods

1. Disposable no. 64 and 15 Beaver (Becton-Dickinson, Franklin Lakes, NJ) blades.
2. Circular radial keratotomy optical zone marker (Bausch and Lomb, Rochester, NY), to mark the diameter of the intended wound.
3. Wire lid speculum (Bausch and Lomb), to hold the eye open in rabbits.
4. Topical Fluress (Akron, Buffalo Grove, IL) fluorescein solution, to document epithelial defects.
5. Guarded 100-μm blade (Alcon, Ft. Worth, TX) and Swarez lamellar dissecting blade (Alcon), to initiate lamellar corneal dissections and extend them across the cornea, respectively.
6. Summit Apex (Summit, Waltham, MA) excimer laser.
7. Hansatome microkeratome (Bausch and Lomb) with disposable stainless steel blades, to produce lamellar corneal flap.
8. Contact lens (Soflens 66 F/M base curve; Bausch and Lomb).

2.4. Microinjection into Stroma

1. Hamilton (Reno, NV) syringe microinjection system with drawn capillary pipets attached to blunt needle with polyethylene tubing.
2. 0.05% Bovine serum albumin (BSA) in phosphate-buffered saline (PBS) (Sigma, St. Louis, MO).

2.5. Tissue Procurement, Cryofixation, and Formaldehyde Fixation

1. Sharp Wescott scissors.
2. Iris scissors.
3. No. 15 Beaver blade.
4. Fine 0.12-mm toothed forceps, for tissue removal. High-quality instruments can be obtained from Bausch and Lomb or Alcon.
5. Cryomolds (Fisher, Fair Lawn, NJ) with OCT solution (Sakura Finetek, Torrance, CA), for embedding rabbit corneas.
6. 37% Buffered formaldehyde (Sigma) and paraffin, to fix and mount whole mouse eyes, respectively.

2.6. Tissue Sectioning

1. Reichert-Jung cryostat (Leica, Deerfield, IL) with a disposable blade holder, to perform cryosections.
2. Microtome, to prepare paraffin sections.
3. Superfrost plus slides (Fisher).

2.7. Histological analysis, TUNEL Assay, and Immunocytochemistry

1. Hematoxylin and eosin (H&E) and propidium iodide (Sigma), for staining.
2. TUNEL assay kit (Intergen, Purchase, NY).
3. Dako (Carpinteria, CA) Universal LSAB + peroxidase kit, for immunocyto-chemistry. Fluorescent kits are also available. The specific kit utilized is selected based on the isotype of the primary antibody.

3. Methods

3.1. Animals

All studies must adhere to the Association for Research in Vision and Ophthalmology Statement for the Use of Animals in Ophthalmic and Vision Research. Animals must be healthy and without evidence of eye infection or trauma. Surgery is typically performed in only one eye of the animal so that it can socialize, eat, and drink normally after anesthesia. There is evidence of contralateral effects of corneal scrape and other surgical manipulations (3). For this reason, we prefer not to use the contralateral eye as a control eye.

3.2. Anesthesia and Euthanasia

Mice are anesthetized by ip injection of 5 mg/kg of xylazine and 50 mg/kg of ketamine intraperitoneally. Adult New Zealand white rabbits are anesthetized by im injection of 30 mg/kg of ketamine hydrochloride and 5 mg/kg of xylazine hydrochloride. These injections are typically given in the rear upper leg. The eye is anesthetized by topical application of a drop of proparacaine or tetracaine just prior to manipulation of either the mouse or rabbit eye with instruments. The cornea is highly innervated, and, therefore, it is critical that the topical anesthetic be applied even though the animal is under general anesthesia (*see* **Note 1**).

Euthanasia is also performed while the animal is under general anesthetic. Rabbits are injected with 100 mg/kg of pentobarbitol via an ear vein. Mice are injected with 100 mg/kg of pentobarbitol intraperitoneally.

3.3. Wounding Methods

Each of these procedures is best performed under direct visualization using a stereo-operating microscope, although corneal epithelial scrape can be performed with the loupes or a magnifying glass.

3.3.1. Scrape

Corneal epithelial scrape injuries are most easily performed by scraping with a no. 64 Beaver blade (rabbit) or a no. 15 Beaver blade (mouse). Typically a 7-mm-diameter wound is made in the rabbit cornea and a 2-mm-diameter wound is made in the mouse cornea, but the size may vary depending on what aspect of the wound-healing response is being studied.

1. After general and topical anesthesia is obtained, place a wire eyelid speculum into the rabbit eye. Gently separate mouse eyelids with the fingers.
2. Press lightly the marker of the appropriate diameter against the corneal epithelium so that an indentation is visible (**Fig. 2A**).
3. Remove all of the epithelium within the mark by gently, but firmly, scraping with the blade edge rotated 45° away from the direction the blade is moved (**Fig. 2B**). This prevents the scalpel blade from cutting into the corneal stroma, which would change the healing characteristics of the wound. Care must be taken to remove all epithelium within the mark down to the smooth stromal surface to increase the uniformity of the injury.
4. Apply topical Ocuflox drops several times a day to help prevent infection if the animal will not be euthanized within 4 h of the injury (*see* **Notes 2** and **3**).
5. Observe and monitor the epithelial wound by placing a single drop of Fluress into the eye, massaging the eyelids together, and illuminating the surface with a cobalt blue filtered light (**Fig. 2C**). The fluorescein in this dye stains exposed basement membrane or stroma.
6. Take photographs for documentation or quantitation of wound area over time with a 35-mm camera using a cobalt blue filter. Constant magnification must be maintained if quantitation is to be performed and, therefore, it is best that the camera be held at a precise distance from the eye by a tripod. Images can be scanned and the area of the wound quantitated using NIH Image software. The typical 7-mm rabbit epithelial wound will heal in 3 to 4 d and the typical 2-mm mouse wound will heal in approx 48 h.

3.3.2. Alternate Methods

3.3.2.1. LASER

In some cases, it is important that the epithelial wounds be highly uniform from animal to animal. This is best attained by using an excimer laser in phototherapeutic keratectomy mode with an ablation diameter of 6 mm (the maximum with most excimer lasers) to remove the epithelium. Excimer lasers are available in many ophthalmology departments. Excimer lasers remove tissue by photodisruption without generating significant heat that would damage the tissue. No laser-related damage is produced in the surrounding tissue. Most excimer lasers can be used for this purpose, but the Summit Apex is optimal because of the optical properties of the laser-microscope system.

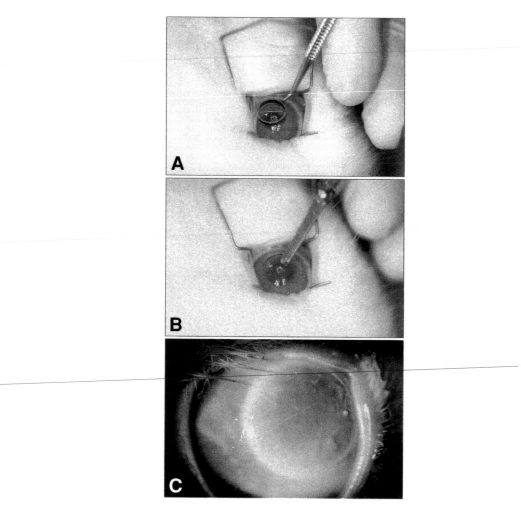

Fig. 2. Forming and monitoring of epithelial defect in rabbit cornea. (**A**) The corneal surface was initially marked with a 7-mm-diameter optical zone marker. (**B**) Note that the blade is turned away from the direction that scrapping is performed to prevent cutting into the stroma. (**C**) After formation of the defect and until complete epithelial healing occurs, the epithelial defect can be observed and photographed by putting a drop of Fluress fluorescein solution into the eye.

Since the 193-nm excimer laser energy bearing on the epithelium fluoresces blue but does not fluoresce (appears black) when bearing on the stroma, the investigator can precisely determine when the epithelium has been completely ablated. The operating microscope is focused so that the reticle appears to rest on the cornea centered on the pupil. The lights are dimmed and the laser is activated. As bursts of the laser are automatically applied at a rate of 10/s, the investigator monitors the blue emitted from the epithelial surface. After approx 200–250 bursts the investigator will begin to note black in the periphery of the area being ablated, indicating that the epithelium has been completely removed at this point. Within a few pulses, the entire ablation circle will appear black, indicating that all epithelium overlying this area has been photoablated. It is important not to extend the ablation further at this point unless deeper extension into the stroma is intended.

Healing of the cornea following this method is similar to that with mechanically scraping the cornea, although the keratocyte apoptosis response is somewhat diminished *(2)* (*see* **Notes 2** and **3**).

3.3.2.2. Lamellar Flap Formation

Another wound type that can be produced in the rabbit cornea is lamellar flap formation. This is similar to the lamellar flap formed as a part of the laser *in situ* keratomeliusis (LASIK) procedure performed in human eyes to correct nearsightedness. Investigators may wish to produce such a flap to investigate the altered wound-healing response that is associated with the LASIK procedure. Alternatively, formation of an epithelial-anterior stromal flap provides access to the central stroma while leaving the central corneal epithelium intact. For example, we use such a flap to directly expose keratocytes in the central stroma to adenoassociated viral vectors that would not penetrate the epithelium. Thus, the investigator can transfer genes coding for growth factors, antiapoptotic factors, and other proteins into the keratocytes and study the effects of these genes on the corneal wound-healing response.

1. With the rabbit under general anesthesia and the eye anesthetized with topical anesthetic, briefly proptose the eye anterior to the lids and place a surgical clamp to hold the lateral upper and lower eyelids together to maintain proptosis of the eye.
2. Place the base of the Hansatome microkeratome (**Fig. 3A**) on the corneal surface and activate suction with the microkeratome power supply.
3. Since the curvature of the rabbit cornea is different from that of the human, the base will not suction onto the eye as it does in the human. For this reason, place a clamp on the suction tubing running from the microkeratome base to the power supply so that the instrument senses suction in the tubing. Otherwise, safety monitors in the power supply will block the automated microkeratome head from cutting the flap.
4. Press the microkeratome base very firmly on the cornea, put the microkeratome head containing the blade (**Fig. 3B**) into position, and depress the forward pedal activating the motor. Maintain posterior pressure of the base against the cornea to simulate suction obtained in the human eye while the head of the microkeratome courses across the gear track to cut the flap.

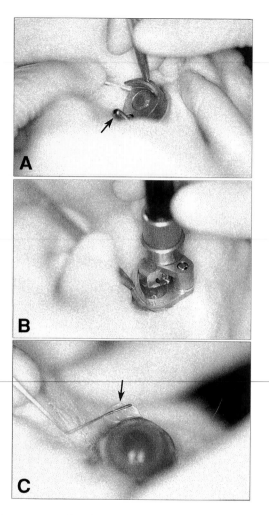

Fig. 3. Use of Hansatome microkeratome to make stromal-epithelial flap. (**A**) The base of the microkeratome is placed on the cornea. The pin (arrow) on which the cutting head pivots during cutting of the flap can be seen. The eye is proptosed anterior to the eyelid. (**B**) The head of the microkeratome is placed into position and engaged with the gear track on the base. (**C**) The flap (arrow) is lifted with a spatula and reflected onto the superior conjunctiva. Note that it remains attached to the cornea by a hinge of tissue.

5. Return the head to its origin by depressing the reverse pedal.
6. Remove the base and head of the microkeratome from the eye.
7. Insert the end of a smooth round spatula into the stromal interface where the cut was made and reflect the flap back against the conjunctiva exposing the bed (**Fig. 3C**).

8. The microkeratome is designed to leave the flap attached to the superior cornea by a hinge. Return the flap to its original position with the spatula once drug or viral vector is applied to the bed and/or the posterior stromal surface of the flap. After 1 min the flap will self-adhere to the cornea.
9. Place a drop of Ocuflox into the eye.
10. The flap can be protected with a contact lens for the first day and the eyelids closed with a temporary suture tarsorrhaphy (*see* **Notes 2** and **3**).
11. The cornea and flap can be analyzed as a unit or the flap can be excised and the flap and remaining cornea analyzed separately when the cornea is processed for histological analysis.

3.4. Microinjection into Stroma

Cytokines and other proteins cannot penetrate into the stroma when the epithelium is intact because of barrier function. Microinjection can be used to analyze the effect of individual cytokines, combinations of cytokines, or other potential modulators on keratocytes in the cornea. For example, we have previously used this method to study the effect of interleukin-1 on keratocytes in vivo (*1*). The Hamilton syringe system (**Fig. 4A**) has the capacity to introduce volumes as small as 1 µL. The needle that is provided with the system cannot be used directly because it is dull and large in bore. Therefore, we attach a glass capillary tube that has been drawn in a flame to produce a fine needle (**Fig. 4B**) to the metal needle of the microinjector with polyethylene tubing. The polyethylene connector tubing is about 5 cm long and also provides the flexibility to manipulate the needle tip. This needle is used to draw up the solution to be injected. Typically, we use a carrier solution that contains 0.05% BSA in PBS since the cytokines and other modulators are present at low concentration and could be absorbed into the glass in the needle.

1. Draw the solution to be injected into the drawn glass needle. We usually inject 1 or 2 µL of the solution. Commonly, we use the mouse since cytokines and other modulators of interest are more likely to be commercially available for this species. Other species can, however, be used when desirable.
2. With the animal under general and topical anesthesia, pass the tip of the freshly drawn needle (so that it is sterile) filled with solution into the central stroma under direct, magnified observation with an operating microscope. It must be remembered that disturbance of the overlying epithelium via needle passage also stimulates stromal changes such as localized keratocyte apoptosis (*1*). Therefore, we pass the needle through the epithelium at the limbus (edge) of the cornea and advance it through stroma to the site of injection. We also include vehicle control eyes for comparison.
3. Withdraw the needle after the injection is completed. Little direct disturbance to the cornea is induced since the glass needle is fine and sharp.

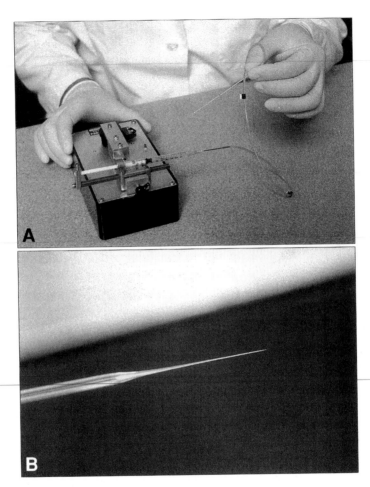

Fig. 4. Hamilton syringe system used for microinjection into corneal stroma: (**A**) entire system including metal needle and motor-driven injector; (**B**) magnified view of end of capillary needle that has been drawn to sharp fine point.

4. At different time points following injection of different concentrations of the substance of interest, euthanize the mouse and process the eye for histology, TUNEL assay, immunocytochemistry, or other analyses that reveal the impact of the modulator on keratocyte cells.

3.5. Tissue Procurement, Cryofixation, and Formaldehyde Fixation

1. Immediately after euthanasia, remove the rabbit cornea while the remainder of the eye remains *in situ*.

2. We prefer to perform the excision a millimeter or so into the sclera. Use sharp Wescott scissors and 0.12-mm forceps to excise the conjunctiva from its insertion into the limbus of the cornea.

3. Use a no. 15 Beaver blade to make an incision into the sclera approx 0.5–1 mm posterior to the limbus. Gently extend this incision deeper and deeper into the sclera until the black of the underlying uvea can be seen in the depth of the incision. The incision must be long enough to admit one of the tips of the sharp Wescott scissors.

4. Insert the lower tip of the scissors into the incision and slide into the potential space between the sclera and the underlying uvea.

5. Make a 360° cut in the sclera circumferential to the cornea while maintaining the lower tip of the scissors's blade in this space.

6. Grasp the scleral edge of the corneoscleral rim with forceps and gently lift from the eye. Iris and other uvea are likely to remain attached; grasp with a second pair of forceps and pull away from the corneoscleral rim. Care must be taken not to traumatize either the epithelium or the endothelium of the cornea during this manipulation. Traumatic injury to either one of these surfaces will induce stromal wound healing at the site of damage.

7. Place the corneoscleral rim epithelium side down in a 12- to 15-mm-diameter cryofixation mold.

8. Fill the mold with OCT solution so that the issue is completely immersed. Care must be taken not to introduce bubbles.

9. Immediately freeze the mold by partially submersing into 2-methyl-butane in a stainless steel bowl resting on a block of dry ice.

10. As soon as the block is frozen, store in aluminum foil at –85°C until the tissue block is sectioned.

11. When necessary, remove the whole mouse eye immediately after euthanizing the animal.

12. Immediately place the eye in 37% buffered formaldehyde solution and allow to fix for a minimum of 24 h. Embed the eye in paraffin block and section.

3.6. Tissue Sectioning

1. Prepare 7-μm sections extending transversely across the central cryopreserved rabbit cornea from frozen tissue blocks maintained at –20°C with a cryostat (*see* **Note 4**) and place on Superfrost plus slides (*see* **Note 5**). These slides are important for tissue adherence during staining.

2. Freeze the slides with sections at –85°C until use.

3. Just prior to staining, fix cryosections with acetone at –20°C for 10 min and then wash with two changes of PBS.

4. Place formalin-fixed mouse eyes in molds with paraffin. We typically prepare these blocks so that two or three eyes are oriented within the block so that sections will contain three complete eye sections extending through the central cornea, lens, and retina of the eye.

6. Cut 5- to 7-µm sections with a keratome and place on the slides.
7. Deparaffinize the sections using standard techniques prior to staining.

3.7. Histological Analysis, TUNEL Assay, and Immunocytochemistry

3.7.1. H&E Staining

H&E staining is performed on either fresh frozen rabbit corneal sections or formalin-fixed mouse whole-eye sections using standard histological methods and light microscopy (**Fig. 1**).

3.7.2. Propidium Iodide Staining

Similar to H&E staining, cell nuclei in fresh frozen rabbit cornea or formalin-fixed mouse whole-eye sections can be stained with 0.05% propidium iodide solution for 10 s. Then wash three times with PBS and once in water. Finally, mount a cover slip and examine the section using a fluorescent microscope and a rhodamine filter (**Fig. 5A**).

3.7.3. TUNEL Assay

The peroxidase-based or rhodamine fluorescent (**Fig. 5B,C**) TUNEL assay is performed according to the manufacturer's instructions to detect fragmentation of DNA associated with apoptosis in fresh frozen rabbit corneal sections or formalin-fixed mouse whole-eye sections (*see* **Note 6**). Counterstain can be excluded in the TUNEL assay to allow more sensitive detection of keratocytes because of the unambiguous localization of the keratocyte cells in the stroma. Corneas that had a flap formed with a microkeratome or have LASIK that includes flap formation and laser ablation of the underlying bed have keratocytes undergoing apoptosis on the anterior and posterior sides of the flap (**Fig. 5D**) (*see* **Notes 7** and **8**).

4. Notes

1. Topical anesthetic should not be reapplied after the initial wounding because of the known effect of anesthetics in retarding corneal epithelial healing. It is rare for animals to exhibit behavior that indicates discomfort after any of the procedures described herein. If lack of socialization, eating, or drinking is noted, animals can be treated with liquid Tylenol or another oral anesthetic. Animals should be euthanized if there appears to be significant discomfort.
2. It is helpful to use a temporary tarsorrhaphy to protect the rabbit eye for the first 24 h following corneal scrape wounding, excimer laser ablation, or flap formation. A temporary tarsorrhaphy may be placed in the rabbit eye with a double-armed 5-0 nylon suture (Alcon). The edge of the central upper eyelid is

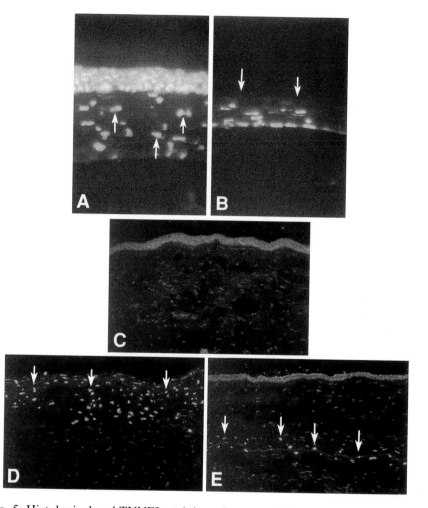

Fig. 5. Histological and TUNEL staining of cornea. (**A**) Propidium iodide staining of normal cornea. Arrows indicate keratocytes in the stroma. (**B**) Propidium iodide staining of rabbit cornea at 4 h after epithelial scrape injury. Arrows indicate the anterior stromal surface. Note that there are fewer keratocytes in the anterior stroma. (**A**) and (**B**) are at the same magnification. The cornea undergoes hydration changes after epithelial removal. (**C**) TUNEL assay of normal unwounded cornea. There is only background staining of keratocytes in the stroma. (**D**) TUNEL assay of rabbit cornea at 4 h after epithelial scrape injury. Note anterior keratocytes stain (arrows), indicating that they are undergoing apoptosis. (**E**) TUNEL assay of rabbit cornea at 4 h after flap formation with microkeratome and laser ablation of underlying bed (LASIK). Keratocytes (arrows) are in the midstroma along the lamellar cut stain, indicating that they are undergoing apoptosis. Magnification: ×400.

grasped with forceps and the needle is passed into the external skin of the eyelid about 1 mm above the margin and directed inferiorly so that it exits in the middle of the eyelid margin. The second arm is passed about 2 mm lateral to the first in the same manner. Both needles are then passed through the lower eyelid by going through the margin directly across from the upper eyelid exit point and out through the skin about 1 mm away from the margin. The two needles are removed and a bow-tie knot is tied. This knot can be untied and the eyelids opened repeatedly. A tarsorraphy must not remain in place for longer than 24 h because the rabbit eye has a tendency to develop bacterial infection.

3. Another method that can be used to protect the eye or the flap for 24 h is suturing of the nictitating membrane (sometimes referred to as the third eyelid of the rabbit) across the cornea to the lateral eyelid. With the animal under general and topical anesthesia, the nictitating membrane is grasped with heavy (0.3-mm) forceps. A single-armed 5-0 nylon suture is passed through the nictitating membrane near the tip. The membrane is drawn across the cornea and sutured to the lateral margin of the eyelids where the upper and lower eyelids connect temporally. The suture is tied so that the nictitating membrane is retained in position across the cornea. The next day, the suture is removed.

4. Cryosectioning of tissue embedded in OCT is an art. It is helpful to obtain training from an experienced operator. Practice should be performed on trial blocks before important tissue samples are used. It is helpful to use a cryostat with a disposable blade holder to ensure that the blade is sharp.

5. There is a tendency for tissue sections to curl as they are cut. This is controlled by altering the temperature within the cryostat in the range of –18 to –20°C and by capturing the section onto the Superfrost microscope slide as they are cut. Once the number of desired sections are cut from a block, it should be returned quickly to –85°C to prevent degradation of the tissue.

6. It is important to include both positive and negative controls when performing the TUNEL assay, to verify that the assay conditions are correct to identify apoptosis without giving nonspecific training. When investigators begin using the TUNEL assay they frequently note nonspecific staining. An excellent control is the unwounded cornea. There should be no staining of the keratocytes or the endothelial cells in the normal unwounded cornea. Conversely, the superficial epithelial cells should stain in an optimal assay since these cells undergo apoptosis as a normal aspect of epithelial maturation and renewal. In some cases, epithelial scrape in the mouse cornea will induce some endothelial cells to die by apoptosis *(1)*. This has not been noted in the rabbit model.

7. One of the advantages of using the cornea as a model is that it is possible to perform counts per unit tissue for quantitation. We have used this to count apoptotic keratocytes following different surgical procedures *(2)*. We have also used it to count the number of keratocyte cells per square millimeter of tissue undergoing mitosis when immunocytochemistry is performed to detect the Ki-67 mitosis-related antigen. We perform measurements by counting the total number of TUNEL-positive or stained cells in 6–10 randomly selected, nonoverlapping

full-thickness columns from the central cornea. The diameter of each column is the diameter of a microscopic field of the microscope being used for the measurements. For example, we commonly use a ×400 microscopic field. The mean is then determined. By using a reticle, these measurements can be converted into the number of cells per square millimeter of tissue *(2)*. These measurements are facilitated by the organization of the cornea and the unambiguous localization of stromal cells.

8. Care must be taken in interpreting TUNEL results more than 18 h after wounding. At this point, inflammatory cells typically appear in the stroma, and these cells likely contribute to apoptosis that is noted in the stroma at this time. Similarly, myofibroblast cells derived from keratocyte proliferation may begin to appear at this time point (detected by α–smooth muscle actin staining on immunocytochemistry) and can contribute to the noted apoptosis. At earlier time points (we typically use 4 h after wounding), one can assume that all of the noted stromal apoptosis is occurring in keratocytes.

Acknowledgments

This work was supported in part by US Public Health Service grant EY10056 from the National Eye Institute, National Institutes of Health, Bethesda, MD; and an unrestricted grant from Research to Prevent Blindness, New York.

References

1. Wilson, S. E., He, Y.-G., Weng, J., Li, Q., McDowall, A. W., Vital, M., and Chwang, E. L. (1996) Epithelial injury induces keratocyte apoptosis: hypothesized role for the interleukin-1 system in the modulation of corneal tissue organization and wound healing. *Exp. Eye Res.* **62,** 325–328.
2. Helena, M. C., Baerveldt, F., Kim, W.-J. and Wilson, S. E. (1998) Keratocyte apoptosis after corneal surgery. *Invest. Ophthalmol. Vis. Sci.* **39,** 276–283.
3. Drubaix, I., Legeais, J. M., Robert, L., and Renard, G. (1997) Corneal hyaluronan content during post-ablation healing: evidence for a transient depth-dependent contralateral effect. *Exp. Eye Res.* **64,** 301–304.

6

Subcutaneous Sponge Models

David T. Efron and Adrian Barbul

1. Introduction

All wounds progress through a well-described series of events that ultimately result in healing. Cellular, biochemical, and molecular changes occur, each characterizing unique phases of the healing process. Scientists have long desired to study both the global process of healing and its individual phases or steps.

Experimental models of healing have been used extensively to better understand the process of wound healing. There are models that preferentially reflect the fibroplastic or the collagen synthetic phase over others. It is important for researchers to understand what the model used can or cannot tell about the various phases of wound healing. Additionally, by better understanding normal healing, one can identify the pathophysiological mechanisms that lead to impaired healing.

The polyvinyl alcohol (PVA) sponge model is an extensively used model for wound-healing studies. It provides (at least in the short term) a relatively biologically inert substance that may be implanted subcutaneously and into which all phases of the healing process are expressed. The PVA sponge was first used in the late 1950s in reconstructive surgery but was soon abandoned clinically because of poor behavior during long-term implantation. Properly employed it can provide information on almost all phases of wound healing, making it a powerful tool for the study of wound healing. Although this chapter deals with PVA sponges, other materials such as viscose cellulose have also been used, albeit much less frequently.

From: *Methods in Molecular Medicine, vol. 78: Wound Healing: Methods and Protocols*
Edited by: Luisa A. DiPietro and Aime L. Burns © Humana Press Inc., Totowa, NJ

1.1. Rationale for PVA Sponge Model

The PVA sponge model belongs to the class of dead-space models used for studying granulation and reparative tissue ingrowth. As opposed to the steel wire mesh cylinder model, it does not have a lag phase and tissue grows within its interstices shortly after implantation. The model is best used for acute studies because it begins to elicit foreign body reaction with giant cell accumulation and fibrosis after about 2 wk in the rat and 4 wk in the mouse. Within these time parameters, it remains a highly reproducible and biologically valid model for studying acute healing responses.

One of the main uses of the PVA sponge implants is to assess reparative wound collagen accumulation by measuring hydroxyproline (OHP) content in sponge acid hydrolysates. Measured collagen deposition correlates well with the breaking strength of incisional cutaneous wounds (**Fig. 1**). The PVA sponge can also provide quantifiable samples of the wound environment for study of wound physiology. Wound cells, wound fluid, extracellular matrix, DNA, and RNA can all be harvested from the sponge for biochemical, immunohistochemical, or molecular analysis. Additionally, this model can reflect the systemic (nutritional, pharmacological) or local (growth factors, gene induction, gene therapy) manipulation of the healing process. Finally, the sponge acts as an in vivo cell culture nidus allowing evaluation of the roles and contributions of all wound cells.

2. Materials

Any species is theoretically usable in this model, but animals with loose skin provide a more accessible implantation. All experiments need to be approved by the animal use committee of the local institution. Given normal biological variability, a minimum of 8–10 animals per group is necessary to achieve statistical significance. This consideration plus cost should guide the choice and appropriateness of the species or strain used.

Because these are survival experiments, the procedure should be carried out in a clean/sterile manner, especially if the animals concerned are immunocompromised. Although rodents are innately highly resistant to wound infection, the reduction of contamination and maintenance of a sterile wound environment allows for more accurate assessment of normal healing.

1. PVA sponge material (PVA Unlimited, Warsaw, IN).
2. Cork bore.
3. Beaker (200 mL).
4. Double-distilled deionized water.
5. Balance.
6. Sterile normal saline.

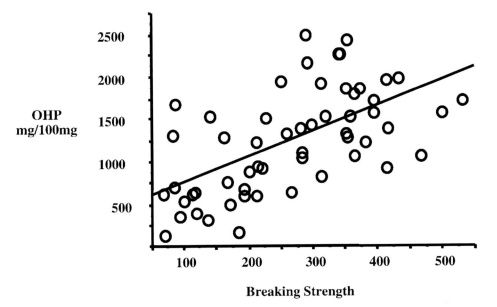

Fig. 1. Correlation between wound breaking strength and sponge OHP content. Data were compiled from 55 animals and four separate experiments. $p < 0.001$; $y = 3.003x + 459.979$; $r^2 = 0.358$.

7. Sterile Petri dishes.
8. Corkboard (or other such operating platform).
9. Sterile drape.
10. Sterile gauze sponges ($4'' \times 4''$).
11. Anesthesia.
12. Hair clipper (we prefer this over depilating agent because there is no effect on the underlying skin).
13. Sterile skin prep solution (organic iodine, chlorhexidine, alcohol).
14. Sterile gloves.
15. Two toothed Adson's forceps $\times$ 2.
16. Scalpel.
17. Scalpel guide.
18. Metzembaum scissors (rounded-point fine scissors are necessary, especially for mice; sharp-tipped (Iris) scissors will cause trauma to the skin while creating the pocket).
19. Suture/needle driver or surgical clips.
20. Heating lamp.
21. Aluminum foil.
22. 1 *N* HCl.
23. Oven.

24. Sterile forceps.
25. Sterile conical 15-mL test tube.
26. Centrifuge.
27. Microfilter (0.22 μm) (Millipore, Bedford, MA).
28. Sterile 50-mL centrifuge tubes.
29. Collagenase (crude collagenase type IV; Sigma, Grand Island, NY).
30. Dulbecco's modified Eagle's medium (DMEM).
31. Fetal bovine serum (FBS).
32. Russian tissue forceps.
33. RPMI-1640 tissue culture medium supplemented with 2 m*M* glutamine, 50 U/mL of penicillin, and 50 μg/mL of streptomycin.
34. Iris scissors.
35. Fine mesh strainer.
36. Ammonium chloride: 0.83% in Tris buffer, pH 7.4.
37. Ficoll-Hypaque (Sigma, St. Louis, MO).
38. Trizol reagent (Life Technologies, Rockville, MD).

3. Methods

3.1. Preparation of Sponges

PVA sponge material is purchased in sheets. Some companies precut the material to a desired thickness; for rodents 2 to 3 mm works best, but up to a 5-mm thickness can be used in rats. The porosity of the material is variable and can influence the ingrowth of granulation tissue. Pore sizes of 90–120 μ permit optimal granulation tissue harvest. Different sheet lots vary greatly in thickness and porosity, and these parameters can have significant consequences on the results and reproducibility of the experiments. Given all these variables, it is important to purchase enough material to complete the proposed experiments as well as carry out possible repeat or follow-up experiments.

1. PVA sponge is often contaminated with preservatives such as formalin. Wash the sponge sheets thoroughly, first overnight with running tap water and then with double-deionized water. Let the sheets air-dry.
2. Cut the sponge sheets into disks of identical diameter using a cork bore, usually 10–12 mm for rats and 5–7 mm for mice. A disk shape is easy to insert and remove from the animal, although square or rectangular shapes have also been used.
3. Once the disks are cut, weigh those to be used for collagen assays and group them by weight within 1 mg. Collagen, assayed as OHP, is normalized per weight of dry sponge and therefore the use of equal-weight sponges allows reproducible measurement and/or comparison of collagen content within varying sponges. Small differences in weight can make large differences in the reported collagen content. Sponges inserted for DNA, RNA, cell, or wound fluid harvest and for histology or immunohistochemistry need not be weighed. We have found that sponges weighing approx 25–45 mg for rats and 15–25 mg for mice provide

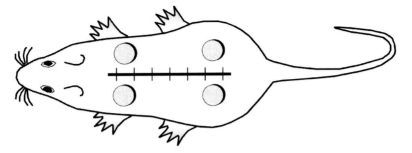

Fig. 2. Diagram of rat wound-healing model shows position of dorsal wound and four PVA sponges inserted into sc pockets.

readily detectable amounts of collagen at 1, 2, and 4 wk postwounding. With these sizes, adult rats can accommodate up to 10 and adult mice 4 sponges implanted along the dorsal incisions.

4. Sterilize the sponges prior to insertion. This may be achieved by gas or steam autoclaving prior to wounding. Alternatively the sponges can be boiled in double-deionized water for 20 min and cooled by soaking in normal saline on the day of insertion.

3.2. Wounding

1. Anesthetize the animal and shave its back from the nape of the neck to the base of the tail. The shaving should extend at least 2 cm laterally on either side from the midline.
2. Secure the animal to the operating surface. Prep the shaved part of the back with organic iodine solution (or other solution of choice).
3. Mark the length of the incision on the back. For a rat we prefer a length of 7 cm (**Fig. 2**).
4. Make a small nick in the midline just cephalad to the tail base and insert the scalpel guide subcutaneously along the spinal column, below the panniculus carnosus.
5. Carry the incision through the skin along the scalpel guide.
6. Create small sc pockets on either side of the wound with Metzembaum scissors, fashioned such that the pockets are separated and the sponges do not touch. In most animals collagen synthesis and wound breaking strength decrease in a cephalad to caudad direction; therefore, it is important to insert the sponges designated for collagen assays in the same sc location in all animals. We preferentially use the most cephalad pockets for this purpose.
7. Close the skin with surgical clips (or suture) placed at regular intervals along the wound (approx 1 cm apart).
8. Allow the animals to recover from anesthesia, preferentially under a heating lamp.

3.3. Retrieval and Analysis of Sponge Samples

3.3.1. Removal of Sponges

When excising the pelt great care must be taken so that the sponge granuloma is not penetrated, which could lead to a loss of wound fluid (*see* **Note 1**). Furthermore, excessive bleeding into the sponges should be avoided because this alters the cellularity of the sponges and the characteristics of the wound fluid.

After the animal is euthanized, harvest the sponges. There are several ways to harvest the sponges. All sponges should be retrieved with minimal handling and trauma so that there is minimal or no loss of wound fluid or cells.

For sponges inserted for the collagen assay, carefully separate the cephalad sponges from the surrounding capsule and granulation tissue since this will affect the values obtained. As mentioned before, OHP is reported per milligram of dry sponge weight, so it is important to harvest only the reparative tissue that grew within the sponge interstices *(1)*. For the sponges inserted for other assays, less meticulous dissection is required.

3.3.2. Collagen Analysis

1. Wrap the retrieved sponges in aluminum foil, label, and place in a –20°C freezer until ready for processing.
2. Carry out an acid hydrolysis. This must be done regardless of the assay method used. We use 6 mL of 1 *N* HCl in sealed Pyrex tubes for each sponge and carry out hydrolysis in an oven at 110°C for 3 h. For OHP assay, we use the colorimetric assay of Woessner *(2)*, which has been readily reproducible in our laboratory (*see* **Note 2**).

3.3.3. Wound Fluid

1. For wound fluid harvest, remove the sponges as described in **Subheading 3.3.1.**, and squeeze the contents with heavy sterile forceps into sterile conical 15-mL test tubes kept on ice.
2. Each ~40-mg sponge will yield between 200 and 250 µL of wound fluid and each ~20-mg sponge gives 50–100 µL. Pool the wound fluid in order to provide a constant and uniform supply for intended assays.
3. Centrifuge the wound fluid at 11,200*g* for 10 min to remove the cells; further centrifuge the supernatant at 8000*g* for 20 min, and then pass it through a 0.22-µm microfilter to remove any remaining cellular debris.
4. Aliquot and store frozen at –70°C (*see* **Note 3**). The wound fluid can then be subjected to enzyme-linked immunosorbent assay, high-performance liquid chromatography, protein fractionation, Western analysis, or used in subsequent cell culture.

3.3.4. Retrieval of Wound Cells

Wounds, as they progress from injury to scar, represent the summation of the cells participating in the process. In turn, when a wound fails, it is owing in some way to a cellular dysfunction. Manipulating wound cell content and/or activity forms the basis of modern wound therapy. Thus, it is imperative to define the characteristics of wound-participating cells, both during normal healing and in response to different therapeutic strategies.

The PVA sponge model is eminently suitable for harvest of wound cells within 10 d postwounding. Later days yield a mostly fibrotic and poorly cellular sponge. Cells released from the sponge-wound matrix at various times postinsertion reflect and vary with the current phase of healing. Retrieved cells may include red blood cells, macrophages, lymphocytes, fibroblasts, and endothelial cells, and they may be separated by various techniques. For all cell harvests, sponges must be harvested using a sterile technique.

3.3.4.1. FIBROBLASTS

1. Significant numbers of fibroblasts appear in the wound around d 3 postinjury, and there are increasing fibroblast numbers until d 14 *(3)*. To release fibroblasts from the sponge interstices, place 10 sponges in each 50-mL sterile centrifuge tube containing 1.5 mL of collagenase (2000 U/mL) and 13.5 mL of DMEM, giving a final concentration of 200 U of collagenase/mL.
2. Incubate the tubes for 15 h at 37°C in a humidified atmosphere of 5% CO_2.
3. At the end of the incubation period, add 20 mL of DMEM medium containing 10% FBS to each tube to inhibit further collagenase activity.
4. Squeeze the sponges repeatedly, using Russian tissue forceps, to release the cells from the interstices, and discard the sponge.
5. Bring the resulting cell solution up to 50 mL with DMEM medium containing 10% FBS and centrifuge at 300g for 8 min.
6. Wash the pellet twice in DMEM, and finally resuspend it in 10–15 mL of DMEM and seed at 1 mL/flask in 75-cm^2 culture flasks.
7. Add 14 mL of DMEM containing 10–20% FBS to each flask. Transfer the culture flasks to a tissue culture incubator and culture at 37°C in a humidified atmosphere of 5% CO_2.
8. Change the media every 4 d by pouring off the old media and adding fresh medium *(see* **Note 4**).
9. Passage the cultured fibroblasts weekly by trypsinization and use in experiments at the first through third passage. We have found that fibroblasts lose their wound phenotype if they undergo more than three passages *(4,5)*. Cells can also be frozen as necessary.

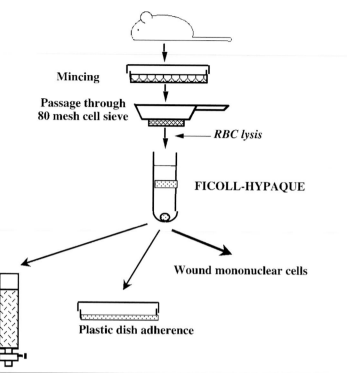

Fig. 3. Schema for wound mononuclear cell harvest and separation.

3.3.4.2. MONONUCLEAR CELLS

1. Macrophages and lymphocytes may also be harvested from wound sponges (**Fig. 3**). Following extraction from the animal, place the sponges in sterile Petri dishes containing 10 mL of supplemented RPMI-1640.
2. Mince the sponges into very fine pieces (<1 mm) with Iris scissors while keeping the dishes on ice.
3. Separate the sponge material using a fine-mesh cell strainer (*see* **Note 5**).
4. Spin and wash the cells three times in RPMI-1640.
5. Lyse the red blood cells from the wound cell preparation using ammonium chloride solution.
6. The mononuclear cell fraction is separated by density gradient centrifugation. Layer the cell suspension over Ficoll-Hypaque and centrifuge at 400g for 30 min at 20°C.
7. Remove the supernatant, wash the cells twice with medium, and finally resuspend in the medium. Macrophages can be purified and/or removed by either plastic dish adherence or nylon wool column adherence (**Fig. 3**).

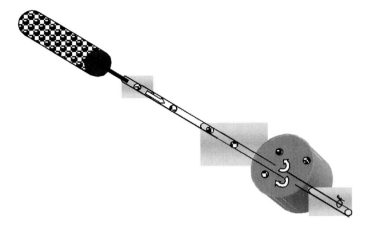

Fig. 4. PVA sponge infusion model.

3.3.5. Preparation of Nucleic Acids

1. Avoid contamination with hair because this may introduce RNases.
2. Perform the harvest in a sterile manner.
3. Remove the sponges as indicated previously and place them in Trizol reagent, a convenient one-step method for nucleic acid extraction. Process according to the manufacturer's directions. The mRNA is now available for reverse transcriptase polymerase chain reaction or Northern blot analysis.

3.4. Alternative Methods

3.4.1. PVA Sponge as a Model for Wound Manipulation

We have recently described a novel method for atraumatic delivery of wound-active substances into PVA sponges at various times throughout the healing process *(6)*. Cut sponges are mounted on small Silastic catheters that have been perforated along the length that traverses the sponge (**Fig. 4**). The constructs are subsequently sterilized and inserted into the animals. They are designed to be connected to an Alzet miniosmotic pump infusing 1 µL/h; higher-volume infusions are likely to dilute the wound environment with detrimental effects. The constructs may be attached to the pumps at the time of insertion (to provide immediate infusion into the sponges), or they may be attached at various times postinsertion. The sponges are harvested in the same manner as described under **Subheading 3.3.4.** Unfortunately, because of size constraints, there is only enough room for one pump-sponge construct per animal (maximum of two depending on the size of the animal, the sponge, and the model pump to be employed in the experiment).

This system has several major advantages over other local infusion methods. First, it allows directed delivery to the wound sponge and the infusion can be commenced or ceased at any time. Second, it is atraumatic and obviates the need for repeated injections into the sponges. This avoids injuring the sponge healing process and minimizes the risk of infection. Third, the construct allows for direct delivery of drugs, DNA, and viruses into the wound module, avoiding host effects seen with systemic administration of wound-active substances.

Controls for this model must include vehicle-infused sponges; saline infusion alone has been shown to significantly increase collagen deposition as compared to noninfused sponges.

3.4.2. Human Sponge Models

The earliest sponge implant model for use in humans was described by Viljanto *(3)*. Using a construct of viscose cellulose rectangles inserted into Silastic tubes, this surgeon has implanted hundreds, if not thousands, of these constructs into pediatric and adult surgical patients and has described the kinetics of cell migration and biochemical changes *(7)*. Most of the catheters are removed within 48–72 h postsurgery, limiting long-term studies.

More recently, a PVA sponge encased in a Silastic tubing model has been described for human use. Allowed to remain in volunteers or patients for up to 14 d, the sponge is retrieved and permits biochemical assessment of wound cellularity, DNA content, OHP measurement, as well as evaluation of collagen subtypes *(8–10)*.

4. Notes

1. If wound breaking strength is to be measured, remove the staples or sutures once the animal is euthanized. Excise the dorsal pelt containing the healing scar with sufficient excess on either side of the wound to allow grasping within the tensiometer.
2. The hydrolysate can also be assayed for α-amino nitrogen, as an index of total protein present in the sponge.
3. Alternatively, in a method described by Albina et al. *(11)*, the sponges are placed in a 5-cc syringe (with the stopper removed), which is then placed into a test tube and centrifuged at 3000g for 10–15 min.
4. While rat wound fibroblasts grow efficiently, mouse wound cells are slow growing and very difficult to culture through multiple passages.
5. An alternative technique uses rapid compression of the sponges using a Stomacher (Tekmar, Cincinnati, OH). By histological and DNA quantification, this technique leads to total and complete cell extraction from the sponge matrix *(11)*.

References

1. Weiner, S. L., Wiener, R., Platt, N., Urivetzky, M., and Meilman, E. (1975) The need for modification of the polyvinyl sponge model of connective tissue

growth: histologic and biochemical studies in the rabbit. *Connect. Tissue Res.* **3,** 213–225.

2. Woessner, J. (1961) The determination of hydroxyproline in tissue and protein samples containing small proportions of this amino acid. *Arch. Biochem. Biophys.* **93,** 440–447.

3. Viljanto, J. (1976) Cellstic: a device for wound healing studies in man: description of the method. *J. Surg. Res.* **20,** 115.

4. Regan, M. C., Kirk, S. J., Wasserkrug, H. L., and Barbul, A. (1991) The wound environment as a regulator of fibroblast phenotype. *J. Surg. Res.* **50,** 442–448.

5. Schäffer, M. R., Efron, P. A., Thornton, F. J., Klingel, K., Gross, S. S., and Barbul, A. (1997) Nitric oxide, an autocrine regulator of wound fibroblast synthetic function. *J. Immunol.* **158,** 2375–2381.

6. Efron, D. T., Most, D., Shi, H. P., Tantry, U. S., and Barbul, A. (2001) A novel method of studying wound healing. *J. Surg. Res.* **98,** 16–20.

7. Viljanto, J. A. (1990) Assessment of wound healing speed in man, in *Clinical and Experimental Approaches to Dermal and Epidermal Repair: Normal and Chronic Wounds. Progress in Clinical and Biological Research*, vol. 365 (Barbul, A., Caldwell, M. D., Eaglstein, W. H., Hunt, T. K., Marshall, D., Pines, E., and Skover, G., eds.), Wiley-Liss, New York, pp. 279–290.

8. Diegelmann, R. F., Lindblad, W. J., and Cohen, I. K. (1986) A subcutaneous implant for wound healing studies in humans. *J. Surg. Res.* **40,** 229–237.

9. Diegelmann, R. F., Kim, J. C., Lindblad, W. J., Smith, T. C., Harris, T. M., and Cohen, I. K. (1987) Collection of leukocytes, fibroblasts, and collagen within an implantable reservoir tube during tissue repair. *J. Leuk. Biol.* **42,** 667–672.

10. Lindblad, W. J. and Diegelmann, R. F. (1984) Quantitation of hydroxyproline isomers in acid hydrolysates by high-performance liquid chromatography. *Anal. Biochem.* **138,** 390–395.

11. Albina, J. E., Mills, C. D., Barbul, A., Thirkill, C. E., Henry, W. L. Jr., Mastrofrancesco, B., and Caldwell, M. D. (1988) Arginine metabolism in wounds. *Am. J. Physiol.* **254,** E459–E467.

7

A Mouse Model of Burn Wounding and Sepsis

Julia M. Stevenson, Richard L. Gamelli, and Ravi Shankar

1. Introduction

Despite major advances in the treatment of critically injured burn patients, sepsis remains a major obstacle to recovery (1–4). In fact, sepsis is a leading cause of morbidity and mortality in this patient population (5–6). Those who survive the initial injury become increasingly susceptible to septic complications during the second week of hospitalization. The majority of these patients show a severe depression of their innate immunity as evidenced by T-cell suppression and functional deficits in neutrophils and monocytes (7–14).

To gain a better understanding of the mechanisms of altered tissue responses in thermal injury and sepsis, one needs a model that adequately reflects many aspects of burn pathology. Much information on the cellular aspects of burn pathology has been gleaned from rodent models, typically mouse or rat. All of them typically involve the introduction of the thermal injury followed by a septic insult.

In this chapter, a standard burn protocol (15) and two separate protocols for introducing sepsis are presented. The first is a model of unimicrobial sepsis in which *Pseudomonas* is seeded onto the fresh burn wound (16). The second of the two protocols, a polymicrobial insult, utilizes a standard cecal ligation and puncture (CLP) technique (17). CLP also allows introduction of the septic insult at a time point removed from the thermal injury itself, a scenario that better reflects the clinical course of the severely burned patient who succumbs to sepsis (*see* **Note 1**).

From: *Methods in Molecular Medicine, vol. 78: Wound Healing: Methods and Protocols*
Edited by: Luisa A. DiPietro and Aime L. Burns © Humana Press Inc., Totowa, NJ

2. Materials

2.1. Animals

1. Male B6D2F1/J mice, 6 to 8 wk old, weighing 22–25 g, which have been acclimatized for 1 wk prior to use. This strain of mice is chosen for their relatively high bone marrow cellularity.

2.2. Induction of Burn Wound

1. Electric hair clipper.
2. Water bath.
3. Template (*see* **Fig. 1**).
4. Watch or clock with second hand.
5. Absorbent laboratory bench paper.

2.3. Introduction of Sepsis (choose one)

2.3.1. Burn Wound Seeding with Pseudomonas aeruginosa

1. 37°C Shaking bacterial incubator.
2. *P. aeruginosa* (ATCC 19960; Rockville, MD).
3. Tryptic soy broth (TSB).
4. Polypropylene tube (50 mL).
5. 1X PBS with glucose (no. 11500-030; Gibco-BRL).
6. 1X PBS without glucose (no. 10010-023; Gibco-BRL).
7. Polypropylene tubes (15 mL).
8. Disposable plastic cuvets.
9. Disposable pipet tips (1 mL).
10. Spectrophotometer.
11. RPMI-1640 medium warmed to 37°C.
12. Three tryptic soy agar (TSA) plates (100 × 15 mm).

2.3.2. Cecal Ligation and Puncture

1. Nonporous surface.
2. Tape.
3. Straight scissors (4 in.) (Roboz, Rockville, MD),
4. Adson's forceps with teeth (Roboz).
5. Adson's forceps without teeth (Roboz).
6. Sterile 3.0 silk ties.
7. Sterile 21-gage needles.
8. Suture clips (9 mm) and clip applier (Becton Dickinson, Sparks, MD).
9. 70% Alcohol in a spray bottle.

2.3.3. Anesthesia and Resuscitation

1. Anesthetics (choose one protocol):
   a. Pentobarbital (Nembutal, Abbott, North Chicago, IL).
   b. Ketamine (Ketaset, Fort Dodge Laboratories, Fort Dodge, IN) and xylazine (Xyla-Ject; Phoenix, St. Joseph, MO).

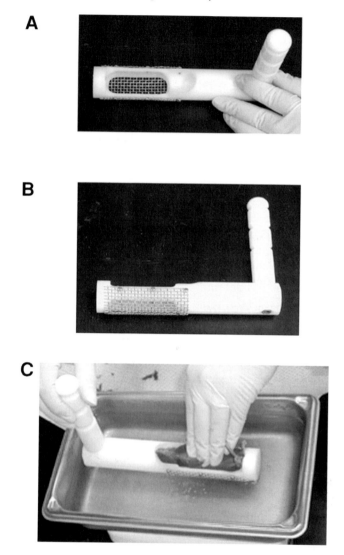

Fig. 1. Burn injury template: (**A**) top and (**B**) side views; (**C**) immersion in water bath for 8 s.

2. Resuscitation fluid: sterile 0.9% NaCl.
3. Disposable 1 cc syringes with 25- or 27-gage 5/8-in. needle.

3. Methods

3.1. Anesthesia

Either pentobarbital or a combination of ketamine and xylazine can be used. The combination of ketamine and xylazine more uniformly produces the required depth of anesthesia, with a shorter induction time and with less respiratory depression than pentobarbital. Either protocol will provide about 1 h of anesthesia. Both protocols are provided; use only one.

1. Pentobarbital: Pentobarbital is available in a 50 mg/mL concentration; the optimal dose, 50 mg/kg, can be achieved by diluting the pentobarbital with saline in a 1:12 ratio (1 mL of pentobarbital plus 11 mL of 0.9% saline) and administering 0.3 mL intraperitoneally (**Fig. 1**) for a 25-g mouse.

2. Ketamine plus xylazine: Ketamine is available in 100 mg/mL and xylazine in 20 mg/mL concentrations. The required dose, 160 mg/kg of ketamine and 4 mg/kg of xylazine, can be achieved by first diluting the ketamine 1:10 (1 mL of ketamine plus 9 mL of 0.9% saline) and the xylazine 1:80 (1 mL of xylazine plus 79 mL of 0.9% saline) and then adding these together in a 1:1 ratio. The resulting solution (10 mg/mL of ketamine and 0.25 mg/mL xylazine) is then administered 0.8 mL intraperitoneally for a 25 g mouse.

3. When the proper plane of anesthesia has been attained, the mouse should not respond to a brisk pinch to its foot or base of the tail (*see* **Note 2**).

3.2. Induction of Burn Wound

1. Once the mice are adequately anesthetized, shave the dorsum with the electric clippers to ensure even burn wounding (**Fig. 3**).

2. Place the mouse on its back in a template constructed of plastic and a metal screen (**Fig. 1A,B**), so that its back is directly over the screen. Immerse mouse and template together into a 100°C water bath for 8 s (**Fig. 1C**). The mouse and template should be far enough in the water so that the portion of the mouse's back that is exposed by the screen is entirely in contact with the water, but so that no other part of the mouse touches the water.

3. Remove the mouse from the template and place the animal on its back on absorbent bench paper to remove any remaining hot water and halt ongoing burning. Turn the mouse over onto its abdomen and allow the animal to cool. If burn-alone controls are to be used, they should be resuscitated at this point without undergoing infection.

3.3. Introduction of Sepsis

Use either the burn wound seeding with *P. aeruginosa* or CLP, but not both.

3.3.1. Burn Wound Seeding with P. aeruginosa

3.3.1.1. PREPARATION OF *P. AERUGINOSA*

This entire portion of the protocol should be done *prior* to wounding of the animal.

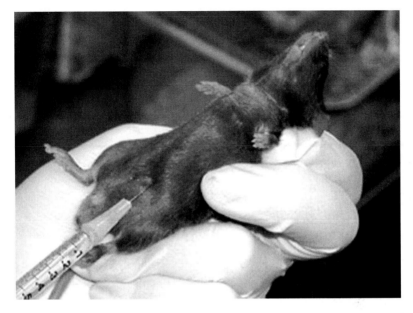

Fig. 2. Anesthesia is administered intraperitoneally into the left lower quadrant of the mouse's abdomen, but high enough to avoid injecting into the bladder. The needle should be inserted only as far as is required to enter the peritoneal cavity.

1. Grow the *P. aeruginosa* overnight in 50 mL of TSB in a 250 mL Erlenmeyer flask for 16–18 h with agitation at 225 rpm and 37°C (*see* **Notes 3–5**).
2. Remove the flask from the incubator, decant the cells and the medium into a 50-mL polypropylene tube, and centrifuge at 1300*g* for 10 min at 4°C.
3. Pour off and discard the supernatant, and resuspend the cell pellet in 20 mL of 1X PBS with glucose. Centrifuge at 1300*g* for 5 min at 4°C. Repeat this washing procedure twice for a total of three washes. Be sure to use 1X PBS without glucose for the final wash to remove any colored PBS before measuring the sample in the spectrophotometer (*see* **Note 6**).
4. After the completion of the third washing step, resuspend the cell pellet in 10 mL of 1X PBS without glucose. Use PBS without glucose for all remaining steps.
5. In a 15-mL tube, make a 1:2 dilution of this cell suspension using 1X PBS (1-mL cell suspension + 1 mL of 1X PBS).
6. From this dilution, make another 1:2 dilution for a serial dilution of 1:4 (1-mL 1:2 cell suspension + 1 mL of 1X PBS).
7. Place three TSA plates in a 37°C bacteria incubator for drying.
8. Blank the spectrophotometer at a fixed wavelength of 665λ using 1 mL of 1X PBS without glucose in a disposable cuvet.

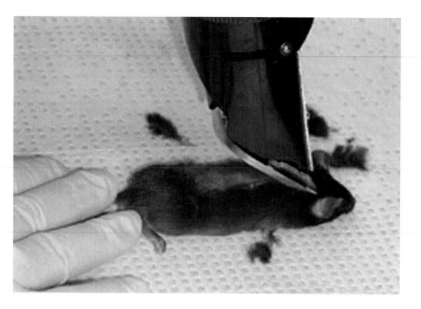

Fig. 3. Shaving dorsum of mouse in preparation for burn wounding.

9. Measure the absorbance of both the 1:2 and 1:4 dilutions in the spectrophotometer using a fixed wavelength of 665λ. Use disposable plastic cuvets, filling each with 1 mL of each sample. Routinely, the target absorbance of 0.4 is used, which should provide approx 30% mortality in the burn-plus-sepsis group of mice. Dilute either the 1:2 or 1:4 accordingly to reach the target absorbance value.

10. Fill five 15-mL polypropylene tubes with 9 mL each of RPMI-1640 media warmed to 37°C, label the tubes 1:10 through $1:10^5$, add 1 mL of the diluted sample to the 1:10 tube, and mix (*see* **Note 7**). Take 1 mL of this 1:10 dilution and add it to the $1:10^2$ tube. Continue serially diluting 1 mL of each tube with the next highest dilution until $1:10^5$ is reached. This final dilution should contain 1000 colony-forming units of *P. aeruginosa* per 250 μL and will be the dose administered to the desired mice with thermal injury.

11. Remove the TSA plates from the incubator, inoculate each plate with 10 μL of the final $1:10^5$ dilution, and plate the bacteria evenly over the plate with a sterile glass rod. Incubate the plates overnight in a 37°C bacteria incubator. To confirm the accuracy of the counts and therefore the inoculum given the mice, there should be approx 40 colonies per plate.

12. Dispose of the plates in an infected waste container.

3.3.1.2. Burn Wound Seeding

1. Allow the burn wound to cool to room temperature (failure to do so may kill some of the bacteria on application).

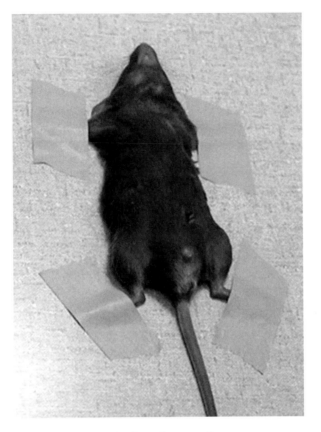

Fig. 4. Positioning of mouse for surgery.

2. Using a clean sterile 1-mL pipet tip, place 250 µL of the diluted bacteria on the wound, releasing the bacteria slowly as you gently drag the pipet tip across and up and down the wound (try to cover as much of the wound with the 250 µL as uniformly possible).
3. Allow the bacteria to soak in before further handling of the animal.

3.3.2. Cecal Ligation and Puncture

1. Ensure that all instruments are sterile at the start of the experiment.
2. Place the anesthetized mouse on its back on a nonporous surface and tape the extremities down (**Fig. 4**).
3. Saturate the abdomen with 70% ethanol.
4. Using the forceps with teeth, pull up on the skin of the abdomen on the midline and use the straight scissors to make a small nick in the skin. Then with the scissors open, cut the skin vertically up and down from the initial nick to create a 1-cm incision (**Fig. 5A**).

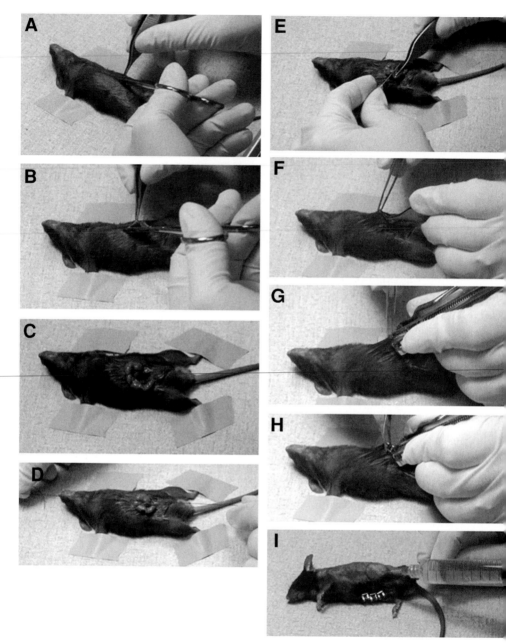

Fig. 5. CLP. (**A**) Skin incision; (**B**) entering abdominal cavity; (**C**) cecum delivered out of abdomen; (**D**) cecal ligation using 3.0 silk tie; (**E**) puncture of cecum with 21-gage needle; (**F**) replacement of cecum into abdomen while tenting up skin and muscle layers; (**G**) placement of first clip; (**H**) placement of second clip; (**I**) sc injection of saline in flank.

5. Repeat the procedure in **step 4** on the muscle layer to enter the peritoneal cavity. Take care not to injure any intraabdominal structures (**Fig. 5B**) (*see* **Note 10**).
6. If performing a laparotomy alone as a control, proceed to **step 9**.
7. If performing a CLP, locate the cecum and gently deliver it up and out of the abdomen using the smooth forceps (**Fig. 5C**) (*see* **Notes 9** and **10**).
8. Using a 3.0 silk tie, tie off the distal 1 cm of the cecum (**Fig. 5D**) and trim the ends (*see* **Note 11**).
9. Using the 21-gage needle, puncture the cecum through both lumens midway between the tie and the distal end of the cecum (**Fig. 5E**) (*see* **Note 12**).
10. Replace the cecum into the abdominal cavity using the smooth forceps (**Fig. 5F**).
11. Using the forceps with teeth, pick up both the muscle and skin layers at the superior aspect of the wound and pull them taut to bring the edges of the wound together. With the other hand, clip the muscle and skin closed with a ligature clip (**Fig. 5G**) (*see* **Note 13**).
12. Remove the forceps and regrab onto the clip just placed, pulling up to again tent up the skin and muscle layers, and place a second clip below the first (**Fig. 5H**). Usually two clips are sufficient; however, a third may be placed in a similar manner if needed to completely close the wound.
13. Remove the restraining tapes.

3.3.3. Resuscitation

1. If you have used the *Pseudomonas* wound-seeding model, you may resuscitate with a 1-mL ip injection of 0.9% saline in the same manner as the anesthesia was administered using a 1-cc syringe with a 25-gage needle.
2. If you have performed a laparotomy or CLP, you must administer the saline subcutaneously at a site that is separate from both the dorsal burn wound and the abdominal incision. We have found the flank to be a convenient location. Use the 1-cc syringe with a 25-gage needle, puncture the skin on the flank at a 45° angle, and insert the needle just under the skin. Inject the saline slowly to create a raised wheal under the skin (**Fig. 5I**).

4. Notes

1. Obviously, the design of control groups is at the discretion of the investigator. Historically, the final design of groups when using the *Pseudomonas* wound-seeding protocol has been sham (nonburned), burn alone, and burn plus sepsis. For the CLP protocol, the animals are usually divided into sham and burn groups; these two groups are then subdivided to undergo either CLP, laparotomy alone, or no surgical intervention. The final result is six groups: sham alone, burn alone, sham plus laparotomy, burn plus laparotomy, sham plus CLP, and burn plus CLP. The animals that are randomized to the sham groups should be handled in a manner as similar as possible to the burn animals. That is, they should be anesthetized, shaved, and dipped in tepid water and resuscitated exactly as the burn animals.

2. Once the anesthesia is administered, wait approx 5 min before assessing the plane of anesthesia. Occasionally, some of the animals do not reach the required depth of anesthesia. If this is the case, give an additional 0.05 mL of pentobarbital or 0.1 mL of ketamine/xylazine and wait another 5 min. Repeat until the proper plane of anesthesia is achieved. Only anesthetize a few animals at a time or those that were handled last will start to awaken. Anesthetize no more than four to eight animals at any time depending on the procedure performed and the skill level of the operator.

3. The strain of *P. aeruginosa* used, the size of the inoculum, as well as the strain of mouse will affect the mortality. It is recommended that a pilot experiment be done to determine the optimal inoculum to reach the desired mortality.

4. *P. aeruginosa* bacteria are stored at –70°C as a stock culture in TSB with 10% dimethyl sulfoxide in 1-mL aliquots. Use an entire 1-mL aliquot in 50 mL of TSB for the overnight incubation. The incubation time should not exceed 16 h.

5. For the preparation of *P. aeruginosa*, first the incubation should be started the day prior to burning the animals and the final concentration arrived at just prior to thermal injury so that the wounds can be seeded immediately after the wound is created.

6. If PBS with glucose (which may have a pink hue owing to phenol red indicator) is used for dilution, the spectrophotometry readings will be incorrect, and, therefore, the inoculum administered will not be consistent. It is necessary to use PBS without glucose (without phenol red) for the final wash and serial dilutions. Do not, however, use PBS without glucose for the steps leading to the final dilutions, because some of the bacteria will likely not survive for long without the glucose, and the result will be a wound seeding with less viable bacteria.

7. It is essential to use a new pipet with each transfer of bacteria during the serial dilution steps, taking care to immerse only the tip and avoiding washing the tip up and down so as to avoid carryover and overinoculation with the bacteria.

8. Often there is a visible white line running down the center of the muscle layer called the linea alba; cutting along this line will minimize pain and bleeding.

9. Some models employing this technique advocate massaging of the cecum to cause spillage of contents. This practice may introduce more variability and undue trauma. Instead, a better approach is to titrate the needle size to arrive at the desired mortality rate (in most cases 30–50%).

10. Never handle any intraabdominal structures with the forceps with teeth, because this will cause excessive trauma to these delicate tissues; also, never pull on any structures with force because this will likely avulse blood vessels and cause undue trauma and bleeding.

11. Knot the tie three to four times to ensure that it will not come undone.

12. One may change the needle size and/or decide to puncture only one lumen, depending on the level of sepsis and mortality desired.

13. It is extremely important to be sure that the clips are securely closing both the skin and muscle layers, and that the wound is completely closed. Failure to do so will almost certainly result in evisceration of the bowel once the mouse

awakens. Conversely, take care not to clip through any intraabdominal contents (i.e., bowel).

References

1. Sparkels, B. G. (1997) Immunological responses to thermal injury. *Burns* **23,** 106–113.
2. Shirani, K. Z., Vaughan, G. M., Mason, A. D. Jr., and Pruitt, B. A. Jr. (1996) Update on current therapeutic approaches in burns. *Shock* **5,** 4–16.
3. Demling, R. H. (1985) Burns. *N. Engl. J. Med.* **313,** 1389–1398.
4. Hansbrough, J. F., Field, T. O. Jr., Gadd, M. A., and Soderberg, C. (1987) Immune response modulation after burn injury: T cells and antibodies. *J. Burn Care Rehab.* **8,** 509–512.
5. Alexander, J. W. (1979) Immunological responses in the burned patient. *J. Trauma* **19(Suppl. 11),** 887–889.
6. Moncrief, J. A. (1973) Burns. *N. Engl. J. Med.* **288,** 444–454.
7. Solomkin, J. S., Nelson, R. D., Chenoweth, D. E., Solem, L. D., and Simmons, R. L. (1984) Regulation of neutrophil migratory function in burn injury by complement activation products. *Ann. Surg.* **200,** 742–746.
8. Stratta, R. J., Warden, G. D., Ninnemann, J. L., and Saffle, J. R. (1986) Immunological parameters in burned patients: effect of therapeutic interventions. *J. Trauma* **26,** 7–17.
9. Miller, C. L. and Baker, C. C. (1979) Changes in lymphocyte activity after thermal injury: the role of suppressor cells. *J. Clin. Invest.* **63,** 202–210.
10. Duque, R. E., Phan, S. H., Hudson, J. L., Till, G. O., and Ward, P. A. (1985) Functional defects in phagocytic cells following thermal injury: application of flow cytometric analysis. *Am. J. Patthol.* **118,** 116–127.
11. Warden, G. D., Mason, A. D. Jr., and Pruitt, B. A. Jr. (1974) Evaluation of leukocyte chemotaxis in vitro in thermally injured patients. *J. Clin. Invest.* **5,** 1001–1004.
12. Eurenius, K. and Brouse, R. O. (1973) Granulocyte kinetics after thermal injury. *Am. J. Clin. Pathol.* **60,** 337–342.
13. Newsome, T. W. and Eurenius, K. (1973) Suppression of granulocyte and platelet production by pseudomonas burn wound infection. *Surg. Gynecol. Obstet.* **136,** 375–379.
14. Miller-Graziano, C.L., Szabo, G., Kodys, K., and Griffey, K. (1990) Aberrations in post-trauma monocyte (MO) subpopulation: role in septic shock syndrome. *J. Trauma* **30(Suppl. 12),** S86–S96.
15. Walker, H. L. and Mason, A. D. Jr. (1968) A standard animal burn. *J. Trauma* **8(6),** 1049–1051.
16. Rosenthal, S. M. (1966) A procedure for measurement of wound healing, with special reference to burns. *Proc. Soc. Exp. Biol. Med.* **123,** 347–349.
17. Wichterman, K. A., Baue, A. E., and Chaudry, I. H. (1980) Sepsis and septic shock—a review of laboratory models and a proposal. *J. Surg. Res.* **29,** 189–201.

8

A Porcine Burn Model

Adam J. Singer and Steve A. McClain

1. Introduction

Not only are burns a leading cause of accidental death, but they also result in considerable morbidity and disfigurement leading to significant functional and social impairment. Fortunately, most burns are minor and relatively small. As a result, research efforts have largely focused on the local care of burn wounds. Because of moral and ethical considerations, the use of human skin for in vivo experiments is limited. Over the years researchers have used a variety of animal models as well as in vitro preparations to study cutaneous burns. We have developed and validated a porcine model for partial-thickness contact burns, using it to successfully evaluate a variety of therapeutic agents *(1)*. This chapter describes in detail the model for assessing burn therapies.

A good burn model is one that is simple, safe, and reproducible; that is, it should create burns that are consistent in their extent and depth. Any description of an animal burn model should include the following elements: the instruments used to create the burn, the temperature and duration of exposure with the inflicting instrument, and the method of applying the thermal injury. For researchers and readers to compare various new therapies for burns, it is important to ensure that the agents are being used on similar types and extents of injury. Thus, any animal model for burns must be reproducible and reliable; that is, whenever the same exposure time and temperature are used, similar injuries should result. Partial-thickness burns are also excellent models for studying the main components of wound healing such as reepithelialization and scar formation.

From: *Methods in Molecular Medicine, vol. 78: Wound Healing: Methods and Protocols*
Edited by: Luisa A. DiPietro and Aime L. Burns © Humana Press Inc., Totowa, NJ

1.1. Choosing the Pig as an Animal Model for Burns

One of the most important aspects of developing an animal model for studying cutaneous burns is choosing an appropriate species. The pig has been favored over other animals for several reasons. First, of all mammals, the skin of the pig most closely resembles that of humans *(2,3)*. The cornified layer and epidermis of the pig is relatively thick, similar to that of the human. Like humans, pig dermis is composed of two zones: the well-defined papillary dermis, with delicate collagen fibers and mucopolysaccharide-rich matrix intermingled with connective-tissue cells; and the dense reticular dermis, where woven collagen bundles and elastic fibers provide the bulk of the cutaneous strength and elasticity. Porcine skin differs from human skin in two main aspects: the absence of sweat (eccrine) glands and fewer elastic fibers in the dermis. The sc region is similar to that found in humans, demonstrating sex and age variability. Porcine sc fat differs slightly from human sc fat in that there are one or two layers of collagenous fascia connected to the dermis above by the fibrous septae in the sc fat.

The hair of the pig is arranged in groups of two to three single hairs. Its sparsely haired coat is also similar to that found in most humans, although the hair shafts are coarser than typical terminal hair in humans. The holocrine sebaceous glands are present in the superficial part of the reticular dermis discharging into the hair canal similar to other mammals. The tubular apocrine glands lie adjacent to the hair follicles and are more numerous than in humans, where they are confined mainly to the axilla and perineum. The subepidermal vascular network is less dense than in humans; however, the pattern of vascularization in the lower region corresponds to that in humans.

Other similarities between porcine and human skin include epidermal enzyme patterns, epidermal tissue turnover time, the character of keratinous proteins, and the composition of the lipid film of the skin surface. A recent study evaluating the crossreactivity between human and porcine cytokeratins and proliferation antigens found that structurally the pig's skin may even be superior as a model to nonhuman primate skin *(4)*.

Second, pigs are of a large enough size to allow creation of multiple burn sites on the same pig, thus increasing the sample size without significantly increasing the cost. The large size also allows creation of multiple burns in each individual pig without resulting in a systemic stress response. Generally, we have limited the total number of burns to <5–10% of the total body surface area. Performance of multiple burns within the same pig also allows each pig to serve as its own control when multiple topical therapies can be studied simultaneously *(5)*. This helps control for any variability in healing among different animals.

The pig's size requires that general anesthesia be used prior to creating burns or performing tissue biopsies. This allows precise and predictable titration of iv and/or inhalational anesthetics that is not possible with smaller animals. As a result, most animals survive surgery, allowing performance of longitudinal studies, with multiple tissue samples taken over intervals of days or weeks.

Third, young pigs are highly resistant to contamination and infection. This may be viewed as an evolutionary advantage given their environmental living conditions. However, this quality can be both an advantage and a disadvantage of using the pig. For example, when studying the effects of contamination on infection, we found that high concentrations of bacteria and removal of the burned, necrotic epidermis were required to consistently result in clinically apparent infections (*6*).

The use of pigs as the animal model has several disadvantages. Pigs are relatively expensive. Furthermore, their large size and the need to administer general anesthesia usually make additional personnel necessary during procedures. Finally, pigs generally do not form blisters between the epidermis and dermis as in humans, and recognizing second-degree burns may be difficult. This is thought to be the result of a diminished superficial dermal vascular plexus, their densely arranged dermis, and the lack of loose areolar tissue that precludes intercellular fluid accumulation. To overcome this problem and simulate second-degree burns in humans that routinely form blisters, we removed the necrotic epidermis by gentle manual rubbing (*6–8*). However, it is important to remember that removal of the necrotic epidermis delays reepithelialization and increases infection rates (*8*).

While the age of the pig may vary, we generally prefer young pigs weighing approx 20 kg at the time of injury. Most partial-thickness burns reepithelialize within 2 wk (*6,8–11*). By then, the pig has grown tremendously, making their day-to-day management difficult. Furthermore, the healing process itself is optimal in young pigs.

1.2. Choosing Burn Site

Our model uses a 6.25-cm² square rigid aluminum bar applied directly to the skin. Site selection is important in order to ensure uniform burn injuries. We have found the thoracic paravertebral zone especially suitable in pigs. When created directly over the vertebral spinous processes or too far laterally over the ribs, it is likely that the burn will be nonuniform. In addition, as the ventral abdominal undersurface is approached, we have found that burns do not heal as well as those adjacent to the paravertebral region. We suspect that this is the result of recurrent trauma to burns located near the pig's undersurface during movement or lying. Davis et al. (*7*) noted that burns located in the caudal portion of the pig heal better than more cephalically located ones. We have not found any difference in the healing of cephalad or caudad burns. Although the optimal distance between burns has not been determined, it is believed that a minimum distance of 2 to 3 cm is required in order to reduce any local effects of the burns on each other *(7)*.

1.3. Choosing Thermal Insult

Two types of thermal insults can be used to create burns. In the scald burn model, heated or boiling water is circulated over the injured area. The major advantage of this method is the ability to cover uniformly an entire area of skin regardless of its uniformity and underlying surface. The major disadvantage is that this model is also technically more challenging than the contact model and exposes the research team to the risk of burning themselves. By contrast, the contact model of injury uses an aluminum (or brass) bar that is preheated in hot water for creating the burn. This model does not require any specialized apparatus and has minimal risk of injury to the investigators.

Brans et al. *(12)* have found that with contact burns, a clear demarcation zone with neutrophilic infiltration between the viable and necrotic tissue is observed in the first 72 h after injury. By contrast, an intermingled pattern of damaged and intact collagen fibers with delayed and progressive vascular injury was noted over the first 72 h with scald burns. They conclude that studies focusing on preventing the progression of dermal injury after burns should probably use scalding water to create the burns, whereas we have found that using our contact burn model, burn depth continues to progress for at least 3 d after injury *(13)*. Davis et al. *(7)* also noted burn progression over the course of several days after infliction of contact burns in pigs.

2. Materials

1. Young female pigs weighing 20–25 kg.
2. Mechanical respirator: We use the ADS1000 Anesthetic Delivery System (Engler, Hialeah, FL). However, any mechanical ventilator or bag valve mask apparatus may be used to ventilate the anesthetized pig.
3. Tiletamine and zolazepam (Fort Dodge Laboratories, Fort Dodge, IA).
4. Metal bar: The burns are created with a 2.5 cm × 2.5 cm by 7 cm, 150-g aluminum or brass bar (Small Parts, Miami Lakes, FL) preheated in hot water. Clearly, any size bar can be used to create the desired area of injury. A durable plastic or wooden handle is attached to one end of the bar to enable the investigator to grasp the bar without getting burned (**Fig. 1**). We drilled and tapped an appropriate-sized hole at one end of the bar into which we attached a threaded, nonconducting plastic rod.
5. Water bath: The metal bar is heated in a water bath (Neslab GP-100; Neslab, Newington, NH) whose water temperature is tightly regulated to the desired

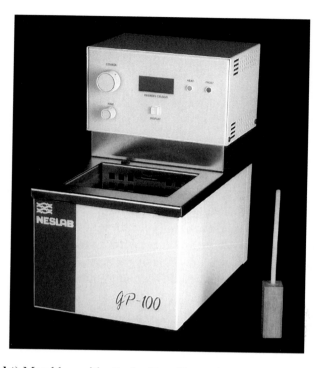

Fig. 1. (**Right**) Metal bar with attached handle used to create burns. (**Left**) The bar is preheated in a thermostatically controlled water bath.

level (**Fig. 1**). We generally use a temperature of 80°C. When the preheated bar is applied to the skin at this temperature for a period of 20 s, a partial-thickness burn is created that damages the upper 30–50% of the dermis *(1)*.

6. Punch biopsies: To obtain tissue specimens for histological evaluation, a disposable 4-mm biopsy punch is used (Miltex, Lake Success, NY). These can be reused until dull, unless infection is being studied.

7. Dressings: Regardless of the type of local therapy, the burns need to be covered and protected from further self-inflicted injuries that result from the animal's normal activity. The burns should be covered with nonadherent gauze dressing (Telfa®, Kendall, Mansfield, MA). To further protect the wounds, the burned areas are then covered with a gauze bandage roll (Conform®, Kendall) and a tough, flexible adhesive elastic bandage (Elastoplast®; Beiersdorf-Jobst, Rutherford College, NC). The edges of the adhesive elastic bandage should be secured to the skin with several skin staples (Proximate Plus MD; Ethicon Endo-Surgery, Cincinnati, OH).

8. 10% Formalin: For routine histopathology, tissue samples should be stored at room temperature in neutral buffered 10% formalin.

9. OCT frozen section mounting medium (Sakura FineTek, Torrance, CA); for frozen sections, tissue samples are snap-frozen in this medium in prelabeled

aluminum foil boats in liquid nitrogen. The aluminum boats are wrapped and stored frozen at −80°C.

10. Hematoxylin and eosin (H&E): One can use a histology service for paraffin embedding, sectioning, and staining with H&E or frozen sections where needed. Specialized stains may be helpful in some studies (e.g., Gram stain for bacterial infection, elastic stains for elastic tissue fibers).

11. Light microscope equipped with a polarized light filter and calibrated ocular micrometer.

3. Methods

3.1. Preconditioning and Anesthesia

Animals should be given a standard diet ad libitum several days prior to the investigation to allow acclimatization to their new surroundings. The pigs should be fasted overnight before any procedures to reduce the risk of vomiting and aspiration during the procedure. Housing and care for animals should be in accordance with the National Research Council guidelines *(14)*.

1. Sedate the pigs with 5 mg/kg of Talazine® intramuscularly. Generally, the onset of sedation will require 5–10 min.

2. Intubate the pigs endotracheally using a straight laryngoscope blade and a no. 7-7.5 endotracheal tube.

3. After their visualization, squire the vocal cords with 2 to 3 mL of 1% lidocaine to reduce the likelihood of laryngospasm and ease the passage of the endotracheal tube.

4. Maintain the animals under a surgical plane of anesthesia with 0.5–2.5% isoflurane in room air. The use of halothane should be avoided in pigs; this agent is associated with a high risk of seizures. A concentration of 2–2.5% isoflurane is usually required for painful procedures such as creating the burns or obtaining biopsies. A concentration of 0.5–1% is usually adequate for nonpainful procedures such as dressing changes (*see* **Note 1**).

3.2. Hair Removal

1. To ensure uniform contact of the metal bar with the skin, the hair is removed prior to creating the burns. Kaufman et al. *(5)* recommend removing the hair with clippers and a depilatory cream at least 24 h before inflicting burns, since clipping and depilation may produce skin edema. However, after experimenting with a variety of depilatory creams, hair removal waxes, and clippers, we have noted that hair removal with electric clippers immediately before the burns is most simple and does not have any appreciable histological effects on healing of the burns. By contrast, shaving the hair with a razor should be avoided, since shaving has been reported to significantly increase the rate of infection in comparison with clipping *(15)*.

3.3. Creation of Burns

1. Preheat the metal bar to the desired temperature by immersing it in a bath of heated water for 3–5 min. The metal bar should be immersed in its entirety, but its handle end should not be in contact with the hot water (*see* **Notes 2–4**).
2. Remove the heated bar from the water bath and blot dry just prior to application, to prevent water droplets from creating a separate steam burn on the skin.
3. Align the bar perpendicular to the skin's surface and apply for a predetermined period of time (usually about 20–30 s) with all pressure supplied by gravity (*see* **Note 5**).

3.4. Application of Dressing

The dressing is very important in order to protect the burns from any further self-inflicted injuries by the animals. While some investigators have constructed a firm hoop made out of metal, plastic, or wood that surrounds the animals and their wounds, we use a multilayered dressing with the outermost layer stapled to the skin at its cephalad and caudad edges at a distance from the burns. The dressing should be wrapped starting below the shoulders and continuing to just cephalad to the hind legs. This will help prevent the dressing from migrating with pig motion (*see* **Notes 6** and **7**).

3.5. Macroscopic Description of Burns

Initially the deep partial-thickness burns have a pale white appearance with a surrounding rim of erythema that subsides within several minutes (**Fig. 2**). Within the next few days the burns become red and develop a thick scab that does not allow direct observation of the reepithelialization underneath the scab. As a result, we rely on tissue biopsies for evaluation of the degree of reepithelialization. This is in contrast to human burns, in which direct visualization of the neoepidermis is usually possible, allowing the observer to follow the progression of reepithelialization. We (as others before) have not observed blister formation in the pig under any of the studied experimental conditions.

3.6. Recommended Outcomes to Measure Healing After Thermal Injuries

A variety of macroscopic and microscopic outcomes can be used to measure healing of burns. Early indicators include infection based on the presence of erythema, purulence, or systemic indicators of infections such as fever. Microscopically, infection is defined by the presence of intradermal neutrophils containing bacteria. While this measure has a high degree of reliability *(6,8,9)*, it does not necessarily indicate clinically relevant infections and may be overly sensitive *(16)*.

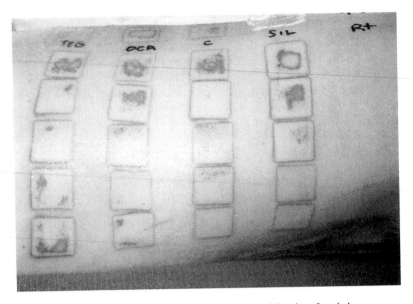

Fig. 2. Macroscopic appearance of burns 30 min after injury.

3.6.1. Reepithelialization

Reepithelialization or the regeneration of neoepidermis occurs from migrating keratinocytes originating in remaining epithelial appendages, mainly hair follicles and apocrine ducts, as well as the surrounding intact epidermis. Reepithelialization of partial-thickness burns usually requires between 7 and 14 d in the pig *(6,8–11)*. Reepithelialization is difficult if not impossible to monitor macroscopically, since visualization of the neoepidermis is not possible beneath the thick crust or scab over the burns. Microscopically, reepithelialization may be measured by two methods.

For the first method we, as well as others *(17)*, measure the length of neoepidermis in a skin section on a slide (prepared from full-thickness biopsies of the healing burn; *see* **Note 8**) and divide this by the length of the section (**Fig. 3**). The advantage of this method is that each burn can be sampled multiple times at various time points. This allows monitoring of reepithelialization over time within the same wound. Furthermore, it allows quantification of the degree of reepithelialization even for wounds that are not completely reepithelialized. Histopathological studies should be done on formalin-fixed, alcohol-dehydrated, xylene-cleared, paraffin-embedded, H&E-stained sections using conventional microscopy (*see* **Note 9**).

The second method is described by Eaglstein and Mertz *(18)*. Thin strips of healing wounds are completely excised with the use of an electrokeratotome.

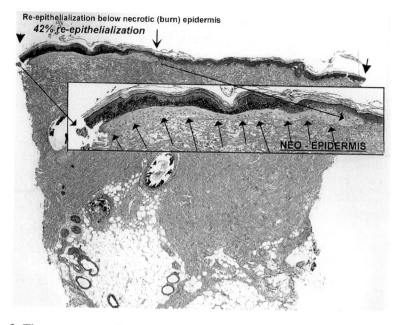

Fig. 3. The percentage of reepithelialization is calculated by dividing the length of the sectioned slide that is covered with neoepidermis (seen at the left end of the slide) by its total length (H&E; ×40).

After incubating the excised wounds in 0.5 mol/L of NaBr overnight, the specimens are separated into epidermal and dermal sheets. The epidermis is then examined macroscopically for defects in the area of the burn wounds. Epithelialization is considered complete when no defects are present in the epidermal sheet. The disadvantage of this method is that the wound may be sampled only once. Therefore, more wounds need to be created in order to evaluate reepithelialization at different time points. Furthermore, the outcome measured (complete reepithelialization) is dichotomous and, thus, less sensitive than the first method used to measure reepithelialization.

3.6.2. Scarring

Cutaneous scarring can be quantified macroscopically using a standard 100-mm visual analog scale ranging from no apparent scar to worst possible appearance *(10)*. Furthermore, it is possible to measure the proportionate amount of reduction in the residual wound surface area by dividing the surface area of the scar by that of a control site (whose dimensions are identical to those of the aluminum bar) marked with a tattoo at the time of the original injury.

Histologically, a scar is characterized by pale-staining, thin collagen bundles, typically oriented parallel to the epidermis. Less complex in structure and containing less collagen than the thick, woven normal dermal collagen bundles, scar collagen appears dark compared to normal dermis by examination under polarized light. The scar appears dark mainly owing to the diminished collagen content and results in less light refraction. The polarizing filters can be rotated to enhance scar detection. However, the more subtle qualities of the scar, such as thin collagen bundles oriented in the same plane as opposed to the woven structure of thicker collagen bundles, can also be recognized without polarized light. We have developed a histological scale that allows quantification of the amount of scarring and its effects on the normal structure of the dermis. For further discussion of this scale, the reader is referred to **ref. *10*.**

4. Notes

1. For short procedures, inhalation anesthesia may be given using only a mask. For brief nonpainful procedures (such as a dressing change), im sedation alone may suffice.
2. We prefer the use of a thermostatically controlled water bath for heating the aluminum bar. However, warming a beaker of water over a hot plate and manually regulating the temperature with an accurate thermometer can be substituted.
3. Both aluminum and brass bars have been used. Aluminum's lower cost is an advantage.
4. Between 60 and 100°C heat transfer and cutaneous injury is proportional to the product of the temperature and duration of exposure. Lower temperatures for longer time periods are equivalent to higher temperatures for shorter time periods in terms of depth or level of injury required by the investigator *(1,19,20)*. We have developed matrices that relate the depth of injury to each of several specific histological elements of the dermis to the temperature and duration of exposure (**Table 1**) *(1)*. Generally, we prefer using lower temperatures (80–90°C) with longer exposure times (20 s rather than 10 s) since the relative errors in exposure time and their influence on burn depth are minimized *(21)*.
5. Whereas some investigators feel that the amount of pressure applied is important, we and others have not found that the depth of injury is dependent on the amount of pressure employed *(22)*. To avoid premature cooling of the bar, the burns should be created immediately after removing the bar from the water bath and blotting it dry.
6. Usually two assistants are required to hold the pig during application of the adhesive dressing to ensure proper placement.
7. In male pigs, care must be taken to avoid encompassing the penis within the dressing, since this may result in obstruction and urinary retention. The use of female pigs maximizes the area available for creating the burns, since the dressing can be wrapped farther caudad. While wrapping the elastic dressing around the animal, care should be taken to avoid excessive compression, which can result in

Table 1
Depth of Injury (in mm, % total dermal thickness)

Temp. (°C)	Collagen dermal discoloration exposure (s)*			Intercollagen discoloration exposure (s)			Endothelial cell exposure (s)			Hair follicle exposure (s)			Mesenchymal cell exposure (s)		
	10	20	30	10	20	30	10	20	30	10	20	30	10	20	30
50	0.0 (0%)	0.0 (0%)	0.0 (0%)	0.0 (0%)	0.0 (0%)	0.0 (0%)	0.0 (0%)	0.0 (0%)	0.0 (0%)	0.0 (0%)	0.0 (0%)	0.0 (0%)	0.0 (0%)	0.0 (0%)	0.0 (0%)
60	0.0 (0%)	0.0 (0%)	0.0 (0%)	0.0 (0%)	0.0 (0%)	0.3 (10%)	0.2 (10%)	0.2 (10%)	0.5 (15%)	0.1 (5%)	0.1 (5%)	0.1 (5%)	0.0 (0%)	0.0 (0%)	0.2 (10%)
70	0.6 (20%)	0.9 (30%)	1.8 (65%)	0.6 (20%)	1.0 (35%)	2.1 (75%)	0.8 (30%)	1.0 (35%)	2.7 (100%)	0.2 (10%)	0.8 (30%)	1.9 (70%)	0.7 (25%)	1.2 (45%)	2.5 (90%)
80	1.0 (35%)	1.6 (55%)	1.5 (48%)	1.0 (35%)	1.6 (55%)	2.1 (80%)	1.3 (45%)	1.9 (75%)	2.3 (85%)	0.7 (25%)	1.4 (50%)	2.2 (90%)	1.0 (35%)	1.6 (60%)	2.5 (90%)
90	0.9 (35%)	1.3 (50%)	2.0 (70%)	0.8 (30%)	1.6 (55%)	2.7 (95%)	1.4 (50%)	2.7 (100%)	2.8 (100%)	1.3 (45%)	2.5 (90%)	2.8 (100%)	1.4 (50%)	2.3 (90%)	2.6 (95%)
100	1.8 (70%)	2.3 (85%)	3.1 (100%)	2.0 (75%)	2.7 (95%)	3.1 (100%)	2.4 (90%)	2.8 (100%)	3.1 (100%)	2.0 (75%)	2.6 (90%)	3.1 (100%)	2.2 (80%)	2.6 (95%)	3.1 (100%)

*"Exposure" refers to the duration of time that the skin was exposed to the heated bar.

colorectal prolapse. This can be accomplished by intermittently unrolling short segments of the adhesive bandage before wrapping the animal.

8. Biopsy punches should be as sharp as possible to avoid damaging the tissue specimen. Generally, 5–10 biopsies can be performed before the blade becomes dull.

9. Some researchers prefer specialized stains (such as Masson's trichrome or S-100 immunoperoxidase stain) and techniques (such as a polarized light filter). We believe that the "standard" H&E staining of 5-μ-thick sections is adequate to visualize all cutaneous structures and its architecture.

References

1. Singer, A. J., Berruti, L., Thode, H. C., and McClain, S. A. (2000) Standardized burn model using a multi-parametric histological analysis of burn depth. *Acad. Emerg. Med.* **7**, 1–6.

2. Montagna, W. and Yun, J. S. (1994) The skin of the domestic pig. *J. Invest. Dermatol.* **43**, 11–21.

3. Meyer, W., Schwarz, R., and Neurand, K. (1978) The skin of domestic mammals as a model for the human skin, with special reference to the domestic pig. *Curr. Probl. Dermatol.* **7**, 39–52.

4. Smith, K. J., Graham, J. S., Skelton, H. G., Hamilton, T., O'Leary, T., Okerberg, C. V., Moeller, R., and Hurst, C. G. (1998) Sensitivity of cross-reacting antibodies in formalin-fixed porcine skin: including antibodies to proliferation antigens and cytokeratins with specificity in the skin. *J. Dermatol. Sci.* **18**, 19–29.

5. Kaufman, T., Lusthaus, S. N., Sagher, U., and Wexler, M. R. (1990) Deep partial thickness burns: a reproducible animal model to study burn wound healing. *Burns* **16**, 13–16.

6. Singer, A. J., Mohammed, M., Tortora, G., Thode, H. C., and McClain, S. A. (2000) Octylcyanoacrylate for the treatment of contaminated partial-thickness burns in swine: a randomized controlled experiment. *Acad. Emerg. Med.* **7**, 222–227.

7. Davis, S. C., Mertz, P. M., Bilevich, E. D., Cazzaniga, A. L., and Eaglstein, W. H. (1996) Early debridement of second-degree burn wounds enhances the rate of epithelization—an animal model to evaluate burn wound therapies. *J. Burn Care Rehabil.* **17**, 558–561.

8. Singer, A. J., Thode, H. C. Jr., and McClain, S. A. (2000) The effects of epidermal debridement of partial thickness burns on infection and reepithelialization in swine. *Acad. Emerg. Med.* **7**, 114–119.

9. Singer, A. J., Berrutti, L., Thode, H. C. Jr., and McClain, S. A. (1999) Octyl-cyanoacrylate for the treatment of partial thickness burns in swine: a randomized controlled trial. *Acad. Emerg. Med.* **6**, 688–692.

10. Singer, A. J., Thode, H. C., and McClain, S. A. (2000) Development of a histo-morphologic scale to quantify cutaneous scars. *Acad. Emerg. Med.* **7**, 1083–1088.

11. Singer, A. J., Mohammed, M., and McClain, S. A. (2000) Octyl-cyanoacrylate versus polyurethane for treatment or burns in swine: a randomized trial. *Burns* **26**, 388–392.

12. Brans, T. A., Dutrieux, R. P., Hoekstra, M. J., Kreis, R. W., and du Pont, J. S. (1994) Histopathological evaluation of scalds and contact burns in the pig model. *Burns* **20(Suppl. 1),** S48–S51.
13. Singer, A. J., Bauch, B., Thode, H. C. Jr., and McClain, S. A. (2000) Predicting healing potential of burns using early histological findings. *Ann. Emerg. Med.* **36,** S24.
14. National Research Council. (1996) *Guide for the Care and Use of Laboratory Animals.* National Academy Press, Washington, DC.
15. Seropian, R. and Reynolds, B. M. (1971) Wound infections after preoperative depilation versus razor preparation. *Am. J. Surg.* **121,** 251–254.
16. Quinn, J., Maw, J., Ramotar, K., Wenckebach, G., and Wells, G. (1997) Octylcyanoacrylate tissue adhesive versus suture wound repair in a contaminated wound model. *Surgery* **122,** 69–72.
17. Winter, G. D. (1962) Formation of the scab and the rate of epithelialization of superficial wounds in the skin of the young domestic pig. *Nature* **193,** 293–294.
18. Eaglstein, W. H. and Mertz, P. M. (1978) New method for assessing epidermal wound healing: the effects of triamcinolone acetonide and polyurethane film occlusion. *J. Invest. Dermatol.* **71,** 382–384.
19. Henriques, F. C. and Moritz, A. R. (1947) Studies of thermal injury I. The conduction of heat to and through the skin and the temperature attained therein: a theoretical and an experimental investigation. *Am. J. Pathol.* **23,** 531–549.
20. Moritz, A. R. and Henriques, F. C. (1947) Studies of thermal injury. II. *Am. J. Pathol.* **23,** 695–720.
21. Rigal, C., Pieraggi, M. T., Serre, G., and Bouissou, H. (1992) Optimization of a model of full-thickness epidermal burns in the pig and immunohistochemical study of epidermodermal junction regeneration during burn healing. *Dermatology* **184,** 103–110.
22. Davies, J. W. L. (ed). (1982) *Physiological Responses to Burning Injury.* Academic, London.

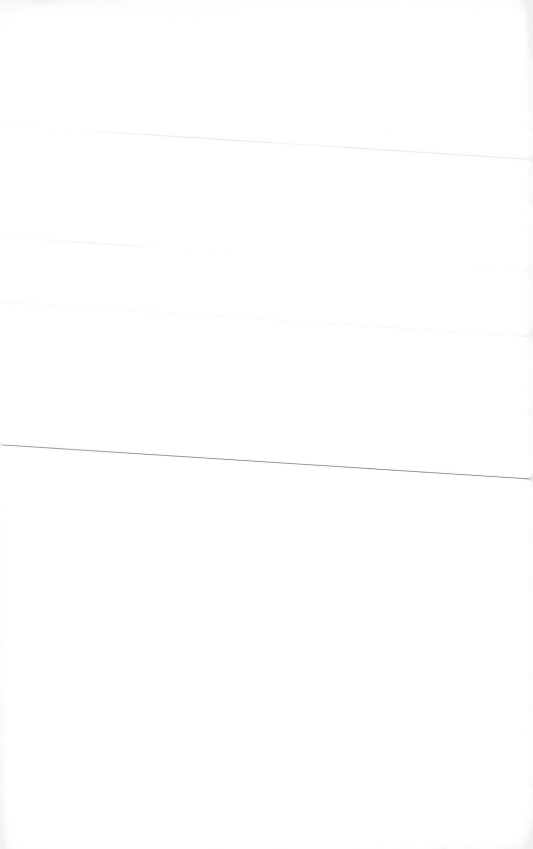

9

Wound Healing in Airways In Vivo

Steven R. White

1. Introduction

The airway epithelium is a target of inflammatory, environmental, and physical stimuli in diseases such as asthma and bronchopulmonary dysplasia. Damage to the epithelium may compromise both the physical barrier and key metabolic functions. Repair involves the migration and spreading of cells over the basement membrane and the proliferation of new epithelial cells. Each step can be modulated actively by growth factors secreted by constitutive cells within the airway, or suppressed by mediators secreted by inflammatory cells that have migrated into the airway. Understanding these steps is essential to gaining insight into the repair process in airway epithelium.

Much of what is known about epithelial repair in vivo is derived from studies in which the epithelium is wounded either with a mechanical probe or with a chemical agent, and the subsequent proliferation, migration, and differentiation into subtype cells is observed over time (reviewed in **refs. *1* and *2***). The removal of epithelial cells from the mucosa, whether by trauma or inflammation, induces prompt extravasation of plasma from the microvascular bed beneath and surrounding the immediate area. Gaps open in and along the junctional stretches between venular endothelial cells, and plasma moves into the injury site and onto the airway surface overlying the basement membrane (*3*). Immediately after injury and after plasma leakage occurs, epithelial cells both adjacent to and remaining in the injury site become activated. Basal cells spread and migrate over the provisional gel until the injured site is completely covered. This process reconstitutes the epithelial barrier to fluid and plasma transport (*3*). Small wounds can be covered completely in <24 h by migration and spreading alone (*1*). Cell proliferation within and adjacent to the site of

From: *Methods in Molecular Medicine, vol. 78: Wound Healing: Methods and Protocols*
Edited by: Luisa A. DiPietro and Aime L. Burns © Humana Press Inc., Totowa, NJ

epithelial injury begins within 24 h and produces a multilayered metaplastic epithelium after 48–72 h. Mitosis and division of normally arrested cells within the epithelium usually begins only after cell migration and spreading have completely covered the site of injury *(4,5)*, although we have demonstrated a regional reflex in which proliferation is also seen in epithelial cells away from the injury site *(6)*. Mitosis continues among the newly migrated cells, producing immature, "indifferent" cells, which differentiate into functional, subtype cells usually within 4–7 d of the original injury *(1)*.

From this sequence of events, it follows that repair after injury involves the coordination and integration of several separate processes. A number of in vitro methods have been developed to examine epithelial cell repair after injury. These generally involve proliferation assays; chemotaxis assays using blind-well chambers; adhesion assays in which cells adhere to extracellular matrix proteins; two-dimensional wound closure assays of cells on a culture dish or cover slip, generally assessed by time lapse video microscopy; and three-dimensional growth and cell activation assays in which two different cell types are grown separated by a gel matrix or a membrane. These methods are extremely useful to examine specific mechanisms under standardized conditions but are limited in their ability to increase the understanding of the in vivo environment, particularly when examining cell-to-cell interactions.

Our laboratory has developed a method that examines airway epithelial cell repair after injury in the in vivo setting *(6,7)*. This method utilizes a standardized mechanical injury to the tracheal mucosal surface in a small mammal such as a mouse, rat, or guinea pig. At time points selected by the investigator, animals can be killed and tracheal epithelial cell wound closure can be assessed by histological techniques. Additionally, the expression of selected genes or proteins can be examined by appropriate *in situ* methods; inflammatory cells can be counted and typed; and the response of other constitutive cells within the airway wall, such as fibroblasts, can be examined. Finally, these responses can be examined in the setting of experimental treatments to the animal given immediately prior to or at selected time points after the tracheal wounding. Thus, the in vivo method may be a useful additional tool by which to examine wound repair and gain insight into basic mechanisms of cell proliferation and migration.

The method of intubation we describe in this chapter is similar to a variety of techniques used by other investigators. Each has, as its core, the direct visualization of the vocal cords. Fiberoptic illumination of the vocal cords with a flexible guide can be used if such a tool is available *(8)*. Costa et al. *(9)* described the fabrication of rodent fiberoptic laryngoscopes specific for each species. Such a light source could be adapted for the method we provide but requires additional fabrication. The use of an otoscope and otoscopic speculum, as we describe, provides ample light at the base of the pharynx and a wide channel through which to pass a metal wand. More important, these tools are inexpensive and can be used within a confined space such as a glove box. Jou et al. *(10)* note the use of a wedge fabricated from the barrel of a 3-mL syringe to aid in intubating small rodents such as rats. Such a wedge facilitates a direct view of the vocal cords but does not provide additional light. Alpert et al. *(11)* note the use of a spatula to elevate the tongue of a rodent and provide direct visualization. With our method, or those methods previously published, a clear view of the vocal cords is required prior to placing a wand into the trachea to create the mechanical injury to the epithelium.

Adaptations of our method can be derived to create tracheal mucosal injury by chemical rather than mechanical means, to instill radioopaque or marker dyes, and for endotracheal intubation followed by mechanical ventilation.

The in vivo method we describe in this chapter is as follows: After proper anesthesia in the test animal, the hypopharynx and vocal cords of the animal are visualized directly using a human otoscope with a medium-sized, disposable speculum. Once seen, a metal wand of suitably small diameter is passed between the vocal cords into the cervical trachea. This wand has a hook at the distal tip; when withdrawn from the trachea under gentle torsion, the hook will remove the epithelial layer without significant damage to the basement membrane and underlying submucosa. Once the tracheal injury is created, the wand and speculum are removed and the animal is allowed to recover from anesthesia. At selected time points, tracheas can be collected and images obtained. Such images (as illustrated in **Fig. 1**, a representative series of images at different time points after tracheal mucosal injury in guinea pigs) then can be processed to meet the goals of the project.

2. Materials

Note that it is incumbent on the investigator to obtain proper approval for the use of animals from the institutional review board of his or her institution.

2.1. Tracheal Injury

1. Appropriate animals for study (mouse, rat, guinea pig).
2. Appropriate anesthetic agents for the animals to be used.
3. Welch-Allyn otoscope, human adult size: The otoscope may have an open (conventional) or closed (fiberoptic) head. In either case, it will have a removable (sliding) magnifying lens. We have used both designs and prefer the closed head.
4. Speculums for otoscope: For guinea pigs, either a 3- or 4-mm speculum may be used.
5. Stylette, appropriately sized for the animal: This is a metal wand that flexes a little to facilitate applying the necessary torsion in the injury process. For guinea

Immediately after   **72 hr**

24 hr   **7 days**

48 hr

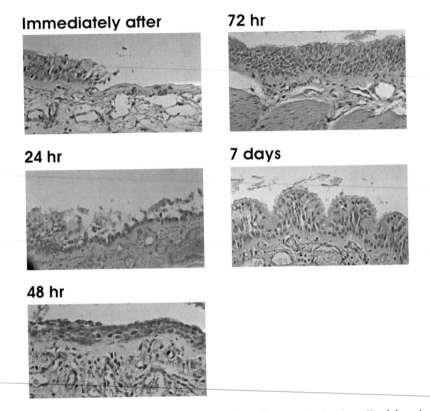

Fig. 1. Representative model in guinea pig using methods described herein for sequence of repair of airway epithelium. The trachea was abraded at time 0 using a metal wand, and tracheas were collected at the indicated time points. In the first phase of repair, there is migration of flattened cells into the injury site. Over time a multiple layer of flattened cells develop. Subsequently, these cells shift their phenotype into the needed terminal cells within the mucosa, such as ciliated and secretory cells. (From **ref. 6**, with permission of the publisher.)

pigs, the wand used is 1.5 mm in diameter. The tip is shaped as shown in **Fig. 2** and is designed to catch the tracheal surface when the wand is pulled backward under torsion. It should be long enough to fit comfortably in one's hand—about 20 cm. For our work, we had these wands fabricated from a surgical grade stainless steel rod in a university machine shop. The length of the wand is milled so that the cross-section, from the hook to the back, is a semicircle. This facilitates the flexing required to torque the wand.

6. Cotton swabs and 2 × 2 cotton sponges.

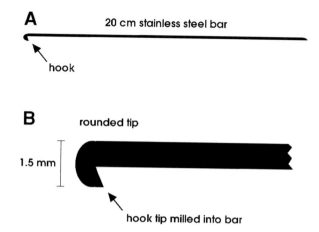

Fig. 2. Schematic of wand used to create tracheal injury. The wand is made from stainless steel. **(A)** The wand is about 20 cm long and 1.5 mm in diameter. **(B)** The wand is milled along its length so that the cross-section is a semicircle down to a hook. The hook is designed to catch the tracheal surface when the wand is pulled backward under torsion. The tip of the wand is rounded so as not to injure the vocal cords or trachea on insertion.

2.2. Digital Imaging of Tracheal Wounds

1. NIH Image software (Wayne Rasband, National Institutes of Health).
2. Macintosh computer capable of running NIH Image (any G3 or G4 Macintosh or Power Macintosh).
3. Good-quality bright-field microscope with an adapter appropriate to the digital camera used.
4. Digital camera with appropriate adapter for microscope (at least 1.3 megapixels, and preferably ≥2.0 megapixels), with appropriate interface to the computer (e.g., USB port or memory card reader).
5. Hemacytometer (for calibration).

3. Methods

We describe the method in guinea pigs. This method can be adapted to either smaller or larger animals using the same principles as described in **Notes 1–6**.

3.1. Tracheal Injury

1. Anesthetize Hartley guinea pigs, 400–700 g in mass, with 40 mg/kg of ketamine and 5 mg/kg of xylazine intramuscularly.

2. Confirm the depth of anesthesia at periodic intervals by monitoring pedal withdrawal and corneal reflexes. To check pedal withdraw, grasp the foot pad and squeeze gently. To check the corneal reflex, use a soft tissue or cotton swab and gently touch the cornea. If the animal withdraws or blinks, more anesthesia is required.

3. Lay the animal on its back on a work table. No restraints should be required with proper anesthesia. You may find it useful to brace the animal with a rolled towel or with foam rubber to prevent the animal from sliding on the table when you intubate it. An alternate method is to have an assistant present the animal to you, abdomen up, cradling the neck.

4. Intubate the animal using the otoscope to visualize the vocal cords. In guinea pigs, we use a 3- or 4-mm disposable speculum on the otoscope. With a gloved hand, open the mouth and grasp the tongue gently. Pull the tongue outward and up; this also lifts the mandible. Using the other hand, insert the tip of the otoscope speculum with the handle of the otoscope facing upward (**Fig. 3**). The tip needs to enter the hypopharynx, and thus go beyond the back of the tongue. Pivot and lift the scope in your hand such that the mandible is lifted. Insert the speculum farther (*gently*) until the vocal cords come into view. The magnifying lens on the otoscope helps substantially in viewing the vocal cords. At this point you can release the tongue. Continue to hold the otoscope firmly throughout the entire procedure.

5. Guinea pigs many times retain food products in the hypopharynx, thus blocking the view of the vocal cords. We find it useful to swab out the hypopharynx using cotton-tipped applicators. Either pull the applicator tip through the speculum or withdraw the speculum and pass the applicator tip by feel to the hypopharynx.

6. If you are still unable to visualize the vocal cords, have an assistant press down gently on the larynx after you have inserted the otoscope speculum. This will help bring the vocal cords into view.

7. Through the otoscope, insert the metal stylette with the shaped tip going first (**Fig. 3B**). This needs to pass between the vocal cords without causing trauma to the cords or the aretinoid cartilage on either side. Trauma can elicit edema and constriction of the larynx and cords with subsequent asphyxiation of the animal.

8. Once the tip is past the vocal cords, insert it about 1–1.5 cm farther into the trachea. Orient the shaped hook of the tip so that it faces downward (dorsally).

9. Torque the wand downward in your hand as you pull back gently to the trachea. The goal is to shave the tracheal mucosa. We generally do this three times. You may rotate the stylette after each attempt if you wish to cause a larger injury. Too much torque can damage not only the epithelium but also the underlying submucosa.

10. Withdraw the stylette and the otoscope. Monitor the animal until it has recovered completely from anesthesia. With appropriate anesthesia and due care to avoid injury, the mortality rate is very low (review **Notes 1** and **2** for some of the complications that may occur with this method).

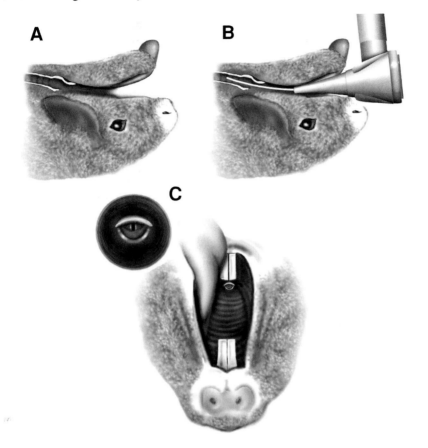

Fig. 3. Drawings of technique for in vivo tracheal injury. (**A**) Lateral view of guinea pig, demonstrating important structures of pharynx. (**B**) Lateral view of guinea pig during intubation with otoscope. An assistant holds the animal, belly up. The tongue is grasped using cotton gauze, and the tongue and jaw are lifted upward. The otoscope speculum is inserted to bring the vocal cords and epiglottis into view. The metal stylette then can be passed through the speculum into the cervical trachea. (**C**) View of vocal cords and epiglottis from pharynx. The inset shows the view of the vocal cords and epiglottis through the magnifying lens of the otoscope. The metal wand is inserted through the otoscope speculum, between the vocal cords, and into the cervical trachea.

3.2. Digital Imaging of Tracheal Wounds

At appropriate time points, animals may be killed and tracheas collected for histological and morphometric analysis. The details of tissue harvest and various staining methods are not covered here. It is appropriate to consider the technique of measuring tracheal injury and repair. We provide a method that will serve as a starting point. This method assumes the prior collection, fixation, and sectioning of an entire trachea in cross-section. While any staining method that provides adequate contrast of the epithelial layer and basement membrane will do, our preference is to work with paraffin-embedded, 5-μm sections stained with hematoxylin and eosin. With such a system, one can collect images of the quality shown in **Fig. 4**.

We use a photomicrography system that employs a good consumer-quality digital camera to obtain images of these airways. This is preferred to either 35-mm photography, owing to the ease and lower cost of image collection, or to video microscopy, owing to the superior resolution of most digital cameras compared to comparably priced, industrial-model video cameras that have been adapted to a microscope (*see* **Notes 7** and **8**). Measurements are made using NIH Image, a popular, free image analysis program. A complete manual is provided with the software; however, the methods given here provide supplemental information on using the program.

1. Calibrate the photomicrography system for morphometric analysis. This is critical to making appropriate measurements of tracheal injury. Using the photomicrography system, photograph the squares of a hemacytometer (shown in **Fig. 5**) at different magnifications. Transfer these images to the computer, and open them in NIH Image. Using the rectangular trace tool, trace the outline of a hemacytometer square and measure its perimeter length and area in pixels. Knowing the millimeter length of this perimeter, one then can derive for that magnification the number of pixels per millimeter and square millimeter. This value is used later to convert measurements made in pixels to absolute units and will provide the investigator with the limit of resolution at a particular magnification.

2. Photograph the tracheal wound slides at appropriate magnifications. We provide examples in **Fig. 4** of how a larger injury may be photographed and montaged to provide a complete image at suitable magnification. Transfer these images to the computer, and open them in NIH Image. Using the freehand trace tool, trace the length of the basement membrane around the tracheal ring or along the airway segment of interest and measure its length, and the area of the airway lumen plus epithelium, in pixels.

3. The tracheal wound should be clearly visible. Using the freehand trace tool, trace the length of the basement membrane at points at which the epithelium is completely or partially denuded. Measure each of these lengths in pixels. Wound width is expressed in pixels and as the percentage of denuded basement membrane for the tracheal ring. Additional measurements relevant to the questions the investigator might ask can be made on the same image, such as the height of the epithelium and the thickness of the basement membrane (**Fig. 4**).

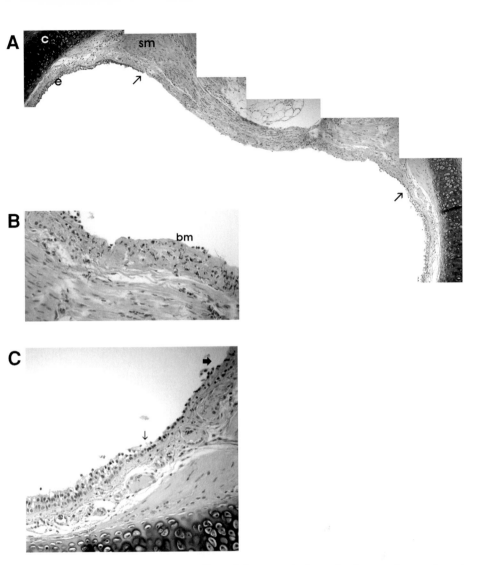

Fig. 4. Representative images collected from typical tracheal wound experiment in guinea pig. (A) Tracheal mucosal wound 24 h after creation in normal guinea pig. This low-power view was collected by an imaging system, and individual frames were montaged to create the final image. The tracheal mucosal wound in this particular animal was approximately one-fourth of the total circumference. When measured by the techniques described in this chapter, the tracheal injury measures approx 1705 pixels, or 407 µm, in length between the two arrows. (B) Higher-magnification view of denuded basement membrane in same tracheal mucosal wound. The epithelium is completely removed, and the basement membrane and underlying connective tissue are not significantly damaged. (C) Higher-magnification view of edge of tracheal mucosal wound shown in (A). Here the edge of the original wound is marked by the thin arrow, and the extent of reepithelialization is marked by the thick arrow. In this image, the height of the normal epithelium is 22.0 µm and that of the new epithelial cells is 4.3 µm. e, epithelium; c, cartilage; sm, smooth muscle; bm, basement membrane.

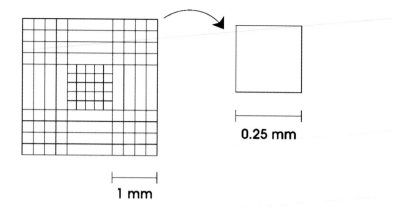

0.25 mm

1 mm

Fig. 5. Grid arrangement on a hemacytometer. The outside corner boxes are subdivided into smaller boxes. The outside corner box has a length of 1 mm, and an inside smaller box has a length of 0.25 mm. The corresponding length in pixels on a digitized image can be used to calibrate dimensions in other images taken with the same imaging system at the same magnification.

4. Notes

1. We have found that there is a learning curve to this procedure. The investigator should plan several practice sessions using animals that are not vital to the overall experimental design (e.g., not precious transgenic animals on the first attempt).

2. There are several important complications to the intubation and tracheal injury that may lead to death of the animal or may preclude the use of the animal in the planned experiment. Among these are the following:

   a. Puncture of the hypopharynx with the otoscope speculum or with the stylette.

   b. Placement of the stylette into the esophagus. This can lead to puncture with a resulting infection of the retrosternal and left pleural spaces.

   c. Puncture of the trachea, which can lead to a pneumomediastinum and infection.

   d. Tracheitis owing to the mucosal injury. The incidence is low if proper clean procedures are employed in creating the injury.

   e. Bleeding owing to the mucosal injury or owing to the intubation. The incidence is very low with proper technique.

3. The procedure may be scaled to larger animals (e.g., rabbits) with relative ease. Instead of an otoscope, one may employ a pediatric laryngoscope with a very short, curved ("Mac") blade, such as those used in the care of human neonates. The stylette to be used may be of the same size as for guinea pigs (1.5 mm in diameter) or may be larger if a larger injury is required. The procedure is otherwise the same.

4. The use of this procedure in rats and mice is more problematic. The problem is the physical size of the pharynx, which many times precludes direct visualization of the vocal cords using the technique we have described—particularly in the mouse. We have had some success in doing blind intubations with a very thin (0.7-mm-diameter) stylette in mice. This stylette has a very small bend at its tip instead of a proper beveled edge. In the anesthetized mouse, one can insert the stylette gently into the mouth and guide it by feel to the hypopharynx. With a finger on the cervical neck over the trachea, one can feel when the stylette has entered the trachea. The stylette then can be torqued and withdrawn. The investigator should be prepared for a substantially higher mortality rate with this procedure. We found that the method of Jou et al. *(10)* can be adapted to perform a blind intubation of a mouse using a 1-mL syringe barrel; tracheal injury then can be done using a very thin metal wand as we describe.

5. Other intubation procedures, such as those suggested in **refs. *8–11***, can be combined with the use of mechanical injury to the trachea as we describe. In adapting other techniques, direct visualization of the glottis and vocal cords is necessary to avoid injuring these structures with the metal wand.

6. Other methods of tracheal injury can be adapted to the method we present. Instead of a metal wand, a catheter of appropriate diameter through which a selected agent (e.g., naphthalene) can be instilled. Alternately, a narrow brush (such as those used for human bronchoscopy) can be employed to create an abrasive injury.

7. The types of digital cameras, microscopes, and computers that may be used in these basic measurements is diverse. Key considerations in building such a system are based on the end points of the work: What are the goals of the investigator, and what other potential uses would a digital photomicrography system have? Microscopes from any good vendor that have a port and an adapter for attaching a digital camera may be used. In considering a digital camera, the limits of the camera's resolution should be ascertained. In our experience, a typical 2 megapixel digital camera photographing a tracheal ring will have a limit of approx 0.1 μm using a ×4 objective and a ×10 camera adapter, and approximately 0.02 μm using a ×20 objective and a ×10 camera adapter. For the types of measurements we describe in this chapter, these limits are more than acceptable. Other issues, including color fidelity, reliability, and other features of the camera should be considered according to the investigator's needs. Finally, we utilized NIH Image since it can make the measurements necessary for this method and is distributed without cost. Other suitable image analysis programs are available for either Windows- or Macintosh-compatible computers.

8. There are other issues that should be considered in morphometric analysis of airway epithelium and of airways in general. A tracheal ring must be oriented in the proper plane on section; deviations from this can lead to progressive error in measurements. A comprehensive analysis of these limitations has been published *(12)*.

Acknowledgments

This work was supported by grants HL-60531 and HL-63300 from the National Heart, Lung and Blood Institute.

I thank John Kim, M.D., and Valerie McKinnis, M.D., for their assistance in developing the tracheal injury technique; Delbert Dorscheid, M.D., Ph.D., for his helpful comments in morphometry analysis; and Karen Dirr for original artwork.

References

1. Keenan, K., Combs, J., and McDowell, E. (1982) Regeneration of hamster tracheal epithelium after mechanical injury. I. Focal lesions: quantitative morphologic study of cell proliferation. *Virchows Arch. Cell Pathol.* **41,** 193–214.
2. Erjefält, I., Erjefält, J., Persson, C., and Sundler, F. (1995) In vivo restitution of airway epithelium. *Cell Tissue Res.* **281,** 305–316.
3. Erjefält, J., Persson, C., and Sundler, F. (1996) Eosinophils, neutrophils, and venular gaps in the airway mucosa at epithelial removal-restitution. *Am. J. Respir. Crit. Care Med.* **153,** 1666–1674.
4. Gordon, R. and Lane, B. (1976) Regeneration of rat tracheal epithelium after mechanical injury. II. Restoration of surface integrity during the early hours after injury. *Am. Rev. Respir. Dis.* **113,** 799–807.
5. Persson, C., Erjefält, J., Erjefält, I., Korsgren, M., Nilsson, M., and Sundler, F. (1996) Epithelial shedding—restitution as a causative process in airway inflammation. *Clin. Exp. Allergy* **26,** 746–755.
6. Kim, J. S., McKinnis, V. S., and White, S. R. (1997) Proliferation and repair of guinea pig tracheal epithelium after neuropeptide depletion and injury in vivo. *Am. J. Physiol. (Lung Cell. Mol. Physiol. 17)* **273,** L1235–L1241.
7. Li, X., Dorscheid, D. R., and White, S. R. (2000) Glycosylation profiles of airway epithelial repair after mechanical injury in vivo in guinea pigs. *Histochem. J.* **32,** 207–216.
8. Thet, L. A. (1983) A simple method for intubating rats under direct vision. *Lab. Anim. Sci.* **33,** 368–369.
9. Costa, D. L., Lehmann, J. R., Harold, W. M., and Drew, R. T. (1986) Transoral tracheal intubation of rodents using a fiberoptic laryngoscope. *Lab. Anim. Sci.* **36,** 256–261.
10. Jou, I.-M., Tsai, Y.-T., Tsai, C.-L., Wu, M.-H., Chang, H.-Y., and Wang, N. S. (2000) Simplified rat intubation using a new oropharyngeal intubation wedge. *J. Appl. Physiol.* **89,** 1766–1770.
11. Alpert, M., Goldstein, D., and Triner, L. (1982) Technique of endotracheal intubation in rats. *Lab. Anim. Sci.* **33,** 78, 79.
12. Kuwano, K., Bosken, C. H., Pare, P. D., Bai, T. R., Wiggs, B. R., and Hogg, J. C. (1993) Small airway dimensions in asthma and in chronic obstructive pulmonary disease. *Am. Rev. Respir. Dis.* **148,** 1220–1225.

10

Murine Models of Intestinal Anastomoses

David L. Williams and I. William Browder

1. Introduction

Wound healing is a physiological process that is essential to the reestablishment of homeostasis (*1–4*). It is generally accepted that wound repair is an immune-mediated event (*5*) that involves a number of cell types such as macrophages, neutrophils, fibroblasts, endothelial cells, and keratinocytes, along with a complex and exquisitely choreographed interaction of wound growth factors (*1,2,4,6,7*). While there have been significant advances in our understanding of wound repair, there are still major gaps in our knowledge of the reparative process. Specifically, the receptors, cell-surface interactions, and intracellular signaling processes critical to wound repair have not been fully deciphered. Over the last decade, there has been a rapid evolution of techniques that can be employed to decipher the cellular and molecular mechanisms involved in diverse physiological processes including microarrays, macroarrays, multiplexed polymerase chain reaction, and surface plasmon resonance.

In reviewing the wound-healing literature, it became apparent that most studies employed rats as the experimental animal (*8,9*) and that the most common wound model is the incisional skin wound (*1*). This is understandable because the skin wound model is easy to reproduce and quantify (*1,10*) and the size of the rat (≥200 g) makes it easy to work with. However, there are two general limitations with this approach. First, in the clinical setting most incisional skin wounds heal normally; consequently, this may not be the most relevant paradigm for studying problematic healing in surgical scenarios. Brasken (*11*), Ikeuchi et al. (*8*), Comert et al. (*12*), and Compton et al. (*10*) have addressed this issue by developing rat models of intestinal anastomoses that are more clinically relevant. Second, most of the reagents available for

From: *Methods in Molecular Medicine, vol. 78: Wound Healing: Methods and Protocols*
Edited by: Luisa A. DiPietro and Aime L. Burns © Humana Press Inc., Totowa, NJ

analyzing cellular and molecular mechanisms have been developed for human and/or murine systems. At present, there are a limited, but growing, number of reagents available for studying cellular and molecular processes in rats. To address these potential limitations, we developed two murine models of intestinal anastomoses, one in the small intestine and one in the colon *(10,13)*. In developing these models, we drew heavily on previous work in the rat intestinal anastomosis models *(8,10–12)*.

An important parameter of wound repair is the tensile strength of the healing wound *(10)*. Many of the tensiometers described in the literature are not well suited to evaluating the tensile strength of murine intestinal anastomoses because they are not sensitive enough to reproducibly quantify such small forces. Tensiometers that have proven sensitive and reproducible enough for this application are frequently prohibitively expensive. Alternately, custom-designed and built tensiometers are not routinely available to or adaptable by many investigators. To address these concerns, we developed a tensiometric system for the study of murine intestinal anastomoses that is sensitive; reproducible; easy to use; inexpensive; and composed of standardized, off-the-shelf components.

2. Materials

1. Animals: ICR/Harlan Sprague Dawley (Indianapolis, IN) mice weighing 18–20 g are employed for the intestinal anastomoses. We use male mice that are age and weight matched. The mice are placed in hanging cages and allowed to acclimate for 1 wk after arrival at the Division of Laboratory Animal Resources, James H. Quillen College of Medicine, East Tennessee State University, an Association for the Assessment and Accreditation of Laboratory Animal Care (AALAC)-accredited facility. They are maintained on a 12-h light/12-h dark schedule and allowed access to water and standard laboratory chow (Harlan/Teklab, Madison, WI) ad libitum (*see* **Note 1**).

2. Liquid diet: During the development of the models it became apparent that maintaining the mice on standard laboratory chow did not provide optimal results. To alleviate this problem we developed a liquid diet. The mice are maintained on the diet for at least 72 h prior to surgery. It consists of Ensure (Ross, Columbus, OH) diluted with 1.5 vol of distilled water. Magnesium citrate, a cathartic, is added to the murine diet to further evacuate the intestine prior to surgery. The final diet consists of 1 part full-strength magnesium citrate to 7 parts diluted Ensure. The diet is prepared fresh each day and delivered to the mice through a drinking bottle placed in the cage in a manner identical to that of the water bottle. The mice quickly adapt to and thrive on the liquid diet. They are maintained on this diet for the duration of the study.

3. Anesthestic: General anesthesia is induced by xylazine (20 mg/kg intraperitoneally) and ketamine (100 mg/kg intraperitoneally).

4. Incubator for recovery: Following surgery the mice are placed in an animal incubator (Barnstead/Thermolyne, Dubuque, IA). The incubator is set at 37°C and supplemented with oxygen-enriched air (25 mL/min flow rate).
5. Povidone solution.
6. Dissecting microscope (Dyonics Woburn, MA).
7. Zeiss fiberoptic illuminator (Zeiss, Thornwood, NY).
8. Metzenbaum scissors.
9. 7-0 Nonabsorbable suture.
10. 6-0 Fast-absorbing plain-gut suture.
11. Isothermic lactated Ringers (McGaw, Irvine, CA).
12. Tenotomy scissors.
13. Buprinex (0.05 mg/kg).
14. Chloral hydrate.
15. Tensiometer: A Comten (St. Petersburg, FL) linear travel, velocity-controlled 900 series tensile tester can be purchased from Cole Parmer (Niles, IL). This instrument is equipped with a tester-controller and a rotating piston hydraulic load cell with a sensitivity range of 3–900 g. The tester-controller establishes the desired speed, determines the direction of force applied, and initiates and terminates testing. It is capable of tensile, compression, and flexural types of testing. Our focus is on tensile testing and the instrument is configured accordingly. The capability of this instrument can be enhanced by attaching it to a CEDM-4 digital monitor/controller (DMC) supplied by Comten. The DMC allows variable speed control, a choice of force display units, load and force limits, and provides a digital readout of the force generated. It is attached via the serial (RS232C) port to a personal computer (PC). The DMC converts the analog data signal from the tester to a digital signal that is acquired by the PC. The DMC-PC interface requires the use of a communications program for data acquisition. We employ a shareware program TELIX (Exis, West Hill, Ontario, Canada). The communications protocol is 1200 baud, 8 data bits, 1 stop bit, no parity, and VT100 terminal emulation. Following acquisition, the data are reduced, analyzed (Microsoft Excel version 2000), and graphed (SlideWrite version 5.0, Advanced Graphics Software, Encinitas, CA) with commercially available software packages.

3. Methods

3.2. Preoperative Preparation

1. Fast the mice for 6 h prior to advancing the liquid diet 72 h prior to surgery.
2. Following anesthetic induction, shave the abdomen, place the mice on their backs with legs lightly secured, and prep the abdomens with povidone solution. To facilitate the surgery, we employ a dissecting microscope with a Zeiss fiberoptic illuminator.

3.2. Small Intestinal Anastomosis (Jejunojejunostomy)

1. Create a 2-cm upper midline laparotomy and identify and isolate a loop of jejunum.

2. Using Metzenbaum scissors, transect the jejunum taking care not to interfere with the blood supply to the area.
3. One of two investigated surgical approaches can be used:
   a. Perform the anastomosis with a 7-0 nonabsorbable suture in a running fashion.
   b. Create a single-layer intestinal anastomosis using 6-0 fast-absorbing plain-gut suture in an interrupted fashion.

   As we evaluated both surgical approaches, we found that 6-0 plain-gut suture applied in an interrupted fashion provided superior results when compared with 7-0 nonabsorbable suture applied in a running fashion. All subsequent studies and the development of the colon anastomosis model employed 6-0 plain-gut suture in an interrupted fashion (*see* **Note 2**).
4. Return the bowel to the abdomen and perform a two-layer abdominal closure using suture (*see* **Note 2**).
5. Place 1 mL/20 g of isothermic lactated Ringers in the peritoneal cavity prior to closing for fluid resuscitation.

3.3. Colon Anastomosis

1. After the induction of general anesthesia, shave and prep the abdomen with povidone solution.
2. Make a 2-cm midline laparotomy incision and identify the cecum. Approximately 0.5–1 cm distal to the cecum, identify and isolate the murine colon.
3. Using tenotomy scissors, transect the colon making sure that the blood supply to the area is not compromised.
4. Perform a single-layer colonic anastomosis using 6-0 fast-absorbing plain-gut suture in an interrupted fashion (four to six stitches as needed).
5. Return the colon to the abdomen and then irrigate the abdominal cavity thoroughly with isothermic sterile lactated Ringers solution. Place 1 mL/20 g of lactated Ringers in the peritoneal cavity prior to closing for fluid resuscitation.
6. Close the abdomen in two layers using suture.

3.4. Postoperative Care

1. Prior to placing the mice in the animal incubator for recovery, administer Buprinex for analgesia.
2. Provide water ad libitum in the postoperative period.
3. Keep the mice in the incubator until they recover, as evidenced by righting reflex, mobility, and intake of water.
4. Inject the mice intraperitoneally with 1 cc/20 g of lactated ringers solution for fluid resuscitation on d 1, and on d 2 slowly advance the liquid diet (*see* **Note 3**).

3.5. Euthanasia and Preparation of Anastomoses for Tensiometry

1. On postoperative d 2, 3, 5, or 7, euthanize the mice with a lethal IP dose of chloral hydrate followed by opening and inspection of the abdomen.

2. Gently identify and resect the anastomosis with ~3.5 cm of intestine on each side of the wound, providing specimens 7 cm in length.
3. Trim away the surrounding adherent tissues and attached mesentery and attach a long loop of 7-0 suture to each end of the specimen to facilitate handling.
4. Transfer the specimen to the tensiometer for tensile strength determination.

3.6. Tensiometry

1. Position the anastomosis between the tensiometer clamps (*see* **Note 4**).
2. Use the 7-0 suture at each end of the specimen to attach the tissue to the upper or lower tensiometer clamps such that the anastomosis is halfway between the upper and lower clamps. The ends of the tissue are not held by the tensiometer clamps because intestinal tissue is rather friable and inappropriate tightening of the clamps on either end of the tissue specimen can lead to disruption at a point close to the clamp during tensiometry. We observed that tissue secured with suture provides superior results.
3. Disrupt the wound at a speed of 2 mm/s. Data are acquired at a rate of 2 data points/s (*see* **Note 5**).

4. Notes

1. We employed mice that were sex, age, and weight matched for all of our studies. In addition, the ICR strain that we used was an outbred strain. The choice of strain was based on our previous experience with the ICR model (*13–15*). We opted to use outbred mice because this more closely mimics the human situation. It is reasonable to argue that using an inbred strain might make the experiments more reproducible and make it easier to decipher complex immunological and/or signaling mechanisms. These are valid points, and there is no substantive reason why one cannot employ inbred strains of mice for intestinal anastomotic studies. However, it has been our experience that the outbred ICR are a more hardy mouse strain that may be better able to withstand the rigors of intestinal resection and anastomoses. This is only an opinion: we did not perform comparative studies. Another important issue is the postoperative survival rate. We found that >95% of the mice survived the surgery and ~90% survived up to d 7, the time at which our experiments were terminated. The survival was owing, in part, to maintaining the mice on the liquid diet. In the absence of the liquid diet, postoperative mortality was much higher, in some cases ~40–50%. We attributed this to rupture of the anastomosis owing to movement of solid waste (preingested food) in the intestine when the mice were allowed access to standard laboratory chow. When the mice were maintained on the liquid diet, survival improved significantly.
2. Selection of suture is critical. In our initial studies, we investigated two surgical approaches to murine jejunojejunostomy. First, we used 7-0 nonabsorbable suture applied in a running fashion. In parallel, we evaluated 6-0 plain gut applied in an interrupted fashion (four to six stitches/wound). In each case, we were able to obtain acceptable levels of survival and wound repair. However, we noted that the force velocity curves in mice treated with 7-0 nonabsorbable suture were arti-

ficially high because the anastomosis ruptured prior to the rupture of the suture. In other words, we saw two peaks on the force velocity curves, the first showing separation of the anastomosis and the second the rupture or tearing of the suture from the surrounding tissue. Thus, the data acquired using nonabsorbable suture are much more complicated and may not accurately reflect the strength of the anastomosis. In addition, the technical skill of the surgeon may play a more significant role when using nonabsorbable suture. This problem was easily solved in intestinal anastomoses that were approximated using an interrupted technique with fast-absorbing 6-0 plain-gut suture. The data from the plain-gut suture model more accurately reflect the tensile strength of the anastomosis, since all of the suture material had been absorbed by postoperative d 3.

3. Our initial attempts at murine intestinal anastomoses were complicated by the disruption of the wound by preingested food, even after a 48-h fast. To alleviate this problem, we incorporated the liquid diet into the model and fasted the mice for 6 h prior to advancing the liquid diet. Mice were maintained on this diet for at least 72 h prior to surgery. In developing the diet, our goal was to use readily available preparations that would provide a diet with adequate caloric intake and one to which the mice would readily adapt. We consulted with the campus veterinarian as well as a dietician regarding available liquid diets and the most appropriate composition. During our initial studies, we observed that the mice preferred chocolate-flavored Ensure. The diet was mixed in quantities of ~500 mL and stored at 4°C for no longer than 1 d prior to use. In most cases, the diet was prepared immediately prior to use. We found that it was important to sterilize the water bottles used to deliver the liquid diet each time the diet was administered, which in our case was daily. This is a routine procedure in most animal care facilities. The necessity of sterilizing the bottle and the nipple relates to the presence of microorganisms that can contaminate the liquid diet, causing it to precipitate or clot. For this reason, it is important to ensure that the mice can access the diet as needed. We routinely checked the mice two to three times daily during the course of the experiment.

4. As discussed in **Note 2**, we observed that tensile strength could be accurately assessed by d 3 postsurgery when the plain-gut suture had been absorbed. We did examine tensile strength on d 2 and found that suture was still present and that it complicated tensiometry. Thus, the minimum time to evaluation of wound tensile strength in our model is d 3. We also observed that by d 7 many of the jejunal and a significant portion of the colonic anastomoses exhibited tensile strength greater than intestine that had not been injured. Hence, the bowel would disrupt at a position other than the anastomosis. This indicated that the best window of opportunity for data acquisition was between d 3 and 7. We did not evaluate tensile strength of the anastomoses beyond d 7.

5. In **Subheading 2, item 15**, we described the tensiometer configuration exactly as it was developed and used. There are several caveats that should be considered when setting up a comparable system. First, virtually any currently available PC will accept the digital output from the DMC controller. Second, there are a

number of communications software programs that can be used to acquire the digital signal from the DMC. In fact, some operating systems such as Windows have integrated communications software that can be employed. The type of software used to acquire the signal should be dictated by availability, ease of use, and type of operating system (such as Windows, Mac, Linux) the user employs. Likewise, many currently available software programs can be used to reduce, analyze, and graph the data. We routinely employ Microsoft Excel (Microsoft, Redmond, WA), SlideWrite version 5.0 (Advanced Graphics Software), SigmaPlot version 5.0 (SPSS Chicago, IL), or Prism version 3.0 (GraphPad, San Diego, CA). The most important consideration is to identify a configuration that works well for the end user and to employ it consistently.

Acknowledgments

We wish to acknowledge the assistance of Drs. Judy Thompson, Ray Compton, Charles Portera, Edward Love, Sebastian Lopez, and Luisa Memore in the development of the models. We also wish to thank Alice Terrell for assistance in finalizing the manuscript. This work was supported, in part, by a Veteran Affairs Merit Review grant.

References

1. Browder, W., Williams, D., Lucore, P., Pretus, H., Jones, E., and McNamee, R. (1988) Effect of enhanced macrophage function on early wound healing. *Surgery* **104,** 224–230.
2. DiPietro, L. A. (1995) Wound healing: the role of the macrophage and other immune cells. *Shock* **4,** 233–240.
3. Cherry, G. (1995) The past, present, and future of wound healing. *Wound Rep. Reg.* **3,** 119–119.
4. Ehrlich, H. P. (1998) The physiology of wound healing: a summary of normal and abnormal wound healing processes. *Adv. Wound Care* **11,** 326–328.
5. Beck, L. S., DeGuzman, L., Lee, W. P., Xu, Y., Siegel, M. W., and Amento, E. P. (1993) One systemic administration of transforming growth factor-β1 reverses age- or glucocorticoid-impaired wound healing. *J. Clin. Invest.* **92,** 2841–2849.
6. Bennett, N. T. and Schultz, G. S. (1993) Growth factors and wound healing: biochemical properties of growth factors and their receptors. *Am. J. Surg.* **165,** 728–737.
7. Bennett, N. T. and Schultz, G. S. (1993) Growth factors and wound healing: part II. Role in normal and chronic wound healing. *Am. J. Surg.* **166,** 74–81.
8. Ikeuchi, D., Onodera, H., Aung, T., Kan, S., Kawamoto, K., Imamura, M., and Maetani, S. (1999) Correlation of tensile strength with bursting pressure in the evaluation of intestinal anastomosis. *Dig. Surg.* **16,** 478–485.
9. Hill, M. J. (1999) Mechanisms of diet and colon carcinogenesis. *Eur. J. Cancer Prev.* **8(Suppl. 1),** S95–S98.

10. Compton, R., Williams, D., and Browder, W. (1996) The beneficial effect of enhanced macrophage function on the healing of bowel anastomoses. *Am. Surg.* **62,** 14–18.
11. Brasken, P. (1991) Healing of experimental colon anastomosis. *Eur. J. Surg. Suppl.* **566,** 1–51.
12. Comert, M., Taneri, F., Tekin, E., Ersoy, E., Oktemer, S., Onuk, E., Duzgun, E., and Ayoglu, F. (2000) The effect of pentoxifylline on the healing of intestinal anastomosis in rats with experimental obstructive jaundice. *Surg. Today* **30,** 896–902.
13. Portera, C. A., Love, E. J., Memore, L., Zhang, L., Mueller, A., Browder, W., and Williams, D. L. (1997) Effect of macrophage stimulation on collagen biosynthesis in the healing wound. *Am. Surg.* **63,** 125–131.
14. Williams, D. L., Ha, T., Li, C., Kalbfleisch, J. H., and Ferguson, D. A. Jr. (1999) Early activation of hepatic NFkB and NF-IL6 in polymicrobial sepsis correlates with bacteremia, cytokine expression and mortality. *Ann. Surg.* **230,** 95–104.
15. Williams, D. L., Ha, T., Li, C., Kalbfleisch, J. H., Laffan, J. J., and Ferguson, D. A. (1999) Inhibiting early activation of tissue nuclear factor-κB and nuclear factor interleukin 6 with (1-3)-β-D-glucan increases long-term survival in polymicrobial sepsis. *Surgery* **126,** 54–65.

11

Murine Model of Peritoneal Adhesion Formation

Andrew E. Jahoda, Mary Kay Olson, and Elizabeth J. Kovacs

1. Introduction

The lining of the organs within the peritoneal cavity consists of a single layer of mesothelial cells with a minimum of underlying connective tissue. This same cellular structure covers the luminal surface of the abdominal wall musculature. Together these mesothelial layers serve as a smooth surface, which allows the organs to glide freely within the peritoneal cavity. Damage to the mesothelial lining, as occurs during abdominal surgery (*1*), results in the exposure of the underlying connective tissue. Leukocytes resident within the peritoneal cavity, as well as those within the circulatory system, are recruited to such sites of exposed connective tissue. There, the leukocytes secrete a host of inflammatory mediators and cytokines. If the damage to the mesothelium is great enough, a cascade of events can be triggered that can ultimately lead to proliferation of fibroblasts and the deposition of large amounts of connective tissue, via the process of fibrogenesis. In extreme cases, thick bands of connective tissue can tighten around internal organs, restricting their function and causing irreversible damage. The deposition of connective tissue in the peritoneal cavity, called peritoneal adhesion formation, can cause severe abdominal pain, infertility, bowel obstruction, and death (*1*).

Several methods have been used to assess adhesion formation in the peritoneal cavity. Two of these are gross visual inspection and scoring (*2*) and the quantitation of thickness of the connective tissue on the luminal surface to the abdominal wall musculature (*3*). The latter method is more accurate and objective, because it relies on a computer-generated assessment of the thickness of the connective-tissue layer (**Fig. 1**). Additionally, this histologically based method affords the investigator the opportunity to examine other parameters

From: *Methods in Molecular Medicine, vol. 78: Wound Healing: Methods and Protocols*
Edited by: Luisa A. DiPietro and Aime L. Burns © Humana Press Inc., Totowa, NJ

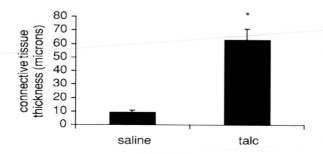

Fig. 1. Quantitative assessment of peritoneal connective-tissue thickness in talc-treated mice. Mice were given an ip injection of 50 mg of talc in saline or saline alone. Fourteen days later, abdominal wall musculature was harvested, fixed, and stained with Masson's trichrome stain, and the abdominal wall connective-tissue thickness was measured in microns using NIH image analysis software. Data shown are mean connective-tissue thickness $\pm$ SEM ($n = 9$ per group). $^*p < 0.01$ from saline-treated mice.

of wound healing besides collagen deposition, such as inflammatory cell infiltration and angiogenesis (*see* **ref. 4** for a review). While several means have been used to induce the formation of adhesions, the present method uses a rodent model in which mice are given a single ip injection of talc (anhydrous magnesium silicate) in sterile saline. Talc has long been known to induce peritoneal inflammation and connective-tissue deposition *(5,6)*. This model is very reproducible and quantitative, thus allowing investigators to test a wide variety of antifibrogenic agents *(7,8)*. An example of the quantitative assessment of abdominal connective-tissue thickness is shown in **Fig. 1**. Note that at the 50-mg dose of talc employed in the present experiment, there is five- to six-fold more connective tissue in the talc-treated vs saline-treated mouse.

2. Materials

1. Adult male and female C57Bl/6 mice 8–10 wk of age (25–30 g): Animals are maintained on a 12-h light/12-h dark cycle and given food and water ad libitum. They are also maintained for a minimum of 5 d prior to initiation of experiments to allow for adjustment to their environment and recovery from the stress of transportation. Mice are randomly assigned to experimental treatment groups.
2. Talc solution: The talc used to inject into the mice is put into suspension in a concentration of 50 mg of talc in 0.5 mL of phosphate-buffered saline (*see* **Note 1**). This suspension can be made in bulk prior to the onset of experiments to ensure consistency throughout the extent of injections. Making 500 mL would provide enough talc suspension to inject almost 1000 mice.

a. Measure 50 g of talc and put in a sterile 500-mL liter graduated cylinder.
b. Fill the cylinder to the 500-mL line with phosphate-buffered saline.
c. Transfer to a bottle and autoclave.

To prepare for administration of talc to mice, estimate the amount of talc solution needed for the experiment. Shake the talc suspension vigorously before use in order to ensure distribution of talc. Using a sterile technique in a laminar flow hood, transfer the appropriate amount to a sterile 50-mL conical tube. To ensure that the suspension remains sterile, place materials under an ultraviolet light in a laminar flow hood with the blower on for 15 min prior to use. Shake the talc suspension vigorously before drawing into a syringe. Prepare 1-cc syringes, with 25- or 27-gauge needles. Fill the syringes with 0.5 mL of sterile talc in saline, or saline alone as a control.

3. Alcohol wipes.
4. Dry ice.
5. Scissors and rat-tooth forceps.
6. Tissue cassettes.
7. Tissue-Tek VIP processor (Sakura, Torrance, CA).
8. 10% Buffered formalin.
9. Xylenes.
10. Paraffin (Ameraffin from Allegiance).
11. Microtome.
12. Oven.
13. Bouin's fixative (Rowley, Donvers, MA).
14. Weigerts Hematoxylin A (Rowley).
15. Weigerts Hematoxylin B (Rowley).
16. Biebrich scarlet-acid fuchsin (Rowley).
17. 1% Biebrich Scarlet (90 mL) (Rowley).
18. 1% Acid fuchsin (10 mL) (Rowley).
19. Glacial acetic acid (1 mL) (Rowley).
20. Phosphotungstic–phosphomolybdic acid (2.5% each) (Rowley).
21. Aniline Blue (2.5% in 2% acidic acid) (Rowley).
22. 1% Glacial acetic acid; make fresh each time.
23. Accu-Mount (Baxter, McGaw Park, IL).

3. Methods

3.1. Animal Handling and Injection of Talc

1. Pick up a mouse by the base of the tail with the right hand. Using the thumb and index finger of the left hand, grasp the skin at the nape of the mouse's neck, near the shoulder blades. Pull the skin so that it is taught and the mouse cannot move its head or front legs.
2. To minimize the chance of injecting into peritoneal contents, tilt the mouse's head downward to shift the bowel superiorly and inject in the inferior aspect of

the peritoneal cavity. Wipe the surface of the skin at the injection site with an alcohol wipe. Insert the needle through the skin and into the peritoneal cavity. Aspirate prior to injecting the talc to ensure that the tip of the needle is not placed within a blood vessel or abdominal organ. Inject the talc (or saline) solution.

3. Immediately after injection, gently massage the abdomen of the mouse to distribute the talc.

4. To distinguish between control mice and talc mice (if not placed in separate cages), mark the base of the tail of one group with a black Sharpie pen. The tails will need to be remarked every 2 to 3 d, since the markings will wear off. Black pen marks last longer than other colors.

5. Return the mice to their cages and check daily to ensure that they are mobile and active.

6. Sacrifice animals between 14 and 21 d for assessment of abdominal connective-tissue deposition (*see* **Note 2**).

3.2. Harvesting of Abdominal Wall Tissue

1. Euthanize the mice by an appropriate method.

2. Perform dissection with a fine pair of curved scissors and rat-tooth forceps (*see* **Note 3**).

3. Wet the fur of the abdomen with alcohol to keep the fur from interfering with the dissection.

4. Grasp the skin and sc tissue with forceps and make a small cut through the skin, taking care not to invade the abdominal musculature.

5. Using the scissors with the curve pointing up, separate the sc tissue from the layer of muscle. Having removed the superficial layer, a midline incision through the abdominal muscle can now be easily performed.

6. After inspecting the peritoneal cavity for any gross changes, harvest the abdominal wall for histological evaluation. The tissue should be about 0.5 cm wide and 0.5–1 cm long. Place the tissue in a plastic tissue cassette prior to fixation. Since the talc has primarily a microscopic effect on the luminal surface of the abdominal wall, it is important to avoid manipulating the peritoneal side of the tissue (*see* **Note 4**).

3.3. Processing, Sectioning, and Staining of Tissue

3.3.1. Processing and Sectioning

1. On removing the sample of abdominal wall, trim the tissue to specification and place in a tissue cassette (*see* **Note 5**).

2. Place the tissue on an automatic tissue processor (Tissue-Tek VIP) in two changes of 10% buffered formalin, dehydrated in graded alcohols from 70% to absolute ethanol, cleared in two changes of xylene and infiltrated in liquid paraffin. This is an overnight procedure.

3. Embed the tissue in paraffin.

4. Section the tissue at 4 μ on a rotary microtome and place in a 60°C oven to melt paraffin and secure the tissue to the slides. Stain the tissue with Masson Trichrome.

3.3.2. Staining

1. Deparaffinize and hydrate the sections in distilled water.
2. Mordant in Bouin's fixative for 30 min at 60°C for 30 min at room temperature.
3. Wash the sections in running tap water for 10 min.
4. Rinse in distilled water.
5. Stain with Working Weigert's Hematoxylin for 7 min (the solution may be saved for 1 wk).
6. Wash in running tap water for 10 min.
7. Stain with Biebrich Scarlet-Acid fuchsin for 2 min (discard the solution).
8. Rinse in distilled water.
9. Tone in phosphotungstic–phosphomolybdic acid for 10–12 min (discard the solution).
10. Rinse in distilled water.
11. Stain in Aniline Blue for 1 min (the solution may be saved).
12. Rinse in distilled water.
13. Treat with 1% glacial acetic acid for 1 min.
14. Rinse in distilled water.
15. Dehydrate, clear, and mount with Accu-Mount.
16. Read the results:
    a. Nuclei: black.
    b. Cytoplasm, keratin, muscle fibers: red.
    c. Collagen, mucus: blue.

3.4. Analysis of Tissue

When viewing the peritoneal wall under a microscope, both the mesothelium and adventitia may have very little connective tissue, making it difficult to determine which side is the mesothelium. The mesothelial side is distinguished by a smooth surface, whereas the adventitia will have very discrete wisps of sc fatty tissue present.

Examination of the luminal surface of the abdominal wall musculature reveals the mesothelial surface. This is a simple squamous epithelium, which will be difficult to visualize under the microscope. By contrast, submesothelial collagen will stain blue and be easy to identify. As shown in black and white in **Fig. 2**, the abdominal wall muscle layers stain darker gray (which would be pink in color), which is easy to distinguish from blue collagen.

The extent of submesothelial connective-tissue deposition is measured with a high-power microscope interfaced with a computer using the NIH Image

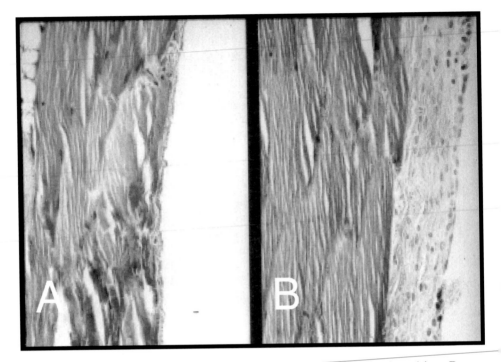

Fig. 2. Histological assessment of peritoneal connective-tissue deposition. Representative Masson's trichrome–stained abdominal wall tissue obtained 14 d after treatment is shown. The lumen of the peritoneal cavity is on the right. (**A**) Saline (as a control). Note the thin layer of connective tissue (collagen) beneath the mesothelium. (**B**) Talc (to induce adhesions). Note the thick band of connective tissue at the luminal surface (magnification: ×400).

Analysis software. This program enables the investigator to select a tool that can take measurements on the screen. By initially measuring a known distance on a slide containing a metered scale, one can then determine a conversion factor to convert NIH measurements to microns.

When measuring the connective tissue of the samples, keeping in mind that it is impossible to measure the entire length of the muscle, caution must be exercised to avoid a bias in the sites chosen to measure. To achieve a nonbiased representation, start at the top of the muscle so that the edge just touches the top of the screen. Then determine the halfway point of the screen and measure the width of connective tissue straight across. Now move the platform of the microscope up until the point at the bottom of the screen is at the top, being sure not to skip or overlap any part of the muscle viewed. Again, take a measurement of the connective tissue directly across at the midway point on the screen. For convenience and to ensure a nonbiased measurement, a thin strip of a Post-it® can be cut and placed on the monitor where one intends to take all of the measurements.

3.5. Data Interpretation and Statistical Analysis

Data are expressed as mean connective tissue thickness (in microns) ± SEM (as shown in **Fig. 1**). To achieve accurate measurements of connective-tissue thickness, 10–30 measurements were made on multiple sections (≥3 per mouse) with six mice per treatment.

4. Notes

1. Earlier studies from our laboratory employed different doses of talc ranging from 20 to 100 mg *(4)*. Those studies revealed a dose-dependent relationship between the amount of talc administered and the amount of connective tissue deposited. Although the highest dose tested yielded nearly a 10-fold increase in connective-tissue deposition, such a high level may make it difficult to accurately test the effects of both pro- and antifibrogenic agents. In subsequent studies, we used either 30 or 50 mg of talc to induce midrange levels of abdominal wall thickening *(7,8)*. This allowed for the determination of treatments that increased or decreased the fibrogenesis *(7,8)*.

2. The assessment of abdominal wall connective-tissue thickness can be made over a period of 2 to 3 wk after administration of talc. A majority of the studies were conducted at d 14. Although connective-tissue thickness is significantly elevated at 7 d post–talc treatment, the connective tissue is more cellular and less fibrous *(8)*. Measurement of connective-tissue thickness after 28 d is not recommended, because collagen content diminishes, possibly owing to tissue remodeling.

3. It is important to be consistent with the harvest location so that the results are not skewed. Some areas will appear more affected than others, so predetermining the area to be harvested beforehand will eliminate any possible bias. In our laboratory, talc is always injected into the lower right quadrant, and tissue is always taken from the lower left quadrant.

4. The tissue can be placed on a piece of thick paper or index card with the luminal side facing up. This decreases curling of the tissue during fixation and processing and ensures the proper orientation of the specimen.

5. Cassettes need to be labeled prior to submerging them in formalin solution. This should be done with either a #2 pencil or a Secure Line Superfrost marker (Allegiance). This is the only type of marking pen that is recommended for labeling cassettes; *all* other marker (including Sharpie and generic laboratory markers) wash off during the processing steps.

Acknowledgment

This work was supported by National Institutes of Health grant GM 55344.

References

1. Ellis, H. (1982) The causes and prevention of intestinal adhesions. *Br. J. Surg.* **69**, 241–243.
2. Kovacs, E. J. and DiPietro, L. A. (1994) Fibrogenic cytokines and connective tissue production. *FASEB J.* **8**, 854–861.
3. Myllarniemi, H., Frilander, M., Turunen, M., and Saxon, L. (1966) The effect of glove powders and their constituents on adhesion and granuloma formation in the abdominal cavity of the rabbit. *Acta Chir. Scand.* **131**, 312–318.
4. Frazier-Jessen, M. R. and Kovacs, E. J. (1993) Abdominal wall thickness as a means of assessing peritoneal fibrosis in mice. *J. Immunol. Methods* **162**, 115–121.
5. Lichman, A. L., McDonald, J. R., Dixon, C. F., and Mann, F. C. (1946) Talc granuloma. *Surg. Gynecol. Obstet.* **83**, 531–540.
6. Eismann, B., Seelig, M. G., and Womack, N. A. (1947) Talcum granuloma: Frequent and serious complications. *Ann. Surg.* **126**, 820–828.
7. Frazier-Jessen, M. R., Mott, F. J., Witte, P. L., and Kovacs, E. J. (1996) Estrogen suppression of connective tissue deposition in a murine model of peritoneal adhesions formation. *J. Immunol.* **156**, 3036–3042.
8. Jahoda, A. E., Albala, D. M., Dries, D. J., and Kovacs, E. J. (1999) Therapeutic intervention for peritoneal adhesion formation. *Surgery* **125**, 53–59.

12

Methods for Investigating Fetal Tissue Repair

Ziv M. Peled, Stephen M. Warren, Pierre J. Bouletreau, and Michael T. Longaker

1. Introduction

This chapter is devoted to a fascinating topic in molecular biology—scarless fetal wound repair. Our understanding of this phenomenon may one day allow us to manipulate the adult wound-healing process to recapitulate the scarless phenotype. To achieve this goal, we must first understand the molecular "blueprint" for scarless repair. In other words, the first question we must ask ourselves is: What cytokines involved in modulating the healing process enable the early gestational age fetal wound to heal skin wounds in a scarless fashion?

In an attempt to answer this question, we have used the Sprague-Dawley rat model, since prior work has demonstrated that there is a transition from scarless to scar-forming cutaneous healing between d 16 and 18 of gestation (term = 21.5 d) *(1,2)*. Using fetal rat skin, our laboratory has characterized the endogenous gene expression levels of several cytokines known to be involved in the adult wound-healing process *(3,4)*. We have also performed similar analyses in fetal dermal fibroblasts, since they are effector cells for scarless repair *(5,6)*. Therefore, we routinely harvest skin and explant fibroblasts from our Sprague-Dawley rats at time points representing both the scarless and scar-forming periods of rat gestation.

In this chapter, we describe, in detail, our methods for anesthetizing and wounding the Sprague-Dawley rat fetuses. Our methods are modifications of the techniques initially described by Whitby and Ferguson in a mouse model *(7)*. We then explain how we harvest these fetal wounds for analyses. Furthermore, since it is essential to study the effector cells in vitro, we illustrate our methods for explanting fibroblasts from fetal rats to establish primary cell lines.

From: *Methods in Molecular Medicine, vol. 78: Wound Healing: Methods and Protocols*
Edited by: Luisa A. DiPietro and Aime L. Burns © Humana Press Inc., Totowa, NJ

2. Materials

2.1. Fetal Wounds

1. Ketamine HCl (100 mg/mL) (Ketaset; Fort Dodge Animal Health, Fort Dodge, IA).
2. Acepromazine maleate (10 mg/mL) (Butler, Columbus, OH).
3. Xylazine-20 (20 mg/mL) (Butler).
4. Luer Lock syringe (3 cc) (Sherwood, St. Louis, MO).
5. 25-Gage needle (Sherwood).
6. Betadine solution (Purdue Frederick, Norwalk, CT).
7. Gauze pads (4 cm × 4 cm).
8. Sterile 1.5-mm dermal biopsy punches (Miltex, Bethpage, NY).
9. Sterile #15 blade scalpel.
10. 7-0 Nylon suture on a tapered needle.
11. 3-0 Vicryl suture on a cutting needle.
12. Four pairs of fine-tipped forceps.
13. Dissecting microscope with ×10 ocular magnification and ×1.5–5 objective magnification (Zeiss, Thornwood, NY).
14. Adjustable light source (Dolan-Jenner, Lawrence, MA).
15. Needle driver.
16. Heat lamp.
17. Absorbent pads.
18. Sterile surgical gloves.
19. Electric clippers.
20. Microscissors.
21. Animal weighing scale.
22. Sterile towels.
23. Bag (250 mL) of sterile normal saline (0.9% NaCl).
24. Blunt probe.
25. India ink.

2.2. Explanting of Fibroblasts

1. Absorbent pads.
2. Sterile #10 blade scalpel.
3. Two pairs of fine-tipped forceps.
4. Betadine solution (Purdue Frederick).
5. Sterile phosphate-buffered saline (PBS).
6. Nonsterile PBS.
7. Five 100-mm Falcon® culture dishes (cat. no. 353003; Becton Dickinson, Franklin Lakes, NJ).
8. One 100-mm Falcon® culture dish with polystyrene coating (cat. no. 353803; Becton Dickinson).
9. Minimum essential medium—alpha medium (α-MEM) (cat. no. 12571-063; Gibco-BRL, Grand Island, NY).

10. Penicillin/streptomycin (cat. no. 15140-122; Gibco-BRL).
11. Fungizone (cat. no. 15295-017; Gibco-BRL).
12. Fetal bovine serum (FBS) (cat. no. 10437-028; Gibco-BRL).

3. Methods

3.1. Fetal Wounds

3.1.1. Preparation

1. Autoclave all of the instruments to be used during this procedure.
2. Prepare a clean area of bench space and line with absorbent pads.
3. Prepare a second clean area of bench space, line with absorbent pads, and place a heat lamp nearby.
4. In a sterile fashion, fill a 3-mL syringe with sterile normal saline.

3.1.2. Anesthesia

1. Weigh the animal on a scale.
2. Mix an "anesthetic cocktail" as follows: 0.5 mL of acepromazine maleate (10 mg/mL), 1.5 mL of ketamine HCl (100 mg/mL), 1.5 mL of xylazine-20 (20 mg/mL).
3. Administer an IP injection (0.5–0.7 mL/kg) of the anesthetic cocktail (*see* **Notes 1–3**).
4. Allow the animal to sit undisturbed for 10–15 min for the anesthetic to take effect.
5. When the animal appears sedated, pick it up gently and place it in the supine position on the absorbent towels.
6. Verify that respirations are easily visible and test the adequacy of anesthesia. Depth of anesthesia can be assessed by gently pinching the forepaw of the animal with a forceps; if no sharp withdrawal reflex is noted, an adequate level of anesthesia usually has been achieved.

3.1.3. Creation of Wounds

1. Carefully shave the abdominal region with the clippers.
2. Carefully brush away all of the loose hair from the abdomen and drape the abdomen with a set of sterile towels.
3. Paint the shaved area with Betadine solution, using a 4 × 4 cm gauze pad and working in a circular motion from the center outward. Repeat two more times allowing the Betadine to dry prior to each subsequent application.
4. Position the heat lamp so that it shines above the area to be incised.
5. Using a toothed forceps, pick up the abdominal skin and make a midline laparotomy incision approx 3 cm in length with the #15 blade scalpel (*see* **Note 4**).
6. Using fine-tipped forceps, exteriorize the bicornuate uterus (*see* **Fig. 1**).

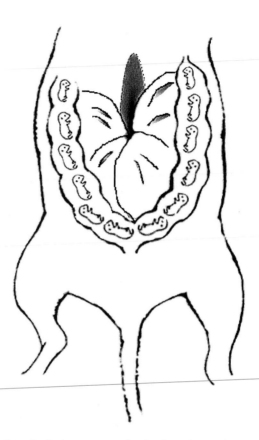

Fig. 1. Line drawing depicting an anesthetized rat in supine position after midline laparotomy incision. The bicornuate uterus has been exteriorized to allow adequate inspection of the individual fetal sacs.

7. Identify one to three fetuses to be wounded near the cervical junction of the uterine horns, and mark the corresponding amniotic sacs with a blunt probe dipped in India ink (*see* **Note 5**) *(8–10)*.

8. Replace the uterus into the abdominal cavity so that one of the selected amniotic sacs is easily seen and manipulated through the laparotomy incision.

9. Place a purse string suture in one of the amniotic sacs using the 7-0 nylon suture on a tapered needle and the fine-tipped forceps (*see* **Note 6** and **Fig. 2A**).

10. Using the microscissors, make a small nick within the purse string suture. At this point, amniotic fluid will escape. The efflux of amniotic fluid is actually desirable because it will facilitate manipulation of the fetus into the necessary position for creation of the wound (*see* **Fig. 2B**).

11. Using the blunt probe, carefully manipulate the fetus so that its dorsum is visible through the incision in the amniotic sac.

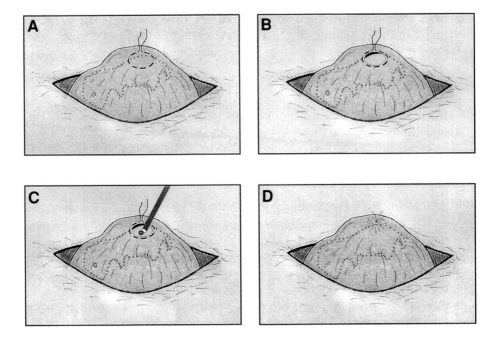

Fig. 2. Steps involved in creation of fetal wound. (**A**) The first step involves placement of a purse string suture into a selected amniotic sac. (**B**) Next, microscissors are used to create an opening within the amniotic sac and within the confines of the purse string suture. (**C**) The fetus is manipulated with a blunt probe so that its dorsum is visible through the opening in the amniotic sac. A punch biopsy is then used to make an excisional wound in the dorsal skin. (**D**) Finally, the purse string is closed after replacement of the amniotic fluid volume with sterile normal saline.

12. Using the punch biopsy, applying gentle pressure make a small excisional wound on the dorsal aspect of the fetus (*see* **Note 7** and **Fig. 2C**).
13. Once the wound is made, dip the tip of the blunt probe into the India ink and dab the area of the wound. This area will immediately take up the ink and there is no need to allow the area to dry. This step facilitates future identification of the wound site, both grossly and histologically.
14. Close the purse string suture. Just prior to complete closure, inject approx 1 to 2 mL of sterile normal saline to replace the lost amniotic fluid volume (*see* **Fig. 2D**) *(10)*.
15. **Steps 8–15** can be repeated up to two more times per pregnant female. In our experience, operating on more than three fetuses per pregnant female leads to a high rate of spontaneous abortion.

16. Once all of the wounds have been made, replace the uterus into the abdominal cavity and close the fascial layers with a 3-0 vicryl suture. In addition, close the skin using a subcuticular 3-0 vicryl suture.
17. Keep the animals under heat lamps and monitor them closely for the next 6–12 h until they awaken and begin to move around.
18. Replace the animals in their cages and return them to the housing facility.

3.1.4. Harvesting of Wounds

1. At a preselected time point postwounding, reanesthetize the pregnant female using the same techniques described in **Subheading 3.1.2.**
2. Open the abdominal incision and reexteriorize the uterus as in **Subheading 3.1.3., steps 5** and **6.**
3. Identify the fetuses that had been wounded. They should be easily identifiable by the nylon sutures on the amniotic sacs (*see* **Fig. 3**).
4. Incise the amniotic sacs with the microscissors and immediately decapitate the fetuses.
5. Under the dissecting microscope and using the microscissors, excise the wound along with as small a margin of unwounded skin as possible. The tissue can then be processed according to the desired use (e.g., immediately snap-frozen for future RNA extraction).
6. Repeat **steps 3–5** for each wounded fetus.
7. Once all the wounds have been harvested, euthanize the adult female via CO_2 narcosis.

3.2. Explanting of Fibroblasts

3.2.1. Preparation

1. Set aside a clean area of the laboratory and cover the benchtop area to be used with absorbent towels.
2. In a laminar flow hood, set up four 100-mm culture dishes. Fill three of them with 10 mL of sterile PBS and the fourth with approx 5 mL of Betadine solution.
3. Also in a laminar flow hood, prepare a polystyrene-coated 100-mm culture dish by etching several lines at the bottom of the plate using a scalpel blade or a Pasteur pipet (*see* **Note 8**).
4. Prepare a bottle of cell culture medium as follows:
   a. Remove 50 mL from a 500 mL bottle of α-MEM.
   b. Add 50 mL of FBS.
   c. Add 5 mL of penicillin/streptomycin.
   d. Add 500 μL of Fungizone.

3.2.2. Harvesting of Skin

1. Euthanize a pregnant female rat with pups at the desired gestational age via CO_2 narcosis.

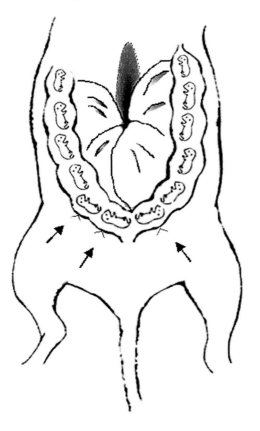

Fig. 3. Line drawing depicting the exteriorized bicornuate uterus after second laparotomy and just prior to harvesting of fetal wounds. Note the three fetal sacs (arrows) that had been previously operated on and their location at the junction of the two uterine horns. These fetal sacs are easily identified intraoperatively by the presence of the closed purse string suture.

2. Shave and prepare the abdominal region of the adult animal as described in **Subheading 3.1.3.**
3. Perform a midline laparotomy incision and exteriorize the uterus as described in **Subheading 3.1.3., steps 5** and **6.**
4. Remove all of the individual fetuses from their respective amniotic sacs and place them in a 100-mm culture dish containing approx 10 mL of PBS. It is humane to immediately decapitate the fetuses to minimize any further pain. This step is especially critical in the later gestational ages (e.g., embryonic day 18 or older).

5. Using a sterile pair of forceps or scissors, carefully harvest the dorsal skin from the caudal-most portion of the forelimbs to the cranial-most portion of the hind limbs.

6. Place the harvested skin in a separate 100-mm culture dish filled with 5–10 mL of PBS.

3.2.3. Explanting of Skin

The following steps are all performed in a laminar flow hood:

1. Take the culture dish containing the harvested skin into a laminar flow hood.

2. Pick up a piece of harvested skin with a sterile forceps and dip into the Betadine solution. Once all of the surfaces of that piece of skin have been coated with Betadine, sequentially dip the skin into the three culture dishes containing sterile PBS. In this way, by the time the skin is dipped into the third culture dish containing sterile PBS, no Betadine should be seen washing away.

3. Place the washed piece of skin on the pre-etched polystyrene-coated culture dish with the dermal side facing down (*see* **Notes 9–11** and **Fig. 4A**).

4. Place a few drops of medium around the pieces of tissue on the plate. Use only enough medium to surround the tissue completely (*see* **Fig. 4B**). Adding excess medium will cause the tissue to float off the plate and prevent cell growth.

5. Culture the tissue overnight in an incubator at 37°C with 5% CO_2.

6. The next day (d 2), gently place another few drops of medium on the tissue. Be careful not to dislodge the tissue from the bottom of the plate, yet add enough medium to keep the tissue moist.

7. Culture the tissue overnight in an incubator at 37°C with 5% CO_2.

8. The next day (d 3), very gently add 3–5 mL of medium to the plate. At this point, the plate can be examined under the microscope, and fibroblasts should be seen arborizing outward from the tissue edges.

9. The following day (d 4), add medium to the culture plate to a total of 10 mL.

10. Allow the cells to grow until a large number are seen emerging from the tissue edges. This process usually takes 3–5 d. At this point, change the medium to a fresh 10 mL, and while doing so, aspirate the tissue off of the culture plate. Then allow the cells to grow for 2 to 3 d more undisturbed.

11. At this point (usually 10–12 d postexplant), treat the cells with trypsin in a standard fashion and transfer onto a new plate. The cells will now be at passage one and on a plate with minimal tissue debris.

12. Expand the cells in culture as desired.

4. Notes

1. We recommend sedating the animals with a short burst of CO_2 prior to administration of the anesthetic cocktail. This step makes the animals easier to handle and seemingly exposes them to less distress from the needle.

2. If CO_2 is not to be used, we recommend calming the animals by leaving them alone in their cages for a few minutes undisturbed after transport to the site of surgery. In our experience, the animals can become quite agitated after being

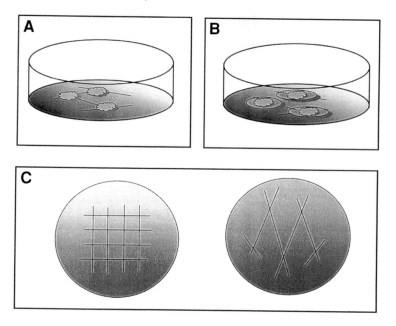

Fig. 4. **(A)** A tissue culture plate with a special polystyrene coating is pre-etched with a scalpel and the harvested tissue is placed with the dermal side down over the pre-etched areas. **(B)** A drop of medium is then placed over each piece of tissue, just enough to keep the tissue moist for 24 h, but not so much that the tissue floats off the bottom of the culture plate. **(C)** Top view of two pre-etched tissue culture plates. The left plate contains a gridlike pattern that may facilitate adherence of the harvested tissue to the plate, but that may ultimately limit cell growth. The right plate contains an "open" pattern of etchings. In our experience, the open pattern not only facilitates tissue adhesion, but also does not limit cell growth.

    carried in their cages to the surgical area, and when in a highly disturbed state, we have noted that the animals suffer a higher rate of anesthetic mortality.

3. An alternative method of administering anesthesia is an IM injection in the perirectal area underneath and slightly lateral to the tail. This approach may be particularly useful during the latter stages of gestation (i.e., after d 18) when the gravid uterus is sufficiently large so as to risk injury to the uterus/fetuses from an IP injection. The perirectal area is well vascularized yet very sensitive, and, therefore, we recommend sedating the animals with a short burst of CO_2 prior to the administration of the anesthetic cocktail in this location.

4. Take care not to injure the gravid uterus while making this initial incision. Instead of a scalpel, some investigators prefer to use a pair of scissors.

5. We have found that it is better to choose fetuses at the central junction of the uterine horns because the fetuses are slightly larger. This may be because of slightly improved blood flow to the middle placentae *(8)*.

6. At this point, it is often helpful to have a second person steady the amniotic sac while the primary surgeon places the purse string suture. Alternatively, if only one person is available for the surgery, two 7-0 nylon stay sutures can be placed laterally in the amniotic sac and held in place with hemostats to steady the selected amnion.

7. Very gentle pressure should be applied at this step, especially when operating on animals at the early gestational age time points (e.g., prior to d 16), since the fetal tissues are very gelatinous.

8. We have found that etching a gridlike pattern onto the bottom of the 100-mm culture plate actually inhibits the growth of the explanted fibroblasts beyond the grid lines. We have therefore adopted an "open" pattern of etchings to allow the maximum possible spread of cells beyond the explanted tissue (*see* **Fig. 4C**).

9. When initially explanting the tissue, it is important to have the piece of skin as dry as possible to facilitate optimal adherence to the culture plate. Therefore, we have found it helpful to remove excess sterile PBS from the washed tissue by gently dabbing it on the inside cover of one of the sterile culture dishes used for washing. Subsequent manipulation of the tissue, so that the dermal side is down, is also facilitated by this step.

10. The tissue should be placed over the pre-etched areas. In addition, use only polystyrene-coated plates. These plates have nitrogen-containing functional groups incorporated onto the surface of the plate that enhance cell attachment and spreading *(12–14)*. Our experience has been that the skin adheres more readily to these areas of the plate.

11. In the Sprague-Dawley rat model, the skin is far more differentiated by d 18 and 21 of gestation compared with d 14 and 16. At the former two time points, the dermal side of the harvested skin is easily distinguishable from the epidermal side, and, therefore, appropriate orientation is easily accomplished. At the latter two time points, however, this difference is not easy to distinguish. Fortunately, the tissue biopsies that are taken from these fetuses are so thin that placement of the tissue on the culture plate without regard to orientation is sufficient for successful cell growth.

References

1. Ihara, S., Motobayashi, Y., Nagao, E., and Kistler, A. (1990) Ontogenetic transition of wound healing pattern in rat skin occurring at the fetal stage. *Development* **110,** 671–680.

2. Mackool, R., Rowe, N., Mehrara, B., Chau, D., McCormick, S., Longaker, M. T., and Gittes, G. K. (1998) Excisional wound healing in the fetal rat. *Surg. Forum* **49,** 463–464.

3. Hsu, M., Peled, Z. M., Chin, G. S., Liu, W., Lee, S., Levinson, H., Gittes, G. K., and Longaker, M. T. (2001) Ontogeny of TGF-B1, TGF-B3, and TGF-B receptors I and II expression in fetal rat fibroblasts and skin. *Plast. Reconstr. Surg.* **107,** 1787–1794.

4. Peled, Z., Rhee, S. J. R., Hsu, M., Chang J., Krummel, T. M., and Longaker, M. T. (2001) The ontogeny of scarless healing II: EGF and PDGF-B gene expression in fetal rat skin and fibroblasts as a function of gestational age. *Ann. Plast. Surg.* **47,** 417–424.

5. Chin, G., Lee, S., Hsu, M., Kim, W., Levinson, H., and Longaker, M. (2001) Discoidin domain receptors and their ligand collagen are temporally regulated in fetal rat fibroblasts in vitro. *Plast. Reconstr. Surg.* **107,** 769–776.

6. Lorenz, H. P., Lin, R. Y., Longaker, M. T., Whitby, D. J., and Adzick, N. S. (1995) The fetal fibroblast: the effector cell of scarless fetal skin repair. *Plast. Reconstr. Surg.* **96,** 1251–1259; discussion 60, 61.

7. Whitby, D. J. and Ferguson, M. W. J. (1991) The extracellular matrix of lip wounds in fetal, neonatal and adult mice. *Development* **112,** 651–668.

8. Padmanabhan, R. and Singh, S. (1981) Effect of intrauterine position on foetal weight in CF rats. *Indian J. Med. Res.* **73,** 134–139.

9. Barr, M. and Brent, R. L. (1970) The relation of the uterine vasculature to fetal growth and the intrauterine position effect in rats. *Teratology* **3,** 251–260.

10. Barr, M., Jensh, R. P., and Brent, R. L. (1970) Prenatal growth in the albino rat: effects of number, intrauterine position and resorptions. *Am. J. Anat.* **128,** 413–428.

11. Lingwood, B. E., Hardy, K. J., Long, J. G., McPhee, M., and Wintour, E. M. (1980) Amniotic fluid volume and composition following experimental manipulations in sheep. *Obstet. Gynecol.* **56,** 451–458.

12. Curtis, A. S. and McMurray, H. (1986) Conditions for fibroblast adhesion without fibronectin. *J. Cell. Sci.* **86,** 25–33.

13. Chilkoti, A., Schmierer, A. E., Perez-Luna, V. H., and Ratner, B. D. (1995) Investigating the relationship between surface chemistry and endothelial cell growth: partial least-squares regression of the static secondary ion mass spectra of oxygen-containing plasma-deposited films. *Anal. Chem.* **67,** 2883–2891.

14. Ramsey, W. S., Hertl, W., Nowlan, E. D., and Binkowski, N. J. (1984) Surface treatments and cell attachment. *In Vitro* **20,** 802–808.

13

Growth of Human Blood Vessels in Severe Combined Immunodeficient Mice

A New In Vivo Model System of Angiogenesis

Peter J. Polverini, Jacques E. Nör, Martin C. Peters, and David J. Mooney

1. Introduction

1.1. In Vivo Models of Angiogenesis

The development of strategies for the treatment of angiogenesis-dependent diseases has been greatly aided by the development of in vivo models of angiogenesis *(1)*. These bioassays provide investigators with tools to visualize vessel architecture and function and to analyze and manipulate various steps in the angiogenic response. Some of the more widely used model systems include the iris and avascular cornea of the rodent eye *(2–4)*, the chick chorioallantoic membrane *(5)*, the hamster cheek pouch *(6)*, the dorsal skin and air sac *(7)*, and several noninvasive imaging techniques to visualize living vascularized tissues *(8,9)*. In recent years, advances in the development of sterile porous matrices as delivery vehicles for genes, proteins, and cells have greatly enhanced the ability of investigators to analyze key cellular and molecular events that govern the angiogenic response *(10–13)*. In addition, naturally occurring and chemically modified matrices such as Matrigel® have proven invaluable for the study of angiogenesis in vivo *(14)*. While all of these methods afford the opportunity to study a number of essential steps in the angiogenic response, investigators are still burdened by the fact that they must draw conclusions about the behavior and function of human microvessels and human angiogenic responses from nonhuman populations of endothelial cells. Moreover, current model systems are greatly limited owing to their inability to capture key cellular and molecular

From: *Methods in Molecular Medicine, vol. 78: Wound Healing: Methods and Protocols*
Edited by: Luisa A. DiPietro and Aime L. Burns © Humana Press Inc., Totowa, NJ

events that occur when human blood vessels are confronted with normal or diseased human tissues and cells.

1.2. Severe Combined Immunodeficient Mouse Model of Human Angiogenesis

Recent interest in the development of novel strategies for tissue and organ reconstruction has been driven by rapid advances in the fields of tissue engineering and stem cell biology *(15–21)*. With continued improvements in the design of biodegradable polymer matrices, it is now possible to maintain transplanted cells in a more optimal physiological environment and thus enhance new tissue growth and organization. Highly porous biodegradable scaffolds fabricated from poly-L-lactic acid (PLLA) and polyglycolic acid are commonly used as temporary scaffolds for tissue engineering *(22,23)*. The use of these polymer matrices in severe combined immunodeficient (SCID) mice has already proven their usefulness in studies designed to investigate the development of human microvessels and the role of survival factors such as vascular endothelial growth factor (VEGF) and survival gene products such as Bcl-2 *(see* **Note 1***)* and A1 in human angiogenesis *(24–26)*. We have reported that human dermal microvascular endothelial cells (HDMECs) transplanted in PLLA scaffolds into SCID mice rapidly organized and differentiated into functional microvessels that anastomosed with mouse microvessels and carried circulating mouse blood cells *(24,26)*.

In this chapter, we describe in detail a novel bioassay recently reported by us—the SCID mouse model of human angiogenesis *(27)*. We show that HDMECs incorporated into polymer matrices rapidly organize into microvessels, express specific markers associated with angiogenesis, undergo differentiation into mature functioning vessels lined by murine smooth muscle cells, and transport murine blood cells. The overall strategy for implanting human endothelial cells into SCID mice is depicted in **Fig. 1**. **Figure 2** is a series of photographs demonstrating the implant procedure and showing examples of vascularized implants. The scaffolds used in this procedure have

---

Fig. 1. *(opposite page)* Diagram depicting the overall strategy for growing human blood vessels into SCID mice. Naive HDMECs or HDMECs **(B)** transduced with a gene **(A)** are applied to the surface of Matrigel-treated PLA scaffold and allowed to infiltrate the scaffold **(C)**. The implants become well vascularized 5–7 d after implantation **(D)**, with a significant number of human microvessels persisting for up to 28 d. Transducing HDMECs with the survival gene *bcl-2* can extend this time frame. Human blood vessels expressing the alkaline phosphatase gene are shown overlying the diagram of a vascularized implant **(D,** inset**)**.

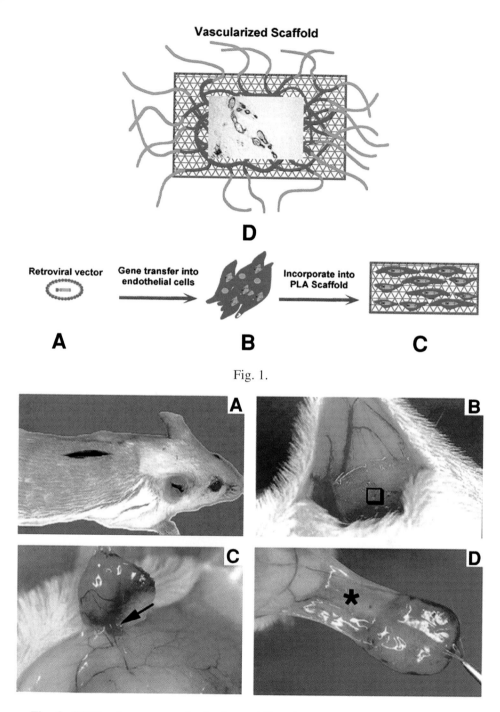

Vascularized Scaffold

D

Retroviral vector

A

Gene transfer into
endothelial cells

Incorporate into
PLA Scaffold

B

C

Fig. 1.

Fig. 2. SCID mice are anesthetized, a midline incision (**A**) is made on the back, and the implants are positioned subcutaneously on the right and left side of the mouse (**B**). (**C**) An ample supply of blood vessels (arrow) can be seen penetrating the fascia surrounding the implant. (**D**) A well-developed fibrous capsule (**✱**) is shown surrounding an implant.

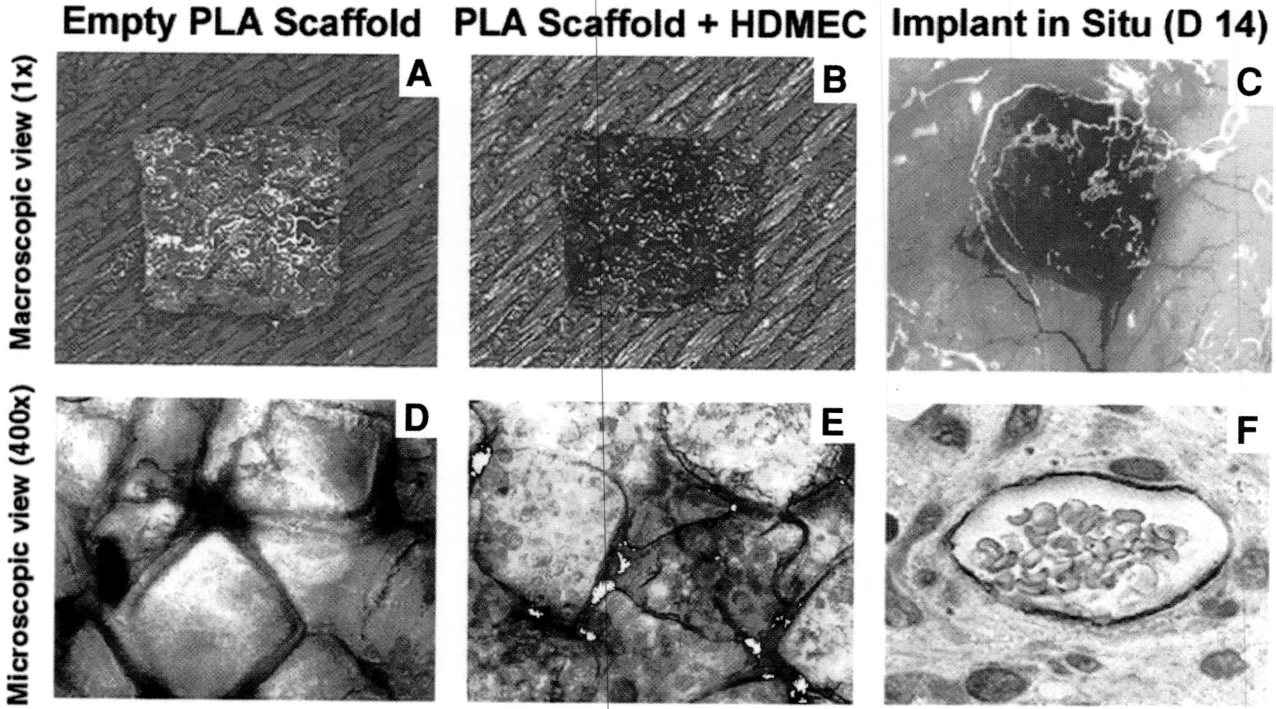

Fig. 3. Highly porous PLA matrices provide a scaffold for transplantation of endothelial cells into SCID mice. (**A,B**) Macroscopic and (**D,E**) phase contrast photographs of PLA scaffolds before (**A,D**) and after (**B,E**) seeding with human endothelial cells are shown. Implants are populated by numerous human blood vessels by d 14 (**C,F**).

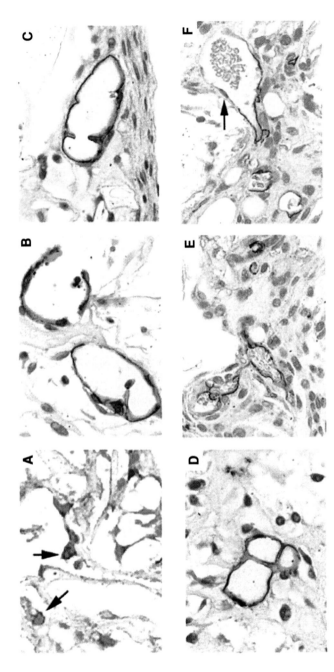

Fig. 4. Stages in development of human microvessels in SCID mice. Antihuman CD34 antibody was used to identify human endothelial cells. HDMECs (arrows) are dispersed throughout the sponge 1 d after implantation (**A**), and form empty cylinders within 5 d (**B–D**). Endothelial cells lining the walls of newly formed blood vessels start to migrate inward at about d 5–7 partitioning blood vessels into two or three smaller vessels (**C,D**). This type of vessel amplification is termed *intussusception*. At 14 d postimplantation, mouse blood cells can be seen in the lumen of most microvessels (**E,F**). The arrow in (**F**) points to a chimeric blood vessel only partially stained with antihuman CD34 antibody. All photomicrographs are at ×1000 magnification.

an average pore diameter of 250 μm, which allows easy penetration and entrapment of endothelial cells (**Fig. 3**). Matrigel is added to serve as an immediate source of growth factors and nutrients for the endothelial cells, and to help retain them in the scaffold during the transplantation process. When examined macroscopically, the implants will appear as highly vascularized, fibrous, encapsulated tissues. By d 7, histological examination will reveal an abundance of highly organized microvessels that are immunoreactive with the endothelial cell–specific markers *(28,29)*, human CD31 and CD34 (**Fig. 3**). Although an array of microvessels can be detected as early as 3 d postimplantation, microvessels are most abundant between d 5 and 7.

1.3. Strategies for Characterizing Human Microvessels in the SCID Mouse

To confirm that the endothelial cells populating the microvessels within the implants are of human origin, several approaches can be used to verify the identity of the endothelial cells lining the microvessels. We recommend performing immunostaining with anti–human CD31 and anti–human CD34 (**Fig. 4**) antibodies. These antibodies only react with endothelial cells from microvessels located inside the implant and not with mouse endothelial cells that populate vessels that have infiltrated the faseia and connective tissue surrounding the implant.

To confirm further that the microvessels in the implant are populated with the transplanted human endothelial cells, we have also used retroviral infection to transduce HDMECs and generate stable clonal populations of cells expressing either the artificial Flag epitope or the alkaline phosphatase (AP) gene. In both cases, only microvessels within the implants should show positive staining for the markers utilized, demonstrating that these microvessels are populated by transplanted human endothelial cells, and not by host cells. In our experience, the microvessels present in the connective tissue that surrounds the implants are invariably negative for markers of human endothelial cells. This is another advantage of this model system. For all practical purposes, the microvessels given rise to by the transplanted endothelial cells are confined almost exclusively within the implanted scaffold and can be readily retrieved for further study *(30)*.

Functional characterization of these microvessels can be achieved by examining the expression of vascular cell adhesion molecule-1 (VCAM-1) and intracellular adhesion molecule-1 (ICAM-1), two mediators of endothelial cell-cell interactions and regulators of angiogenic responses *(31,32)*. VCAM-1 is an inducible endothelial cellular adhesion molecule that is expressed in stimulated HDMECs *(33)*, and ICAM-1 is a regulated ligand for lymphocyte-endothelial cell adhesion *(34)*. We have found that at 7 d, approx 60% of the microvessels in the implants expressed these adhesion molecules, while at 14 d this proportion was reduced to approx 25% (**Fig. 4A**). The decrease in expression of these two adhesion molecules in microvessels over time can be explained, at least in part, by the fact that their expression levels seem to be reduced in more mature or quiescent blood vessels *(35)*.

1.4. Stages in Organization of Transplanted Human Endothelial Cells into Functioning Microvessels

The temporal and spatial events involved in the development of a human microvascular network within the transplanted scaffolds can be evaluated by microscopic examination of implants at various time intervals using CD31 as a marker to identify HDMECs. Five days after implantation, one may expect to see a substantial number of nonfunctional tubular structures devoid of circulating blood cells. Starting on d 7, and at time intervals thereafter, an increasing number of these rudimentary vessels will contain circulating blood in their lumens. From d 7 to 14, there is often a significant drop in the number of nonfunctional microvessels, and by d 21 they will essentially disappear. Approximately 20% of the tubular structures that developed initially anastomose with the mouse vasculature and differentiate into functional microvessels.

Representative histological fields illustrate the progression from isolated endothelial cells at d 1 to functional microvessels at d 14. One day after implantation all endothelial cells are dispersed throughout the scaffolds (**Fig. 4A**). At d 5, tubular structures in stages of development ranging from rudimentary vascular channels to completely open cylinders are seen throughout the implants (**Fig. 4B**). Two days later, cells located along the walls of the newly organized sprouts appear to migrate toward the center of the vascular channels (**Fig. 4C**), where they partition the vessels into two to three smaller lumens (**Fig. 4D**). This process of vessel assembly, in which groups of cells are introduced into the lumens of the newly formed microvessels, is termed *intussusception (36)*. At 14 d, the majority of the tubules seen in histological sections are functional microvessels that contain circulating mouse blood cells (**Fig. 4E,F**). Interestingly, we have observed that some of the microvessels located at the periphery of the implants contained both cells that were positive and others that were negative for anti–human CD34. We believe that these areas represented chimeric microvessels where human and murine vessels have joined and communicated with host vessels (**Fig. 4F**).

To determine whether the human microvessels become invested with mouse perivascular smooth muscle cells, immunostaining can be performed using anti-α–smooth muscle actin antibody. Seven days after implantation, empty tubular structures lined by endothelial cells are seen throughout the implants (as already described) and often do not show immunoreactivity with smooth muscle actin. At 14 d, one should expect to see weak α–smooth muscle actin staining in a handful of microvessels. However, 3 wk after implantation most microvessels are invested by an interrupted layer of perivascular smooth muscle α-actin-positive mouse cells.

Four weeks after implantation, some of the HDMECs lining the walls of human microvessels appear apoptotic. Interestingly, the total number of microvessels (determined by staining with von Willebrand factor) inside the implants remains relatively constant. We have previously reported that 14 d after implantation, the proportion of microvessels lined with human endothelial cells was 90–100%, whereas after 28 d this proportion had decreased to 50–65%. Taken together, these data suggest that apoptotic HDMECs are gradually replaced by mouse endothelial cells that maintained the integrity and density of the microvessels within the implanted scaffold.

1.5. Advantages of the SCID Mouse Model of Human Angiogenesis

The SCID mouse model of human angiogenesis is simple, reproducible, and applicable for the study of both physiological and pathological angiogenic responses. Its most obvious advantage is that it allows the study of the human angiogenic response in a murine host using defined populations of normal or pathological human cells. Some of the potential applications of this model system include studies of how endogenous or exogenous genes that target endothelial cell functions can influence neovascularization, testing of the effects of antiangiogenic agents on pathological angiogenic responses such as tumor growth, and evaluation of how the survival of endothelial cells can be genetically manipulated to enhance neovascularization of engineered tissues.

A major limitation facing tissue engineers, particularly in the initial phases of tissue or organ reconstruction, is the lack of a reliable strategy that will ensure a sustained vascular supply. We believe that this novel model of human angiogenesis is ideally suited as a system for the delivery of vascular cells or angiogenic factors at sites of newly transplanted tissues or organs. Cotransplantation of cells that overexpress and secrete soluble angiogenic factors may enhance the vascularization of engineered tissues. These cells may also serve as "short-term delivery devices" for angiogenic stimuli to enhance initial vascularization of engineered tissues. Alternatively, the efficacy of a modified scaffold containing angiogenic factors such as VEGF or basic fibroblast growth factor in its composition may be tested with this model system.

In summary, the SCID mouse model of human angiogenesis is ideally suited for the development of strategies designed to enhance our understanding of key features of the human angiogenic response. In addition, it may provide a unique opportunity for studying the effects of genes and proteins delivered via the vasculature on tissues and organs by engineering human endothelial cells and assessing their efficacy before implementing therapeutic strategies in humans.

2. Materials
2.1. Fabrication of Biodegradable Polymer Scaffolds

1. PLLA (Medisorb, Cincinnati, OH).
2. Chloroform.
3. NaCl.
4. Distilled water.
5. Absolute ethanol.
6. Phosphate-buffered saline (PBS).

2.2. Incorporation of Endothelial Cells into Scaffolds and Transplantation into SCID Mice

1. HDMECs (Clonetics, San Diego, CA) are cultured in Microvascular Endothelial Cell Growth Medium (EGM-MV; Clonetics). HDMECs are transduced with the pLAPSN retroviral vector (a gift from D. Miller) and selected in medium supplemented with 250 µg/mL of G418 sulfate (Mediatech, Herndon, VA) to generate stable clones expressing the AP protein. The generation of clones expressing HDMEC-Bcl-2-Flag and HDMEC-LXSN (empty vector control) is performed as previously described by us *(21)*.
2. Matrigel (Collaborative Biomedical, Cambridge, MA).
3. Human oral squamous carcinoma cells (OSCC-3; a gift from M. Lingen) and a human dermal Kaposi's sarcoma cell line (SLK; a gift from Dr. Gabriel Nunez) are cultured in Dulbecco's modified Eagle's medium and RPMI-1640 medium (Gibco-BRL, Grand Island, NY) supplemented with 10% fetal bovine serum, respectively.
4. Scaffold.
5. SCID mice, male 3 to 4 wk old (CB.17.SCID; Taconic, Germantown, NY).
6. Ketamine and xylazine.
7. Calipers.
8. Balance, to weigh implants.
9. 10% Buffered formalin.
10. Superfrost glass slides (Fisher, Pittsburgh, PA).

2.3. Analysis of Human Microvessels in SCID Mice

2.3.1. Immunolocalization of VCAM-1, ICAM-1, CD31, CD34, Flag, and von Willebrand Factor

1. Pressure cooker (Decloaking Chamber; Biocare, Walnut Creek, CA).
2. Citrate buffer: 2.94 g/L of sodium citrate dihydrate, pH 6.0.
3. Rabbit serum.
4. PBS.
5. Sniper (Biocare).
6. Polyclonal goat anti–human VCAM-1 (R&D Systems, Minneapolis, MN).
7. Polyclonal goat anti–human ICAM-1 antibodies (R&D Systems).
8. Streptavidin–horseradish peroxidase (HRP) (Biocare Medical).
9. Monoclonal anti–human CD31 (JC/70A; Dako, Carpinteria, CA).
10. Monoclonal anti–human CD34 (QBEnd/10; Lab Vision, Freemont, CA).
11. Rabbit anti–human von Willebrand factor (Dako).
12. Anti–flag M2 monoclonal antibody (MAb) (Sigma, St. Louis, MO).
13. Lincoln Label 4$^+$ Detection System (Biocare).
14. DAB 500 Chromogen System (Biocare).
15. 3-Amino-9-ethyl carbazole (Sigma).
16. N,N-Dimethylformamide (Sigma).

2.3.2. Staining for AP

1. 10% Buffered formalin.
2. PBS.
3. AP buffer: 100 mM Tris-HCl, pH 8.5, 100 mM NaCl, 50 mM MgCl$_2$.
4. 5-Bromo-4-chloro-3-indolyl-phosphate (BCIP) (Boehringer Mannheim, Indianapolis, IN).
5. Nitroblue tetrazolium chloride (NBT).
6. 0.02% NP40 (Sigma).
7. 0.01% Sodium deoxycholate (Sigma).
8. 20 mM EDTA.

2.3.3. Immunolocalization of α-Smooth Muscle Actin

In addition to the reagents outlined in **Subheading 2.3.**, the following are required:

1. Dakoark kit (Dako).
2. Monoclonal mouse anti-α–smooth muscle actin (1A4; Dako).

2.3.4. Double Staining of Microvessels for CD31 Expression and Apoptosis

1. Sniper (Biocare).
2. Monoclonal anti–human CD31 (JC/70A; Dako).
3. PBS.

4. Biotinylated anti–mouse IgG (Biocare).
5. Avidin-Texas Red conjugate (Vector, Burlingame, CA).
6. ApopTag Fluorescein *in situ* apoptosis detection kit (Intergen, Purchase, NY).
7. Confocal microscope (Bio-Rad MRC-600 CLSM; Bio-Rad, Hercules, CA).

3. Methods
3.1. Fabrication of Biodegradable Polymer Scaffolds

Porous PLLA scaffolds are fabricated as described by Mooney et al. *(23)*.

1. Dissolve the PLLA in chloroform to yield a solution of 5% polymer (w/v), and load 1.67 mL of this solution into siliconized glass beakers packed with 2.3 g of NaCl particles.
2. Evaporate the solvent, and immerse the scaffolds for 16 h in distilled H_2O to leach the salt and to create an interconnected pore structure with an average pore diameter of 250 μm.
3. Sterilize by gamma radiation.
4. The day before transplantation, soak the scaffolds in 100% EtOH for 2 h, wash twice with PBS, and then leave overnight in fresh PBS.

3.2. Incorporation of Endothelial Cells into Scaffolds and Transplantation into SCID Mice

1. Just prior to transplantation, resuspend 1×10^6 naive HDMECs, HDMECs overexpressing Flag-tagged Bcl-2, HDMECs overexpressing AP, or empty vector controls in 36 μL of a 1 : 1 mixture of EGM-MV: growth factor–reduced Matrigel and allow to adsorb into the scaffolds (*see* **Notes 1** and **2**).
2. Incubate the loaded scaffolds for 30 min at 37°C to allow the gelation of the Matrigel (*see* **Note 3**).
3. Anesthetize male SCID mice with ketamine and xylazine and implant two scaffolds subcutaneously in the dorsal region of each mouse.
4. Sacrifice the mice 1–28 d after transplantation, retrieve the implants, and immediately measure with calipers and weigh on an electronic balance.
5. Fix the implants overnight in 10% buffered formalin at 4°C, embed in paraffin, section, and mount on Superfrost glass slides for histological examination.

3.3. Analysis of Human Microvessels in SCID Mice

3.3.1. Immunolocalization of VCAM-1, ICAM-1, CD31, CD34, Flag, and von Willebrand Factor

1. Deparaffinize histological sections of polymer implants, and process for antigen retrieval by pressure cooking the sections at 120°C for 2 min in citrate buffer.
2. To prepare the sections for immunostaining with VCAM-1 and ICAM-1, first block the sections for 5 min with 10% rabbit serum in PBS, then with Sniper for an additional 5 min.

3. Incubate the samples overnight at 4°C with polyclonal goat anti–human VCAM-1 or polyclonal goat anti–human ICAM-1 antibodies diluted in Sniper at 1:250 and 1:300 dilutions, respectively.
4. Incubate the sections with appropriate secondary antibodies for 30 min, followed by incubation with streptavidin-HRP.
5. To prepare sections for immunostaining with CD31, CD34, and von Willebrand factor, block the tissue sections with Sniper for 5 min and incubate overnight at 4°C with 41 μg/mL of monoclonal anti–human CD31, 10 μg/mL of monoclonal anti–human CD34, or 28 μg/mL of rabbit anti–human von Willebrand factor diluted in PBS.
6. To visualize the Flag epitope, incubate the tissue sections with 44 μg/mL of anti–flag M2 MAb for 1 h at 37°C.
7. Apply the appropriate secondary antibody for 30 min, followed by processing with the Lincoln Label 4+ Detection System. To visualize bound antibodies, treat the sections with the DAB 500 Chromogen System or a solution of 0.014 g of 3-amino-9-ethyl carbazole in 2.5 mL of *N,N*-dimethylformamide.

3.3.2. Staining for AP

1. Section the scaffolds retrieved from mice in bread loaf fashion and fix overnight in 10% buffered formalin.
2. Following fixation, wash the scaffolds three times in PBS at room temperature and once in PBS at 65°C for 30 min to inactivate any endogenous phosphatase activity.
3. Wash the samples in AP buffer for 10 min at room temperature.
4. Stain the sections in a solution of 100 μg/mL of BCIP, 0.5 ng/mL of NBT, 0.02% NP40, and 0.01% sodium deoxycholate in AP buffer overnight at room temperature in the dark.
5. Stop the reaction with 20 mM EDTA in PBS, and embed the slices in paraffin for histological evaluation.

3.3.3. Immunolocalization of α-Smooth Muscle Actin

1. Deparaffinize histological sections of polymer implants, and process for antigen retrieval by pressure cooking the sections at 120°C for 2 min in citrate buffer.
2. Use the Dakoark kit to minimize background in the sections stained for α–smooth muscle actin.
3. Incubate the sections with a 1:50 dilution of monoclonal mouse anti-α–smooth muscle actin for 30 min at 37°C.
4. Incubate the sections with appropriate secondary antibodies for 30 min, followed by incubation with streptavidin-HRP.
5. To visualize bound antibodies treat the sections with the DAB 500 Chromogen System or a solution of 0.014 g of 3-amino-9-ethyl carbazole in 2.5 mL of *N,N*-dimethylformamide.

3.3.4. Double Staining of Microvessels for CD31 Expression and Apoptosis

1. Deparaffinize the tissue sections and perform antigen retrieval as described in **Subheading 3.3.1.** Block the sections with Sniper for 5 min, and incubate them overnight at 4°C with 41 µg/mL of monoclonal anti–human CD31 diluted in PBS.
2. Incubate the sections with biotinylated anti–mouse IgG for 30 min, followed by a 30-min incubation with 3 µg/mL of avidin–Texas Red conjugate at room temperature.
3. After a 10-min rinse in PBS, use the ApopTag Fluorescein *in situ* apoptosis detection kit according to manufacturer's instructions (*see* **Note 4**).
4. Visualize the labeled cells by confocal microscopy at ×1000.

4. Notes

1. The percentage of cells that are actually retained in the scaffold is approx 68% (±4%). Therefore, when 1×10^6 cells are seeded into a $6 \times 6 \times 1$ mm scaffold, on average 6.8×10^5 (±4.3×10^4) are retained in the scaffold and are available for transplantation.
2. Additionally, the influence of endothelial cells on tumor growth can be examined by seeding 0.9×10^6 HDMECs along with 0.1×10^6 OSCC-3 cells or only 0.1×10^6 OSCC-3 cells in PLLA scaffolds (*26*). We have shown that cotransplantation of human endothelial cells and tumor cells has a profound effect on tumor neovascularization and progression (*26*). Twenty-one days after cotransplantation of endothelial cells with two different tumor cell lines, OSCC-3 and SLK, we observed the rapid growth of large encapsulated tumors in the implanted scaffolds, further confirming the role of angiogenesis in tumor growth and progression (*26*). The role of enhanced endothelial cell survival on tumor progression was recently demonstrated by our group when we cotransplanted endothelial cells overexpressing Bcl-2 together with tumor cells and found that these tumors grew more rapidly and were significantly larger after 21 d compared with tumors that developed following cotransplantation of empty vector control HDMECs or naive endothelial cells with tumor cells (*26*). In the same experiment, we found a significantly smaller number of apoptotic microvessels, and a concomitant enhancement in intratumoral microvascular density, when endothelial cells overexpressing Bcl-2 were incorporated into scaffolds. The ability to preprogram the cells that comprise the angiogenic and tumoral compartments enhances the ability to study the impact that each one of these cell populations has on the overall progression of tumors. Furthermore, it allows one to genetically modify these cells, characterize them in vitro, and then study their behavior in vivo.
3. An additional application of this model system is in the study of the effects of proangiogenic or antiangiogenic factors that are produced by cells incorporated

into the implant or following the local or systemic administration of these mediators. For example, we have cotransplanted fibroblasts genetically engineered to
secrete high levels of the angiogenesis inhibitor thrombospondin-1 (TSP1), or
truncated forms of this protein, with endothelial cells to evaluate the biological
effect of this inhibitor in our human angiogenesis model system *(37)*. We have
shown a significant inhibition of angiogenesis in implants containing HDMECs
and fibroblasts overexpressing TSP1, or derivatized forms of TSP1 as compared
to implants populated by HDMECs and normal control fibroblasts. The decrease
in the microvascular density of the implants was associated with enhanced
apoptosis of endothelial cells lining implanted human endothelial cell–derived
microvessels. These findings further demonstrated the utility of this model system
for the study of the effect of secreted factors on angiogenesis in vivo.

4. A clear limitation of our model system is the increasing accumulation of mouse
   microvessels in the implants over time. This is most likely owing to the fact
   that some of the transplanted human endothelial cells undergo apoptosis. This
   phenomenon is more noticeable 28 d after implantation and thereafter, when
   a significant proportion of the microvessels either contain TUNEL[+] HDMECs
   or no longer stain for the markers used to identify the human endothelial
   cells. Because of this shortcoming, we believe that our model system is best
   suited for the study of the early active stage of physiological or pathological
   neovascularization. Despite this limitation, the survival of endothelial cells in
   implants can be dramatically enhanced by overexpressing antiapoptotic genes in
   these cells. We have previously demonstrated that Bcl-2 overexpression mediated
   by retroviral transduction of human endothelial cells enhances the survival of
   human microvessels in SCID mice *(21)*. These findings have been corroborated
   by Schechner et al. *(38)*. Although Bcl-2 overexpression certainly increases
   intraimplant microvascular density over time, the genetic manipulation of
   the endothelial cells prior to implantation may interfere with one's ability to
   unambiguously assess the functional properties of normal human microvessels.
   Therefore, we believe that naive, untransduced endothelial cells should be used
   whenever the objective of the investigation is to understand the mechanisms of
   physiological angiogenesis.

Acknowledgment

This work was supported in part by National Institutes of Health grants
HL39926, CA64416, and DE13161.

References

1. Auerbach, R., Auerbach, W., and Polakowski, I. (1991) Assays for angiogenesis:
   a review. *Pharmacol. Ther.* **51,** 1–11.
2. Gimbrone, M. A. Jr., Leapman, S. B., Cotran, R. S., and Folkman, J. (1973) Tumor
   angiogenesis: iris neovascularization at a distance from experimental intraocular
   tumors. *J. Natl. Cancer Inst.* **50,** 219–228.

3. Gimbrone, M. A. Jr., Cotran, R. S., Leapman, S. B., and Folkman, J. (1974) Tumor growth and neovascularization: an experimental model using the rabbit cornea. *J. Natl. Cancer Inst.* **52**, 413–427.

4. Muthukkaruppan, V. and Auerbach, R. (1979) Angiogenesis in the mouse cornea. *Science* **205**, 1416–1418.

5. Auerbach, R., Kubai, L., Knighton, D., and Folkman, J. (1974) A simple procedure for the long-term cultivation of chicken embryos. *Dev. Biol.* **41**, 391–394.

6. Klintworth, G. K. (1973) The hamster cheek pouch: an experimental model of corneal vascularization. *Am. J. Pathol.* **73**, 691–710.

7. Folkman, J., Merler, E., Abernathy, C., and Williams, G. (1971) Isolation of a tumor factor responsible or angiogenesis. *J. Exp. Med.* **133**, 275–288.

8. Jain, R. K., Safabakhsh, N., Sckell, A., Chen, Y., Jiang, P., Benjamin, L., Yuan, F., and Keshet, E. (1998) Endothelial cell death, angiogenesis, and microvascular function after castration in an androgen-dependent tumor: role of vascular endothelial growth factor. *Proc. Natl. Acad. Sci. USA* **95**, 10,820–10,825.

9. Li, C. Y., Shan, S., Huang, Q., Braun, R. D., Lanzen, J., Hu, K., Lin, P., and Dewhirst, M. W. (2000) Initial stages of tumor cell-induced angiogenesis: evaluation via skin window chambers in rodent models. *J. Natl. Cancer Inst.* **92**, 143–147.

10. Andrade, S. P, Fan, T. P., and Lewis, G. P. (1987) Quantitative *in vivo* studies on angiogenesis in a rat sponge model. *Br. J. Exp. Pathol.* **68**, 755–766.

11. Madsen, S. and Mooney, D. J. (2000) Delivering DNA with polymer matrices: applications in tissue engineering and gene therapy. *Pharm. Sci. Technol. Today* **3**, 381–384.

12. Lee, K. Y., Peters, M. C., Anderson, K. W., and Mooney, D. J. (2000) Controlled growth factor release from synthetic extracellular matrices. *Nature* **408**, 998–1000.

13. Kim, B. S. and Mooney, D. J. (1998) Development of biocompatible synthetic extracellular matrices for tissue engineering. *Trends Biotechnol.* **16**, 224–230.

14. Grant, D. S., Kleinman, H. K., Goldberg, I. D., Bhargava, M. M., Nickoloff, B. J., Kinsella, J. L., Polverini, P. J., and Rosen, E. M. (1993) Scatter factor induces blood vessel formation *in vivo*. *Proc. Natl. Acad. Sci. USA* **90**, 1937–1941.

15. Langer, R. and Vacanti, J. P. (1993) Tissue engineering. *Science* **260**, 920–926.

16. Vacanti, J. P. and Langer, R. (1999) Tissue engineering: the design and fabrication of living replacement devices for surgical reconstruction and transplantation. *Lancet* **354 (Suppl. 1)**, SI32–SI34.

17. Caplan, A. I. (2000) Tissue engineering designs for the future: new logics, old molecules. *Tissue Eng.* **6**, 1–8.

18. Stock, U.A. and Vacanti, J. P. (2001) Tissue engineering: current state and prospects. *Annu. Rev. Med.* **52**, 443–451.

19. Matsui, Y., Zsebo, K., and Hogan, B. L. M. (1992) Derivation of pluripotential embryonic stem cells from murine primordial germ cells in culture. *Cell* **70**, 841–847.

20. Watt, F. M. and Hogan, B. L. (2000) Out of Eden: stem cells and their niches. *Science* **287**, 1427–1430.

21. Fuchs, E. and Segre, J. A. (2001) Stem cells: a new lease on life. *Cell* **100,** 143–155.
22. Putnam, A. J. and Mooney, D. J. (1996). Tissue engineering using synthetic extracellular matrices. *Nat. Med.* **2,** 824–826.
23. Mooney, D. J., Sano, K., Kaufmann, P. M., Majahod, K., Schloo, B., Vacanti, J. P., and Langer, R. (1997) Long-term engraftment of hepatocytes transplanted on biodegradable polymer scaffolds. *J. Biomed. Mater. Res.* **37,** 413–420.
24. Nör, J. E., Christensen, J., Mooney, D. J., and Polverini, P. J. (1999) Vascular endothelial growth factor (VEGF)-mediated angiogenesis is associated with enhanced endothelial cell survival and induction of Bcl-2 expression. *Am. J. Pathol.* **154,** 375–384.
25. Gerber, H. P., Dixit, V., and Ferrara, N. (1998) Vascular endothelial growth factor induces expression of the antiapoptotic proteins Bcl-2 and A1 in vascular endothelial cells. *J. Biol. Chem.* **273,** 13,313–13,316.
26. Nör, J. E., Christensen, J., Liu, J., Peters, M., Mooney, D. J., Strieter, R. M., and Polverini, P. J. (2001) Up-Regulation of Bcl-2 in microvascular endothelial cells enhances intratumoral angiogenesis and accelerates tumor growth. *Cancer Res.* **61,** 2183–2188.
27. Nör, J. E., Peters, M. C., Christensen, J. B., Sutorik, M. M., Linn, S., Khan, M. K., Addison, C. L., Mooney, D. J., and Polverini, P. J. (2001) Engineering and characterization of functional human microvessels in immunodeficient mice. *Lab. Invest.* **84,** 53–63.
28. Vermeulen, P. B., Gasparini, G., Fox, S. B., Toi, M., Martin, L., McCulloch, P., Pezzella, F., Viale, G., Weidner, N., Harris, A. L., and Dirix, L. Y. (1996) Quantification of angiogenesis in solid human tumours: an international consensus on the methodology and criteria of evaluation. *Eur. J. Cancer* **32A,** 2474–2484.
29. Miettinen, M., Lindenmayer, A. E., and Chaubal, A. (1994) Endothelial cell markers CD31, CD34, and BNH9 antibody to H- and Y-antigens evaluation of their specificity and sensitivity in the diagnosis of vascular tumors and comparison with Von Willebrand factor. *Mod. Pathol.* **7,** 82–90.
30. Khan, M. K., Linn, S. A., Sutorik, M., Addison, C. L., Lawrence, T. S., Hanash, S. M., and Polverini, P. J. (2000) Modification of an *in vivo* SCID mouse model of human angiogenesis that allows for the differential genomic molecular analysis of RNA and protein levels in endothelial cells undergoing angiogenesis. *Int. J. Radiol. Oncol. Biol. Physics* **48,** 270.
31. Koch, A. E., Halloran, M. M., Haskell, C. J., Shah, M. R., and Polverini, P. J. (1995) Angiogenesis mediated by soluble forms of E-selectin and vascular cell adhesion molecule-1. *Nature* **376,** 517–519.
32. Polverini, P. J. (1996) Cellular adhesion molecules: newly identified mediators of angiogenesis. *Am. J. Pathol.* **148,** 1023–1029.
33. Swerlick, R. A., Lee, K. H., Li, L. J., Sepp, N. T., Caughman, S. W., and Lawley, T. J. (1992) Regulation of vascular cell adhesion molecule 1 on human dermal microvascular endothelial cells. *J. Immunol.* **149,** 698–705.

34. Dustin, M. L. and Springer, T. A. (1988) Lymphocyte function-associated antigen-1 (LFA-1) interaction with intercellular adhesion molecule-1 (ICAM-1) is one of at least three mechanisms for lymphocyte adhesion to cultured endothelial cells. *J. Cell Biol.* **107,** 321–331.
35. Strömblad, S. and Cheresh, D. A. (1996) Cell adhesion and angiogenesis. *Trends Cell Biol.* **6,** 462–468.
36. Patan, S., Munn, L. L., and Jain, R. K. (1996) Intussusceptive microvascular growth in a human colon adenocarcinoma xenograft: a novel mechanism of tumor angiogenesis. *Microvasc. Res.* **51,** 260–272.
37. Nör, J. E., Mitra, R. S., Castle, V., Mooney, D. J., and Polverini, P. J. (2000) Thrombospondin-1 inhibits angiogenesis by activating caspase-3 and inducing endothelial cell apoptosis. *J. Vasc. Res.* **37,** 209–218.
38. Schechner, J. S., Nath, A. K., Zheng, L., Kluger, M. S., Hughes, C. C., Sierra-Honigmann, M. R., Lorber, M. I., Tellides, G., Kashgarian, M., Bothwell, A. L., and Pober, J. S. (2000) *In vivo* formation of complex microvessels lined by human endothelial cells in an immunodeficient mouse. *Proc. Natl. Acad. Sci. USA* **97,** 9191–9196.

I

EXPERIMENTAL MODELS OF WOUND HEALING

B. REVIEWS OF SPECIFIC MODEL SYSTEMS

14

Tissue Repair in Models of Diabetes Mellitus

A Review

David G. Greenhalgh

1. Introduction

Diabetes mellitus is a major cause of impaired tissue repair. Patients with this disease not only have a propensity to develop wounds, but when they do, they tend to have difficulty healing those wounds. Simple wounds often become chronic and infectious wound complications are not uncommon. Unfortunately, the amputation rate for diabetics is much higher than for the nondiabetic population. Because healing problems are so common and devastating, several models of tissue repair have been developed in animals that are "made" diabetic or have a genetic predisposition for diabetes mellitus. The goal of this chapter is to review these models and to try to relate their similarities to human diabetes mellitus. It must be remembered, however, that diabetes mellitus is a very complex spectrum of diseases and that no animal model completely represents all human forms. It is important to choose a model that answers the question that the investigator is asking. By understanding how the various models relate to different aspects of human diabetes mellitus, the investigator can choose the correct model for the proposed studies.

Before choosing an animal model, one must have an understanding of how wound healing is altered in human diabetes mellitus. Many factors are involved in the development of the classic "diabetic" ulcer that develops on the sole of the foot beneath the head of the first or second metatarsal (*1–4*). First of all, diabetic patients frequently have peripheral vascular disease that interferes with blood supply to the feet. In addition to the macrovascular disease, the microvasculature is also affected so that there is altered blood flow to the foot.

From: *Methods in Molecular Medicine, vol. 78: Wound Healing: Methods and Protocols*
Edited by: Luisa A. DiPietro and Aime L. Burns © Humana Press Inc., Totowa, NJ

There are also changes in the basement membrane of the capillaries that lead to perfusion problems. Another key factor is the neuropathy of diabetes mellitus. The lack of sensation can lead to deeper wounds by allowing persistent damage owing to a loss of protective actions. In addition, neuropathy leads to muscle wasting that leads to the loss of the normal arch of the foot. The loss of the normal arch positioning causes increased pressure over the head of the metatarsals. The loss of autonomic nerves leads to decreased sweating, and dry, cracking skin that causes the skin to have an increased risk of breakdown. Finally, diabetes mellitus leads to impaired immune function so that a small wound has a higher propensity for infection. One can see that the many factors that predispose diabetics to healing problems are difficult to completely reproduce in an animal model. Investigators should choose the model that most closely resembles the problem that they wish to study.

2. Models of Diabetes Mellitus

Animal models of diabetes mellitus can be divided into four categories: surgically induced diabetes, chemically induced diabetes, genetic insulin-dependent diabetes, and genetic insulin-resistant diabetes. The positive and negative aspects of each type of model are discussed next.

2.1. Surgically Induced Diabetes Mellitus

The great benefit of the use of animals in biomedical research can be exemplified by the early studies on the effects of insulin on diabetes mellitus (5). Insulin's function was discovered in dogs that had their pancreas removed surgically. Investigators were able to reverse the animals' severe diabetes by treating them with insulin isolated from pancreatic extracts, eventually revolutionizing the treatment of diabetes. These techniques of surgically removing the pancreas can be performed in larger animals to produce insulin-dependent diabetes. It is conceivable that wound-healing studies could be performed after these procedures, but surgical excision of the pancreas is rarely, if ever, used for tissue repair studies, because much simpler animal models of diabetes mellitus are available. It is obvious that a pancreatic excision is a major stress on an animal that not only causes "brittle" diabetes, but also pancreatic exocrine dysfunction. These complicating factors make the use of surgically induced diabetes mellitus impractical.

2.2. Chemically Induced Diabetes Mellitus

Two agents, alloxan and streptozotocin, selectively attack the β-cells of the islets of Langerhans and induce insulin-dependent diabetes mellitus (IDDM) (6–8). Chemically induced diabetes mellitus has been induced in mice, rats, guinea pigs, hamsters, dogs, and monkeys. While the agents are specific for β-cells, not all animals develop the same degree of diabetes. Investigators usually test the animals for hyperglycemia prior to including each animal in a study. The animals may also develop mild damage to other organs, such as the kidneys, liver, and exocrine pancreas. Investigators have also found that there is some damage to α-cells (producing glucagon) and potentially other endocrine cells in the pancreas *(6–8)*. In my experience, the animals often lose weight while developing diabetes. This weight loss could influence wound healing, since short-term weight loss may have significant effects on healing.

The methodologies for chemically induced diabetes mellitus are simple. Three types of strategies can be used *(8)*. First, a single, large dose is administered that causes acute β-cell death. For example, the agent is administered to rodents by IP injection (approximate dose: 240 mg/kg in mice, 45 mg/kg in rats). The animals are allowed to recover for a few weeks. Those animals that are found to be hyperglycemic are used for diabetic studies. Wound-healing studies are then performed using any desired model of tissue repair. Second, low doses of streptozotocin are administered for 4 to 5 d to produce an insulitis that involves cell-mediated immunity and a permanent diabetes. Third, a single lower dose (half the large dose) is used to cause a gradual onset of diabetes mellitus over 10–60 d. At least 80% of the islet cells must be eliminated prior to having a drop in insulin levels.

The advantages of using these agents are that the technique is easy and it produces an insulin-dependent form of diabetes mellitus. Healing studies have demonstrated many forms of tissue-healing impairment that are at least partially reversible by insulin treatment *(9–14)*. The applicability of these models is illustrated by the great number of studies that use this technique. The disadvantages include the use of a chemotherapy agent that may have more systemic effects than desired. The weight loss, as described earlier, suggests that other, less specific effects are also induced.

2.3. Genetic or Spontaneous Diabetes Mellitus Models

Diabetes mellitus develops in many, if not all, species of mammals. Just as with people, there are those animals that have a predisposition for diabetes. These genetically or spontaneously induced models have been used extensively for all kinds of research, including studies of tissue repair. The genetic models can be divided into insulin-dependent models and insulin-resistant models. Frequently, the models are divided into nonobese or obese models, since most insulin-resistant models occur in animals that have a tendency for obesity. Each type of diabetes has at least some but not all characteristics of the corresponding human form of diabetes.

2.3.1. IDDM Models

There are several animals that spontaneously develop IDDM (15–23). These animals develop diabetes that results from autodestruction of the islet cells to produce an abnormally low amount of insulin. These animals include the nonobese (NOD) mouse, BB Wister rat, Chinese hamster, South African hamster, many guinea pigs, Yucatan miniature pig, golden retrievers and keeshond dogs, and many primates. The rodent models (NOD mouse and BB Wister rat) have been extensively used in studies that examine the pathophysiology of diabetes mellitus since rodents develop an insulitis that has many similarities to the development of human juvenile IDDM (23). There have not been as many wound-healing studies performed in these animals, perhaps because using the chemical agents in normal strains is cheaper and because the maintenance of these genetically altered animals is probably more difficult. In addition, a majority of patients that have wound-healing problems have adult-onset, insulin-resistant diabetes mellitus. The studies that have been performed do reveal that there are abnormalities in tissue repair.

2.3.2. Insulin-Resistant Obese Models of Diabetes Mellitus

There are several strains of species that develop insulin resistance (24–27). The list includes the obese (ob/ob) mouse, diabetic (db/db) mouse, Agouti (yellow) mouse, Fat mouse, Tubby mouse, Adipose mouse, New Zealand obese (NZO) mouse, spiny mouse, Japanese KK mouse, Zucker obese ("fatty") rat, and Djungarian hamster (see **Table 1**). The expression of diabetes mellitus depends on the strain of the mouse in which the gene defect occurs. The most frequently used model of diabetes mellitus for wound-healing studies has been the genetically obese, insulin-resistant (db/db) diabetes mouse.

The discovery and development of the obese mouse strains is an interesting story of scientific discovery. Dr. Coleman, at Jackson Laboratories (Bar Harbor, ME), noticed that some C57BL mice developed obesity and profound hyperglycemia. The obesity was found to be the result of an insatiable hunger. The animals literally ate continuously, gaining two to three times the weight of littermates. In addition to obesity, the animals developed insulin-resistant diabetes. Breeding studies demonstrated that the animals were sterile, but that normal littermates carried the gene (28). Coleman and Hummel (29) did parabiosis studies, in which obese animals were connected to normal animals through their blood supply. In one strain, the ob/ob mouse, the obese mouse would lose weight to match the normal attached animal. Coleman surmised that a satiety hormone was missing from the mutated ob/ob mouse. In another strain, the db/db mouse, the attached "normal" animal essentially starved itself to death, whereas the obese animal continued to eat massive amounts. A

Table 1
Genetically Diabetic and Obese Rodents *(24–27)*

Name of rodent	Gene symbol	Inheritance	Chromosome
Mouse			
Obese	ob	Autosomal recessive	6
Diabetic	db, db^{2j}, db^{3j}, db^{ad}	Autosomal recessive	4
Yellow (Agouti)	A^y, A^{vy}, A^{iy}	Autosomal dominant	2
Fat	fat	Autosomal recessive	?
Tubby	tub	Autosomal recessive	7
Adipose	Ad	Autosomal dominant	7
New Zealand (NZO)		Polygenic	
Japanese KK (KK)		Polygenic	
Rat			
Fatty (Zucker)	fa, fa^k		

receptor defect for the same hormone was suspected. These studies eventually led to the discovery of the satiety hormone leptin, which has been found to be one of several recently discovered mediators of body mass composition *(30)*. The ob/ob mice lack the gene to produce leptin and thus are never satiated. There is a rare human form of diabetes mellitus that involves a lack of leptin that is owing to a lack of the ob gene *(31)*. The db/db mouse, however, lacks the receptor for leptin in the hypothalamus *(32)*. These experiments have led to the new field of the hormonal regulation of body mass composition.

Several investigators have utilized either the ob/ob or db/db mice for wound-healing experiments. Goodson and Hunt *(33,34)* used the ob/ob mouse to demonstrate impaired healing compared with controls. Several investigators, including myself, have used the db/db mouse for multiple tissue-repair studies *(35–40)*. The benefit of these db/db animals is that the heterozygous (db/+) littermates are completely normal and can be used as controls. The initial purpose of our studies was to develop a clinically relevant but simple model of impaired healing for the study of growth factors. Recombinant techniques had just been developed, and there was a great push to demonstrate growth factor efficacy in clinically relevant preclinical trials. We decided to create a relatively large wound (1.5 × 1.5 cm) on the backs of the animals *(35)*. The purpose of the large wound was to try to allow a longer time to demonstrate a growth factor effect that could occur with the rapid contraction of rodent wounds. In addition, we wished to develop a system that allowed for the delivery of growth factors, so the wounds were covered with a transparent polyurethane dressing that allowed for injection of the agent onto the wound. In addition, the extent of wound closure was measurable through the transparent dressing.

The studies demonstrated that the rate of wound closure was markedly delayed in the homozygous animals when compared with the heterozygous littermates (35). Histology revealed that there was a marked delay in the entry of the normal inflammatory cells into the wound. In essence, the animals had a prolongation of the inflammatory or lag phase of healing. Once the macrophages arrived in the wound, collagen deposition proceeded relatively normally. This healing abnormality was ideal for testing growth factors since these agents are designed to increase the chemotaxis and proliferation of inflammatory cells, fibroblasts, and capillaries into the wound. The use of the model has been quite extensive in demonstrating that many agents (growth factors) have been found to accelerate healing in the db/db animal (35–40). In addition, the model has been used to determine potential mechanisms of altered healing in diabetic animals. For instance, one hypothesis is that there is a deficiency in growth factor synthesis in wounds that do not heal. Studies in the db/db animals confirm that there is a delay in expression of several different growth factors (41–43). Another theory is that increased expression of proteases may destroy the factors that stimulate healing. Indeed, studies have demonstrated that there is an increase in several matrix metalloproteases in the db/db wounds (44). In conclusion, there have been many benefits of the use of the genetically diabetic and obese mice.

All models have some deficiencies and the db/db mouse has some problems. Clearly, no rodent model can completely translate to the clinical situation. The db/db mouse has some similarities to human insulin-resistant diabetes but does not completely reproduce it. As far as wound-healing studies go, the rodent model always has the issue of contraction; wound contraction occurs to a greater extent in rodents than in humans. Fortunately, the wounds of the db/db mouse do not contract to the same extent as those of nonobese rodents (35). Whether this is owing to a diabetic defect or to the "tightness" of the skin resulting from the obesity is not clear. In addition, at least one study demonstrated that the polyurethane dressing interfered with wound closure (45). This delay in healing may be related to the stiffness of the polyurethane dressing or it may be related to the composition of the dressing. In the growth factor studies, these delays were desired to allow for an extended "window" that would allow a greater chance for improvement, which was not observed in nondiabetic littermates. Infection is another problem in these animals. Because of the hyperglycemia and possibly a lower resistance to bacterial invasion, the db/db animals developed infection in 3–5% of cases. Interestingly, a mild infection tended to lead to an augmentation of healing, presumably by stimulating an inflammatory reaction. Occasionally, however, the animals would develop an invasive infection that destroyed the wound *(46)*. In addition, the diabetic animals were less resistant to some stress and had a higher mortality than controls. As for any model, the potential problems need to be balanced with the benefits of the model.

3. Conclusion

The models described herein have several characteristics that can help the investigator answer questions related to the relationship between diabetes mellitus and wound healing. The investigator should choose the model that has the best chance of answering the question being sought. Of all the preclinical growth factor trials, only one agent has been approved for the topical treatment of chronic wounds. Recombinant PDGF-BB (Regranex [Becaplermin]; Ortho-McNeil) has been approved for the treatment of diabetic ulcers. No other wound type has a recombinant protein approved by the Food and Drug Administration for its treatment. The many animal models of diabetes have assisted in the development of that product.

References

1. McMurry, J. F. Jr. (1984) Wound healing with diabetes mellitus. *Surg. Clin. North Am.* **64,** 769–778.
2. Goodson, W. H. III and Hunt, T. K. (1979) Wound healing and the diabetic patient. *Surg. Gynecol. Obstet.* **149,** 600–608.
3. Economides, P. A. and Veves, A. (2000) Etiopathogenesis of foot ulceration in diabetes. *Wounds* **12,** 3b–6b.
4. Boulton, A. J. and Vileikyte, L. (2000) Pathogenesis of diabetic foot ulceration and measurements of neuropathy. *Wounds* **12,** 12b–18b.
5. Engerman, R. L. and Kramer, J. W. (1982) Dogs with induced or spontaneous diabetes as models for the study of human diabetes mellitus. *Diabetes* **31,** 26–29.
6. Catanzaro-Guimaraes, S. A. (1968) Histometric determination of collagen fibers in granulating wounds of alloxan diabetic rats. *Experentia* **24,** 1168,1169.
7. Rerup, C. C. (1970) Drugs producing diabetes through damage of insulin secreting cells. *Pharmacol. Rev.* **22,** 485–518.
8. Grodsky, G. M., Anderson, C. E., Coleman, D. L., et al. (1982) Metabolism and underlying causes of diabetes mellitus. *Diabetes* **31,** 45–53.
9. Goodson, W. H. III and Hunt, T. K. (1977) Studies of wound healing experimental diabetes mellitus. *J. Surg. Res.* **22,** 221–227.
10. Seifter, E., Rettura, G., Padawer, J., et al. (1981) Impaired wound healing in streptozotocin diabetes: prevention by supplemental vitamin A. *Ann. Surg.* **194,** 42–50.
11. Grotendorst, G. R., Martin, G. R., Pencev, D., et al. (1985). Stimulation of granulation tissue formation by platelet-derived growth factor in normal and diabetic rats. *J. Clin. Invest.* **76,** 2323–2329.

12. Andreassen, T. T. and Oxlund, H. (1987) The influence of experimental diabetes and insulin treatments on the biomechanical properties of rat skin incisional wounds. *Acta Chir. Scand.* **153,** 405–409.

13. Soriano, F. G., Virag, L., Jagtap, P., et al. (2001) Diabetic endothelial dysfunction: the role of poly(ADP-ribose) polymerase activation. *Nat. Med.* **7,** 108–113.

14. Riley, W. J., McConnell, T. J., McClaren, N. K., et al. (1981) The diabetogenic effects of streptozotocin in mice are prolonged and inversely related to age. *Diabetes* **30,** 718–723.

15. Coleman, D. M. (1982) Other potentially useful rodent models for the study of human diabetes mellitus. *Diabetes* **31,** 24,25.

16. Stauffacher, W., Orci, L., Cameron, D. P., et al. (1970) Spontaneous hyperglycemia and/or obesity in laboratory rodents. *Recent Prog. Hormone Res.* **27,** 41–95.

17. Leiter, E. H., Prochazka, M., and Coleman, D. L. (1987) Animal model of human disease: the non-obese diabetic (NOD) mouse. *Am. J. Pathol.* **128,** 380–383.

18. Lieter, E. H. (1989) The genetics of diabetes susceptibility in mice. *FASEB J.* **3,** 2231–2241.

19. Like, A. A., Butler, L., Williams, R. M., et al. (1982) Spontaneous autoimmune diabetes mellitus in the BB rat. *Diabetes* **31,** 7–13.

20. Gerritsen, G. C. (1982) The Chinese hamster as a model for the study of diabetes mellitus. *Diabetes* **31,** 14–23.

21. Phillips, R. W., Panepinto, L. M., Spangler, R., and Westmoreland, N. (1982) Yucatan swine as a model of human diabetes mellitus. *Diabetes* **31,** 30–36.

22. Howard, C. F. Jr. (1982) Nonhuman primates as models for the study of human diabetes mellitus. *Diabetes* **31,** 37–42.

23. Rabinovitch, A. (2000) Autoimmune diabetes mellitus. *Sci. Med.* **7,** 18–27.

24. Coleman, D. L. (1982) Diabetes-obesity syndromes in mice. *Diabetes* **31,** 1–6.

25. Bray, G. A. and York, D. A. (1979) Hypothalamic and genetic obesity in experimental animals: an autonomic and endocrine hypothesis. *Physiol. Rev.* **59,** 719–791.

26. Spiegelman, B. M. and Flier, J. S. (1996) Adipogenesis and obesity: rounding out the big picture. *Cell* **87,** 377–389.

27. Caro, J. F., Sinha, M. K., Kolaczynski, J. W., et al. (1996) Leptin: the tale of an obesity gene. *Diabetes* **45,** 1455–1462.

28. Coleman, D. L. and Hummel, K. P. (1967) Studies with the mutation diabetes in the mouse. *Diabetologia* **3,** 238–248.

29. Coleman, D. L. and Hummel, K. P. (1969) Effects of parabiosis of normal with genetically diabetes in mice. *Am. J. Physiol.* **217,** 1298–1304.

30. Zhang, Y., Proenca, R., Maffei, M., et al. (1994) Positional cloning of the mouse obese gene and its human homologue. *Nature* **372,** 425–432.

31. Considine, R. V., Considine, E. L., Williams, C. J., et al. (1996) Mutation screening and identification of a sequence variation in the human Ob gene coding. *Biochem. Biophys. Res. Commun.* **220,** 735–739.

32. Tartaglia, L. A., Dembrski, M., Weng, X., et al. (1995) Identification and expression cloning of a leptin receptor, OB-R. *Cell* **83,** 1263–1271.

33. Goodson, W. H. III and Hunt, T. K. (1979) Deficient collagen formation by obese mice in a standard wound model. *Am. J. Surg.* **138,** 692–694.
34. Goodson, W. H. III and Hunt, T. K. (1986) Wound collagen accumulation in obese hyperglycemic mice. *Diabetes* **35,** 491–495.
35. Greenhalgh, D. G., Sprugel, K. H., Murray, M. J., and Ross, R. (1990) PDGF and FGF stimulate wound healing in the genetically diabetic mouse. *Am. J. Pathol.* **136,** 1235–1246.
36. Albertson, S., Hummel, R. P. III, Breeden, M., and Greenhalgh, D. G. (1993) PDGF and FGF reverse the healing impairment in protein malnourished diabetic mice. *Surgery* **114,** 368–373.
37. Greenhalgh, D. G., Hummel, R. P. III, Albertson, A., and Breeden, M. P. (1993) Synergistic actions of platelet-derived growth factor and the insulin-like growth factors *in vivo*. *Wound Rep. Reg.* **1,** 69–81.
38. Brown, R. L., Breeden, M. P., and Greenhalgh, D. G. (1994) PDGF and TGF-α act synergistically to improve healing in the genetically diabetic mouse. *J. Surg. Res.* **56,** 562–570.
39. Tsuboi, R. and Rifkin, D. B. (1990) Recombinant basic fibroblast growth factor stimulates wound healing in healing-impaired db/db mice. *J. Exp. Med.* **172,** 245–251.
40. Klingbeil, C. K., Cesar, L. B., and Fiddes, J. C. (1991) Basic fibroblast growth factor accelerates tissue repair in models of impaired wound healing. *Prog. Clin. Biol. Res.* **365,** 443–458.
41. Werner, S., Breeden, M., Greenhalgh, D. G., Hofschneider, P. H., and Longaker, M. T. (1994) Induction of keratinocyte growth factor is reduced and delayed during wound healing in the genetically diabetic mouse. *J. Invest. Dermatol.* **103,** 469–472.
42. Frank, S., Hubner, G., Breier, G., Longaker, M. T., Greenhalgh, D. G., and Werner, S. (1995) Regulation of vascular endothelial growth factor expression in cultured keratinocytes. *J. Biol. Chem.* **270,** 12,607–12,613.
43. Brown, D. L., Kane, C. D., Chernausek, S. D., and Greenhalgh, D. G. (1997) Differential expression and localization of IGF-I and IGF-II in cutaneous wounds of diabetic versus nondiabetic mice. *Am. J. Pathol.* **151,** 715–724.
44. Neely, A. N., Clendening, C. E., Gardner, J., and Greenhalgh, D. G. (2000) Gelatinase activities in wounds of healing-impaired mice versus non-healing-impaired mice. *J. Burn Care Rehabil.* **21,** 395–402.
45. Ksander, G. A., Ogawa, Y. A. M., Chu, G. H., et al. (1990) Exogenous transforming growth factor-beta 2 enhances connective tissue formation and wound strength in guinea pig dermal wounds by secondary intent. *Ann. Surg.* **211,** 288–294.
46. Holder, I. A., Brown, R. L., and Greenhalgh, D. G. (1997) Animal models to study wound closure and topical treatment of infected wounds in the healing impaired and normohealing host. *Wound Rep. Reg.* **5,** 198–204.

15

Wound Healing Studies in Transgenic and Knockout Mice

A Review

Richard Grose and Sabine Werner

1. Introduction

Wound healing is a highly ordered and well coordinated process that involves inflammation, cell proliferation, matrix deposition, and tissue remodeling *(1)*. During the past few years, a series of candidate key players in the wound-healing scenario have been identified. These include not only a variety of different growth factors and cytokines, but also molecules that are involved in cell-cell and cell-matrix interactions, and proteins responsible for cell stability and cell migration. In most cases, the suggested function of these molecules is based on descriptive expression studies and/or functional in vitro studies. By contrast, their in vivo function in wound repair has been poorly defined.

The development of transgenic mouse technologies has already provided new insights into the function of many different genes during embryonic development. These technologies allow gain-of-function experiments (overexpression of ligands and receptors) as well as loss-of-function experiments (gene knockouts by homologous recombination in embryonic stem cells or overexpression of dominant-negative-acting molecules). Although many unconditional knockout and transgenic animals die during embryonic development, spatial and temporal control of gene ablation and overexpression, using both inducible and cre-lox technologies, makes it possible to investigate the functions of proteins formerly precluded owing to developmental lethality. A large number of viable genetically modified mice are now available that should not only be useful in determining the role of the targeted or overexpressed genes in normal

From: *Methods in Molecular Medicine, vol. 78: Wound Healing: Methods and Protocols*
Edited by: Luisa A. DiPietro and Aime L. Burns © Humana Press Inc., Totowa, NJ

physiology, but also for different types of repair processes. Indeed, the past 5 yr have seen an exponential growth in the number of transgenic mice used for wound-healing experiments, and these studies have provided interesting and, in many cases, unexpected results concerning the in vivo function of growth factors, extracellular matrix molecules, proteinases, and structural proteins in wound repair. The list of transgenic wound-healing studies continues to expand, and in an attempt to retain an overview of the field, we have therefore established a regularly updated "Compendium of Genetically Modified Mouse Wound Healing Studies." http://icbxs.ethz.ch/members/grose/woundtransgenic/home.html.

In this chapter, we focus on the studies in which genetically modified mouse models have helped elucidate the roles that many soluble mediators play during wound repair. We begin by covering the fibroblast growth factor (FGF) family, move on to the transforming growth factor-β (TGF-β) superfamily, and then address the data from cytokine and chemokine studies. Finally, **Table 1** summarizes all of the currently published data in this rapidly growing field.

2. Fibroblast Growth Factors

FGFs comprise a growing family of structurally related polypeptide growth factors, currently consisting of 22 members (reviewed in **ref. 2**). During embryogenesis, FGFs play key roles in regulating cell proliferation, migration, and differentiation. In adult tissues, FGFs have a diverse range of effects, including mediating angiogenesis, and neuroprotection, in addition to their stimulatory effects during wound repair (reviewed in **ref. 3**). FGFs transduce their signals through four high-affinity transmembrane protein tyrosine kinases, FGF receptors 1–4 (FGFR1–4) (reviewed in **ref. 4**). Many of the FGFs and their receptors show specific expression patterns in both developing and adult skin (3), where they are particularly involved in the regulation of hair growth (5). Being potent mitogenic and chemotactic factors, FGFs are clear candidates for contributing to the wound-healing response. This hypothesis has been corroborated by a number of studies in which local application of FGFs stimulated tissue repair (6).

2.1. Keratinocyte Growth Factor

2.1.1. Epidermal Expression of a Dominant-Negative Keratinocyte Growth Factor Impairs Wound Reepithelialization

Keratinocyte growth factor ([KGF], FGF-7) binds exclusively to a splice variant of FGF receptor 2 (FGFR2IIIb), a transmembrane protein tyrosine kinase receptor that is present only on epithelial cells (7). In previous studies, a strong upregulation of KGF expression has been observed after skin injury in mice and humans (8,9), with mouse studies revealing KGF mRNA levels more than 150-fold higher compared with the basal levels at d 1 after injury *(8)*. KGF expression at the wound site is restricted to dermal fibroblasts and γδ T cells, and, thus, it was hypothesized to act in a paracrine manner, stimulating keratinocytes to proliferate and migrate and thereby effect wound reepithelialization. By targeting expression of dominant-negative FGFR2IIIb to the epidermis, we could block KGF receptor signaling at the wound site and clearly demonstrate a reepithelialization defect in transgenic mice. The mutant receptor lacks a functional tyrosine kinase domain *(10,11)* and, on ligand binding, forms nonfunctional heterodimers with full-length wild-type receptors, thereby blocking signal transduction *(10–12)*. The truncated form of the KGF receptor is known to bind KGF; FGF-10; FGF-1; FGF-3; and, although with lower affinity, FGF-2 *(7,13,14)*. Therefore, it should inhibit the action of all these ligands.

Although the transgenic mice generated by Werner et al. *(15)* appeared macroscopically normal, a histological analysis of their skin revealed epidermal atrophy, disorganization of the epidermis, abnormal hair follicle morphology, and a 60–80% reduction in the number of hair follicles. Finally, these mice revealed dermal hyperthickening with a gradual replacement of adipose tissue by connective tissue. Histological analysis of full-thickness excisional wounds, where back skin was excised to the level including the panniculus carnosus muscle, revealed a severe delay in wound reepithelialization in the transgenic mice compared with control littermates *(15)*. On d 5 after injury, the number of proliferating keratinocytes in the hyperproliferative epithelium was 80–90% reduced compared with control mice. These results demonstrated an important role for KGF receptor signaling in wound repair, although the type of KGF receptor ligand responsible for this defect was not defined.

2.1.2. KGF-Deficient Mice Show No Defect in Wound Healing

To determine further the role of KGF in development and in repair processes, Guo et al. *(16)* used embryonic stem cell technology to generate mice lacking KGF. The obtained knockout mice revealed no obvious defects, with the exception of the fur, which appeared matted and greasy, especially in male animals. Although KGF is widely expressed during development and in the adult animal, no histological defects could be detected in the KGF knockout mice. Most surprising, even the healing process of full-thickness incisional wounds was normal. Thus, no histological differences could be determined between normal mice and those lacking KGF, and the proliferation rate of the keratinocytes at the wound edge was not altered. These data demonstrate that incisional wounds can heal in the absence of KGF. It would, however, be interesting to study the healing process of excisional wounds in these animals, since the extent of reepithelialization is much higher in excisional than in incisional wounds.

Table 1
Wound-Healing Studies on Transgenic and Knockout Mice[a]

Gene	Strategy	Reference
Activin A	Overexpressor—Keratin 14 promoter	*59*
BMP-6	Overexpressor—Keratin 10 promoter	*62*
BPAG1	Knockout	*85*
Cathepsin G	Knockout	*86*
CD44	Antisense knockdown—Keratin 5 promoter	*87*
CXCR22	Knockout	*75*
EGFR	Knockout	*88*
eNOS	Knockout	*96*
FGF-2	Knockout	*27*
Fibrinogen	Knockout	*89*
HGFL	Knockout	*90*
IL-6	Knockout	*66*
IL-10	Knockout	*77*
iNOS	Knockout	*97*
β5-Integrin	Knockout	*91*
IP-10	Overexpressor—Keratin 5 promoter	*72*
Keratin 6a	Knockout	*92*
Keratin 8	Knockout	*80*
KGF	Knockout	*16*
KGFR	Dominant negative—Keratin 14 promoter	*15*
MMP-1	Overexpressor—haptoglobin promoter	*93*
MMP-3	Knockout	*94*
Nf-1	Knockout	*95*
Osteopontin	Knockout	*98*
PAI-2	Knockout	*99*
PAR-1	Knockout	*100*
Plasminogen	Knockout	*101*
Plasminogen/fibrinogen	Double knockout	*89*
Selectins P and E	Double knockout	*102*
Skn1a/i	Knockout	*103*
SLPI	Knockout	*104*
Smad-3	Knockout	*54*
Stat-3	Knockout—Keratin 5 specific	*68*
Syndecan-4	Knockout	*105*
Tenascin-C	Knockout	*106*
TGF-α/KGF	Double knockout	*16*
TGF-β-1	Knockout	*40*
TGF-β-1	Knockout Scid–/– background	*46*
TGF-β-1	Overexpressor—albumin promoter	*47*

Table 1 *(continued)*

Gene	Strategy	Reference
Thrombomodulin	Knockout	*107*
Thrombomodulin	Overexpressor—Keratin 14 promoter	*108*
Thrombospondin-1	Overexpressor—Keratin 14 promoter	*109*
Thrombospondin-2	Knockout	*110*
tPA/uPA	Double knockout	*111*
tPA/uPAR	Double knockout	*112*
Transglutaminase 1	Knockout	*113*
Vimentin	Knockout	*78*
Vitronectin	Knockout	*114*

*a*A regularly updated version is available online at http://icbxs.ethz.ch/members/grose/woundtransgenic/home/html

The lack of obvious phenotypic abnormalities in the KGF knockout mice is in contrast to the results obtained with the dominant-negative KGF receptor (*see* this section, above). Although it might be possible that KGF is indeed not involved in these processes, this seems highly unlikely, since the pattern of KGF expression correlates very well with its postulated functions in normal and wounded skin. The most likely explanation for the discrepancies between the knockout and the dominant-negative receptor results is a redundancy in ligand signaling. Although KGF might normally be the most important KGF receptor ligand in normal and wounded skin, the lack of this gene in KGF knockout mice might be compensated for by other known KGF receptor ligands. More recent data from our laboratory and from others' suggest that FGF-10 is the principal candidate for effecting this compensation since it is also expressed in the mesenchyme of normal and wounded skin *(14,17)*. Studies using neutralizing KGF and/or FGF-10 antibodies during wound repair should help to clarify this issue further. Furthermore, the tissue-specific knockout of the KGF receptor splice variant of FGFR2 as well as double knockouts of different ligands of this receptor will shed light on the role of the KGF receptor and the various types of FGF in normal and wounded skin.

2.2. Wound Healing in Mice Deficient in TGF-α

As already described, the inhibition of KGF receptor signaling in basal keratinocytes of transgenic mice caused a severe delay in reepithelialization *(15)*. However, the wounds in these animals finally healed (unpublished finding), demonstrating the presence of other epithelial mitogens in the wound that can at least partially compensate for the defect in KGF receptor signaling.

One of these factors might be TGF-α, a strong mitogen and chemoattractant for many different cell types, including epidermal keratinocytes (18). Furthermore, expression of TGF-α is strongly upregulated in the wound tissue on d 1 after injury (16), and addition of exogenous TGF-α to a wound has been shown to enhance epithelial wound healing (19).

To determine the role of endogenous TGF-α in wound repair, two groups generated mice lacking this growth factor (20,21). Surprisingly, these mice appeared normal with the exception of eye abnormalities and waviness of whiskers and fur. By contrast, the epidermis of these mice was indistinguishable from that of control mice. Most interesting, no significant wound-healing abnormalities were observed in these mice, whereby two different wound-healing models (full-thickness back skin excisions and wounds generated by tail amputation) were used. However, one group observed more variability in the rate of wound closure in TGF-α null mice (21), suggesting that the lack of this mitogen can be compensated for to a variable extent by other growth factors. Such a compensation could be achieved by growth factors that, like TGF-α, bind to the epidermal growth factor (EGF) receptor. The most likely candidates are EGF and heparin-binding EGF, which are present at high levels in wound fluid (22). This hypothesis is supported by the severe phenotypic abnormalities of mice lacking the EGF receptor (23,24) and by transgenic mice expressing a dominant-negative EGF receptor in the epidermis (25), although the wound-healing process in these animals has not been analyzed yet. By contrast, the lack of TGF-α is unlikely to be compensated for exclusively by KGF, since incisional wound healing also appeared normal in mice lacking both TGF-α and KGF (16).

2.3. Mice Lacking FGF-2 Show Delayed Reepithelialization

In contrast to the restricted pattern characteristic of many of the FGFs, FGF-2 is expressed in many different tissues and cell types. It exerts a plethora of effects, both in vivo and in vitro, including mitogenic, chemotactic, angiogenic, and developmental activities. Thus, it is reported to act as a survival factor in many models of tissue repair, ranging from neural injury models to corneal and skin wounds (26). Surprisingly, considering the myriad of potential functions, mice lacking FGF-2 appeared superficially indistinguishable from wild-type littermates. However, when these mice were challenged by full-thickness excisional wounding, they showed delayed healing (27). In addition to a retardation in the rate of reepithelialization, mice null for FGF-2 show reduced collagen deposition at the wound site and also have thicker scabs. Expression of FGF-2 is known to be enhanced following injury (8,28), and topical application of FGF-2 has been reported to accelerate both dermal and epidermal repair (29–31). In addition, neutralizing antibodies to FGF-2 were shown to inhibit granulation tissue formation in sponges implanted into rats *(32)*. Taken together, these findings suggest a specific role for FGF-2 during wound healing that, despite the apparent redundancy of FGF signaling, cannot be covered for by other FGF family members.

3. TGF-β Superfamily Members and Downstream Signaling Molecules

The TGF-β superfamily encompasses a diverse range of proteins, many of which play important roles during development and differentiation. Mammalian members include TGF-β1-3, bone morphogenetic proteins (BMPs), Mullerian inhibiting substance, inhibins, and activins (reviewed in **ref. 33**). Their biological effects are mediated by heteromeric receptor complexes, which signal via activation of intracellular Smad signaling pathways (reviewed in **ref. 34**). TGF-β is one of the most studied molecules in the wound-healing scenario. This growth and differentiation factor is found in large amounts in platelets and is also produced by several cell types that are present in a wound, including activated macrophages, fibroblasts, and keratinocytes *(35)*. Three TGF-β isoforms (TGF-β1, TGF-β2, and TGF-β3) are present in mammals and have both distinct and overlapping functions. In vitro, these molecules have been shown to be mitogenic for fibroblasts, but they inhibit proliferation of most other cells. Furthermore, TGF-βs modulate differentiation processes and are very potent stimulators of the expression of extracellular matrix (ECM) proteins and integrins *(33)*. Therefore, they have the properties expected of wound cytokines. Indeed, a series of studies has demonstrated a beneficial effect of exogenous TGF-β for wound repair *(35)*. Furthermore, endogenous TGF-β is likely to play an important role in wound healing, since all three types of mammalian TGF-β are expressed during repair, with each isoform having a characteristic distribution in the wound tissue *(36,37)*. TGF-β induction is modulated in a complicated manner by systemic glucocorticoid treatment of wild-type mice, suggesting that aberrant expression of TGF-β1, TGF-β2, and TGF-β3 is associated with the wound-healing defect seen in these mice *(37)*. Additionally, TGF-β is particularly important for the scarring response; it has been shown that TGF-β1 and TGF-β2 induce cutaneous scarring, whereas TGF-β3 seems to inhibit this effect *(38,39)*.

3.1. TGF-β1-Deficient Mice Show Severely Impaired Late Stage Wound Repair

To clarify further the role of the TGF-β1 isoform in wound repair, Brown et al. *(40)* wounded transgenic mice deficient in TGF-β1 owing to a targeted disruption of the TGF-β1 gene *(41,42)*. These mice exhibit no obvious developmental abnormalities and appear phenotypically normal. However, at approx

3 wk of age, they develop a severe wasting syndrome, which is accompanied by a pronounced multifocal inflammatory response and tissue necrosis, resulting in multisystem organ failure and death *(41,42)*. To overcome this problem, the animals were wounded at d 10 after birth.

Full-thickness excisional wounds were created on the backs of TGF-β1 null mice and control mice and covered with a nonabsorbent dressing. The percentage of wound closure was determined at different time points after injury. Mice were sacrificed at d 10 after wounding and the wounds were analyzed histologically. Surprisingly, early wound healing proceeded almost normally in the TGF-β1-deficient mice, suggesting that other TGF-β isoforms or even different growth factors can compensate for the lack of TGF-β1 *(40)*. Alternatively, maternal rescue *in utero* by transplacental transfer of TGF-β1 and postnatally by transmission in the milk *(43)* might explain the lack of abnormalities in early wounds. However, the lack of TGF-β1 ultimately caused a severe inflammatory response in the wound, as well as in many other tissues and organs, which is likely to be responsible for the wound-healing abnormalities seen at later stages. Thus, histological analysis of the wounds at d 10 after injury revealed a thinner, less vascular granulation tissue in the knockout mice, which was dominated by a marked inflammatory cell infiltrate. Furthermore, decreased reepithelialization and decreased collagen deposition were observed in mutant animals when compared with control mice *(40)*. These defects in wound repair are likely to be a secondary effect of the severe wasting syndrome observed in these mice. Malnutrition and weight loss have been associated with impaired wound healing *(44,45)*, and the weight loss that accompanies the inflammatory response is likely to exert an adverse effect on repair.

In summary, Brown et al. *(40)* study demonstrated that the lack of TGF-β1 can be compensated in the early stage of wound repair. However, the severe inflammation seen in the mice ultimately caused a severe wound-healing defect.

3.2. Immunodeficient Mice Lacking TGF-β1 Show Retarded Healing

To try to dissect the TGF-β1-dependent wound-healing defects from the effects of severe inflammation, Crowe et al. *(46)* crossed TGF-β1 null mice onto the immunodeficient Scid–/– background *(46)*. Scid–/– mice lack T- and B-cells and therefore do not have the machinery to mount the large inflammatory response seen in nonimmunocompromised mice lacking TGF-β1 *(40)*. In contrast to what was predicted, the absence of inflammation in TGF-β1–/– Scid–/– mice resulted in a major delay in all the primary phases of repair by around a week compared to TGF-β1+/+ Scid–/– controls. This delay was not singly owing to either the lack of TGF-β1 or the lack of lymphocytes, but to the combination of the two. This suggests that TGF-β1 and lymphocytes may affect compensatory pathways during repair. Alternatively, the delay may be a side effect of the absence of TGF-β1 in wounds leading to delayed expression of the other two TGF-β isoforms, TGF-β2 and TGF-β3. Although unable to distinguish between which of these hypotheses may be true, Crowe et al.'s *(46)* study presents an elegant method for bypassing a knockout phenotype that would otherwise mask a defect in wound repair.

3.3. Mice Overexpressing TGF-β1 Show Severely Impaired Late Stage Wound Repair

In contrast to the knockout approaches described above, Shah et al. *(47)* investigated the effect of excess levels of TGF-β1 on wound repair. Their hypothesis was that elevated levels of circulating TGF-β1 would accelerate healing but also enhance scarring. Mice with elevated plasma levels of active TGF-β1 were generated by cloning a modified porcine TGF-β1 construct, generating constitutively active TGF-β1, downstream of the mouse albumin promoter region. Using a dorsal incisional wounding model, complemented by ventral sc implantation of polyvinyl alcohol (PVA) sponges, Shah et al. *(47)* were able to study both normal cutaneous wound repair and cellular infiltration as a model of granulation tissue formation.

Surprisingly, these investigators found that, while the PVA sponges yielded the expected results, with increased cellularity, granulation tissue formation, and collagen deposition in transgenic animals, local TGF-β1 levels were lower in the incisional wounds of transgenic mice than in their control littermates. As such, the data show that increased circulating levels of TGF-β1 do not necessarily lead to increased levels of TGF-β1 at the wound site. Concomitant with the decreased TGF-β1 level in transgenic wounds, an increase in levels of TGF-β3 and type II TGF-β-receptor at the wound site were observed, and this resulted in an improved neodermal architecture in the healed transgenic wounds.

3.4. Smad3 Null Mice Show Accelerated Cutaneous Wound Healing with Increased Rate of Reepithelialization and Reduced Inflammation

TGF-βs and activin, both of which regulate key cellular functions during cutaneous wound repair, are known to require the nuclear transcriptional activators Smad2 and Smad3 for their intracellular signaling functions *(48–50)*. Smad2 and Smad3 proteins are recruited to ligand-bound TGF-β and activin receptor complexes, where they are phosphorylated by the type I receptor. The phosphorylated Smads 2 and 3 undergo a conformational change, which allows them to bind to cytoplasmic Smad4, after which they are able to translocate to the nucleus and activate their downstream targets (reviewed in **ref. 51**).

In contrast to Smad2 null mice, which die during embryogenesis *(52)*, mice lacking functional Smad3 survive into adulthood *(53)*. Following full-thickness incisional wounding, Smad3 null mice show a marked augmentation in repair. This accelerated healing was shown to be characterized by an increased rate of reepithelialization and a reduced local inflammatory infiltrate *(54)*. In addition to neutrophils and monocytes being almost absent in the Smad3 knockout wounds, there was a dramatic decrease in granulation tissue formation, resulting in an overall decrease in wound area. Wounds of Smad3 knockout mice were found to have significantly lower levels of TGF-β expression, likely owing to the decreased monocyte concentration, since these cells form a major supply line delivering TGF-β to the early wound.

To determine whether the lack of TGF-β was a cause of rather than an effect of the lack of inflammatory response, exogenous TGF-β1 was applied to the wounds of control and Smad3 null mice. While this treatment resulted in an augmented neutrophil infiltration into the wounds of control mice, it failed to rescue the inflammatory response in Smad3 null animals, indicating that Smad3 signaling may underpin TGF-β1-mediated inflammatory cell chemotaxis. Contrastingly, exogenous TGF-β1 did rescue the granulation tissue phenotype, resulting in a stimulation of matrix production in the wounds of Smad3 null mice, though the fibroblast numbers were not increased. Thus, TGF-β1-dependent matrix deposition seems to function in a Smad3-independent fashion in these mice, in agreement with previous studies suggesting a c-Jun-dependent pathway *(55)*.

Overall, the data suggest that Smad3 signaling plays an inhibitory role during wound repair, since its abrogation leads to enhanced reepithelialization and contraction of wound areas, at least in an incisional wound-healing scenario. As with the KGF knockout mice, it would be interesting to see how efficiently Smad3 null mice manage to repair full-thickness excisional wounds, where the granulation tissue formation is thought to play a more important role.

3.5. Overexpression of Activin A in Basal Keratinocytes Stimulates Wound Repair

Activin A, a TGF-β superfamily member, is a homodimeric protein comprising two activin βA monomers connected by disulfide linkage. That it might play a role in the skin was first suggested by knockout mouse studies, of activin βA *(56)* and of the activin antagonist follistatin *(57)*, which both showed clear phenotypes in hair follicle development. Further studies from our laboratory demonstrated activin βA to be strongly induced following wounding *(58)*.

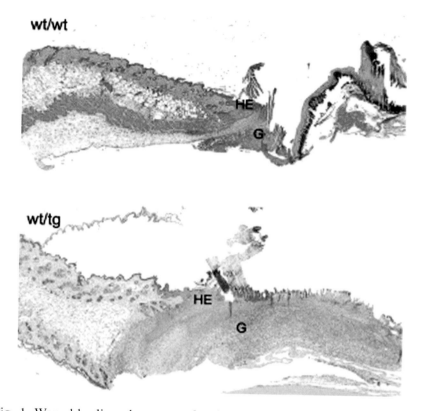

Fig. 1. Wound-healing phenotype of activin-overexpressing mice. Full-thickness excisional wounds were made on the back of 3-mo-old female transgenic mice (wt/tg) and female control littermates (wt/wt). Mice were killed on d 5 after injury. Sections (6 μm) from the middle of the wound were stained with hematoxylin and eosin. G, granulation tissue; HE, hyperproliferative epithelium. Note the larger area of granulation tissue in the transgenic mice. Magnification: ×25. (Reprinted from **ref. 59.** Copyright 1999 Oxford University Press.)

Therefore, mice overexpressing the human activin βA chain in the epidermis, under the control of the keratin 14 promoter, were generated to further investigate its role in tissue repair *(59)*.

A study by Munz et al. *(59)* found that unwounded mice overexpressing activin displayed epidermal hyperthickening and dermal fibrosis. Following full-thickness excisional wounding, the mice also showed enhanced granulation tissue formation and more rapid wound reepithelialization (**Fig. 1**). This augmentation of the granulation tissue was accompanied by an earlier increase in expression of the ECM molecules fibronectin and tenascin-C, although collagen expression remained unaffected. Thus, in addition to revealing novel activities of activin in keratinocyte differentiation and dermal fibrosis, this study implicates activin as a stimulatory factor during wound repair.

3.6. Epidermal Overexpression of BMP-6 Inhibits Wound Reepithelialization

BMP-6 is strongly expressed in the developing murine epidermis, with mRNA levels falling after 6 d postpartum to a low level in adult skin *(60)*. As such, it is closely associated with the most active phases of skin proliferation. To address further the role of BMP-6 in the skin, Blessing et al. *(61)* engineered transgenic mouse lines overexpressing BMP-6 in the suprabasal layers of the epidermis, using the keratin 10 promoter. Different lines with varied patterns of transgene expression showed completely opposite skin phenotypes. Strong and uniform expression of the BMP-6 transgene inhibited cell proliferation but had little effect on differentiation, whereas weak and patchy expression evoked strong hyperproliferation and parakeratosis in adult epidermis and severe perturbations of the usual pattern of differentiation, resulting in a psoriasis-like phenotype.

Since BMP-6 was found to be upregulated in human skin ulcers, where it may be involved in the inhibition of reepithelialization, the same laboratory decided to investigate wound repair in these mice strongly overexpressing BMP-6 *(62)*. Although all the major phases of tissue repair could be observed in transgenic mice, they showed significant delays in eschar detachment, reepithelialization, and granulation tissue maturation. Thus, BMP-6 may well be a causal factor in the failure of repair seen in chronic wounds.

4. Cytokines and Chemokines

Cytokines are small, secreted proteins of up to 20 kDa that affect the behavior of immune cells as well as other cells. They include the interleukins; lymphokines; and several related signaling molecules, such as tumor necrosis factor-α (TNF-α), TNF-β, and interferons. Chemokines are a subset of cytokines that stimulate chemotaxis and extravasation of immune cells via binding to G-protein-coupled receptors on the surface of target cells. It has long been thought that the proinflammatory cytokines, including interleukin-1α (IL-1α) and IL-1β, IL-6, and TNFα, play an important role in wound repair. They likely influence a series of crucial biological effects at the wound site, including stimulation of keratinocyte and fibroblast proliferation, synthesis and breakdown of ECM proteins, fibroblast chemotaxis, and regulation of the immune response.

4.1. IL-6 Knockout Mice Show Severe Deficits in Cutaneous Repair

IL-6 expression is rapidly upregulated following wounding, being produced mainly by keratinocytes, but also by macrophages, Langerhans cells, and fibroblasts *(63)*. A mitogen for keratinocytes *(64)*, its overexpression is associated with several skin pathologies, including psoriasis *(65)*. Using a full-thickness punch biopsy wounding model on IL-6 knockout mice, Gallucci et al. *(66)* showed that IL-6 is essential for reepithelialization, inflammation, and granulation tissue formation.

Excisional wounds to IL-6 null mice took up to three times longer to heal than those of wild-type controls and were characterized by a dramatic delay in reepithelialization and granulation tissue formation. This impaired phenotype was completely rescued by administration of recombinant murine IL-6 protein 1 h prior to wounding. Thus, it appears that IL-6 is crucial for kick-starting the wound response, both via its mitogenic effects on wound edge keratinocytes and via its chemoattractive effect on neutrophils, the first inflammatory cells to reach the clot.

4.2. Stat-3-Mediated Transduction of IL-6 Signaling Is Essential for Tissue Repair

STATs (signal transducers and activators of transcription) are cytoplasmic molecules that transduce signals from a variety of growth factors, cytokines, and hormones. Once activated by tyrosine phosphorylation, they dimerize and translocate to the nucleus, where they bind to specific DNA elements and thus activate target gene expression *(67)*. Stat-3 is activated by IL-6 signaling and is thus a likely candidate for a role in wound repair. Since Stat-3 null mice die during embryogenesis *(68)*, Sano et al. *(69)* used a Cre-lox approach to knock out Stat-3 in keratinocytes. Consistent with a low level of IL-6 expression in normal skin, they saw no effect on skin morphogenesis. However, following full-thickness excisional wounding, the healing process was severely compromised, with dramatically reduced reepithelialization (**Fig. 2**), showing clear similarities to the reepithelialization phenotype of the IL-6 knockout mice. The overall effect on repair was less dramatic than in the IL-6 null mice, since the cell types involved in both the inflammatory response and granulation tissue formation were unaffected by the tissue-specific approach.

4.3. Epidermal Overexpression of IP-10 Delays Wound Repair

Interferon-γ-inducible protein-10 (IP-10) is a chemokine that is detected at high levels in several chronic inflammatory conditions, including psoriasis. It is a member of the CXC family of chemokines and acts primarily in the recruitment of neutrophils and lymphocytes (reviewed in **ref. 70**). It is also one of a group of several chemokines that are upregulated following wounding, with an expression pattern that correlates well with recruitment of inflammatory cells to the wound site *(71)*. To determine whether IP-10 could modulate an in vivo inflammatory response, Luster et al. *(72)* engineered mice that

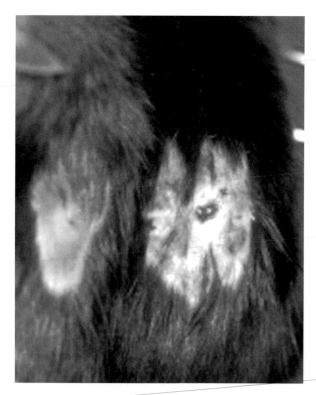

Fig. 2. Retardation of skin wound healing in Stat3-disrupted mice. A comparison of skin wound healing in a Stat3-disrupted mouse (–/–, **right**) and a control littermate (+/+, **left**) is shown. The photograph was taken on d 8 after wounding. (Figure courtesy of Prof. Junji Takeda. Reprinted from **ref. *69*** by permission. Copyright 1999 Oxford University Press.)

constitutively express IP-10 in keratinocytes. These mice showed no obvious abnormalities, until they were subjected to full-thickness excisional wounding. Following injury, IP-10-overexpressing mice showed a more intense inflammatory phase, delayed reepithelialization, and a prolonged, disorganized granulation phase with impaired angiogenesis compared with control littermates. These data suggest that IP-10 is able to inhibit wound repair by disrupting the normal development of the granulation tissue.

4.4. CXCR2 Null Mice Show Multiple Defects in Wound Healing

IP-10 exerts its biological effects via binding to the CXCR3 chemokine receptor. This receptor is reported to antagonize the signal transduction pathway downstream of another chemokine receptor, CXCR2 *(72)*. CXCR2 receptors are expressed on keratinocytes, neovascularizing endothelial cells, and neutrophils and bind the chemokines MIP-2 and KC, both of which are upregulated in mouse wounds *(73)*. To determine their role in wound repair, Devalaraja et al. *(74)* made full-thickness excisional punch biopsy wounds in mice lacking CXCR2. Following wounding, these mice exhibited defective neutrophil recruitment, delayed monocyte recruitment, and decreased secretion of the proinflammatory cytokine IL-1β. Histologically, they also showed delayed reepithelialization and decreased neovascularization *(75)*.

4.5. IL-10 Causes Scarring in a Model of Fetal Wound Repair

Fetal wound healing is characterized by rapid reepithelialization, minimal inflammation, and scar-free repair (reviewed in **ref. 76**). Fetal wounds also show diminished expression of the proinflammatory cytokines IL-6 and IL-8, a phenomenon that was hypothesized to be owing to their negative regulation by the antiinflammatory cytokine IL-10. To test this hypothesis, Liechty et al. *(77)* wounded embryonic skin from IL-10 null mice that had been grafted onto strain-matched adult mice. Wounds of control embryonic skin grafts showed little inflammation and normal restoration of dermal architecture. However, wounded IL-10 null grafts showed significantly higher inflammatory cell infiltration and collagen deposition more akin to the scarring associated with adult repair. This study suggests that IL-10 plays an important role in regulating the expression of proinflammatory cytokines at the fetal wound site, and thus modulates downstream matrix deposition that leads to scar-free repair.

4.6. Embryo Studies Address Roles for Intermediate Filaments in Wound Repair

In a further study into the mechanisms behind the perfect healing that occurs in the embryo, Eckes et al. *(78)* wounded midgestational mouse embryos lacking the intermediate filament protein vimentin. Embryonic day 11.5 mouse embryos are capable of healing an excisional hind leg amputation wound within 24 h *(79)*. Another study, using the same model, had revealed that one of the major intermediate filaments in early embryonic skin, keratin 8, was not essential for normal embryonic repair *(80)*. Using DiI-labeling of wound margin mesenchymal cells, Eckes et al. *(78)* showed that, while reepithelialization proceeded normally, vimentin null embryos failed to contract the mesenchyme of their wound bed (**Fig. 3**). Thus, vimentin is essential for the generation of the tractional forces that drive mesenchymal contraction in the embryonic wound. This defect in repair was also seen in adult wounds to vimentin null mice, again in a defect limited to the connective tissue, which displayed delayed granulation tissue formation and contraction.

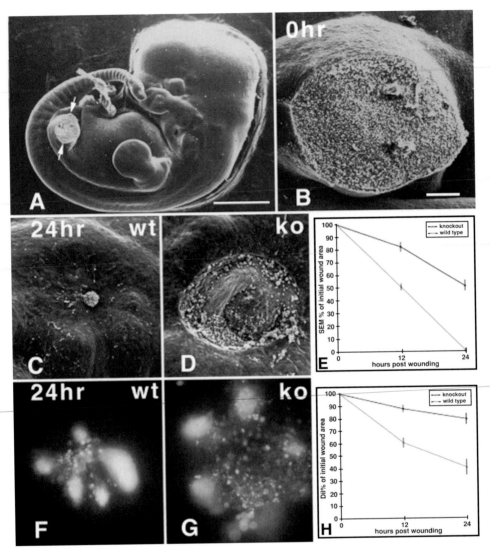

Fig. 3. Wound closure in wild-type and vimentin-deficient embryos. (**A**) Scanning electron micrograph of embryonic day 11.5 mouse embryo with left hind limb bud amputated to leave oval-shaped excisional wound (arrows). (**B**) Higher magnification detail of this 0-h wound. (**C**) After 24 h the wild-type wound is closed. (**D**) By contrast, at 24 h postwounding the vimentin-deficient wound is still open. (**E**) Graphic representation of wound closure (reepithelialization + connective-tissue contraction) as measured from scanning electron micrographs. Shaded and solid symbols indicate area measurements in wild-type and vimentin-deficient embryos, respectively, during the 24-h culture period. Error bars are SEMs. (**F**) Twenty-four hours postwounding, the wild-type controls have significantly contracted their DiI-marked wound mesenchyme.

5. Conclusion

Studies of wound healing using genetically modified mice have already revealed crucial roles for several genes in the repair process. However, some of the normal functions of the genes targeted might not be revealed owing to redundancy or compensation. This hypothesis is supported by the lack of obvious wound-healing abnormalities in various knockout mice, such as mice deficient in KGF or TGF-α *(16)*. Although it cannot be excluded that these proteins are indeed not important for wound repair, their strong induction in healing skin wounds supports their functional significance. In the case of TGF-α and KGF, other growth factors, which bind to the same receptor, might compensate for the lack of these mitogens. Wound-healing studies using animals deficient in two or more homologous molecules, as well as studies with dominant-negative-acting molecules that can inhibit the function of several members of a protein family, will be very useful in answering these areas of question.

At the other extreme, secondary effects, which are owing to systemic defects caused by the transgene, or to transgene-mediated defects in nonwounded skin, might obscure the normal function of a gene in wound repair. Thus, it has long been known that the wound-healing process is significantly impaired by systemic abnormalities such as malnutrition, weight loss, impaired oxygenation, and ageing *(44,45)*. This was also the case in the TGF-β1 knockout mice, which developed a severe wasting syndrome at approx 3 wk of age, accompanied by a severe inflammatory response in various tissues and organs, including the wound. These abnormalities are likely to be responsible for the impaired wound healing seen in these mice, making it impossible to study the local effects of the lack of TGF-β1 on wound repair in this model. One approach to circumvent this problem, as mentioned under **Subheading 3.2.**, was to cross the mice onto an immunodeficient background. However, these problems might also be solved by the generation of mice that have a tissue-specific knockout or tissue-specific overexpression of a transgene *(81)*. Ideally, inducible systems that allow the induction of a transgene or the deletion of an endogenous gene in a time- and tissue-specific manner should be used. Such systems thus allow

---

Fig. 3. *(continued)* **(G)** By contrast, at the same time point, the vimentin-deficient wound has barely contracted. **(H)** Graphic representation of connective-tissue contraction component of wound closure as measured from DiI-marked specimens. Shaded and solid symbols indicate area measurements in wild-type and vimentin-deficient embryos, respectively, during the 24-h culture period. Error bars are SEMs. Scale bars: (A) 1 mm; (B, C, D, F, G) 100 μm. (Figure courtesy of Dr. Paul Martin. Reprinted from **ref. 78** by permission. Copyright 2000 Company of Biologists Ltd.)

the study of the role of a particular gene under specific conditions such as during wound repair.

The first successful results with inducible systems in the skin have recently been published. Two have adopted an estrogen receptor–based approach, where Cre recombinase was fused in frame with the tamoxifen-responsive hormone-binding domain of the estrogen receptor. This fusion protein was expressed under the control of the Keratin 5 promoter *(82)* or Keratin 14 promoter *(83)*. Cre-mediated recombination of loxP sites flanking the target gene thus results in temporally and spatially restricted knockout of the target gene. In a different approach, Wang et al. *(84)* have used topical application of antiprogestin to induce expression of target genes. This method works via skin-specific expression of a fusion protein, under the control of the loricrin promoter, containing a truncated progesterone receptor fused to the yeast GAL4 transcription factor. Thus, by engineering a GAL4-binding domain, normally absent in mammalian cells, upstream of the target gene, transcription can be activated in a tissue-specific and temporally controlled manner. Use of these types of systems promises to yield extremely valuable data on the actions of many genes crucial to wound repair, but formerly impossible to study.

Acknowledgments

We are particularly grateful to Prof. Anita Roberts, NIH Bethesda; Prof. Junji Takeda, Osaka University Medical School; and Dr. Paul Martin, University College London, for kindly providing **Figs. 1–3**. We also thank Prof. Manfred Blessing and Dr. Gillian Ashcroft for critical reading of the manuscript, and our coworkers for providing unpublished data. Work in Sabine Werner's laboratory is supported by the ETH Z¸rich, the Swiss National Science Foundation (grant no. 31-61358.00), the German Ministry for Education and Research (BMBF), and the Stiftung Verum.

References

1. Clark, R. A. F. (1996) Wound repair: Overview and general considerations, in *The Molecular and Cellular Biology of Wound Repair*, 2nd ed. (Clark, R. A. F., ed.) Plenum, New York, pp. 3–50.
2. Ornitz, D. M. and Itoph, N. (2001) Fibroblast growth factors. *Genome Biol.* **2**, 3005.1–3005.12.
3. Werner, S. (1998) The role of fibroblast growth factors in skin morphogenesis and wound repair, in *Epithelial Morphogenesis in Development and Disease* (Birchmeier, C. and Birchmeier, W., eds.), Harwood Academic, GMBH, Chur, Switzerland, p. 233.
4. Johnson, D. E. and Williams, L. T. (1993) Structural and functional diversity in the FGF receptor multigene family. *Adv. Cancer Res.* **60**, 1–41.

5. Rosenquist, T. A. and Martin, G. R. (1996) Fibroblast growth factor signalling in the hair growth cycle: expression of the fibroblast growth factor receptor and ligand genes in the murine hair follicle. *Dev. Dyn.* **205,** 379–386.

6. Abraham, L. A. and Klagsbrun, M. (1996) Modulation of wound repair by members of the fibroblast growth factor family, in *The Molecular and Cellular Biology of Wound Repair*, 2nd ed. (Clark, R. A. F., ed.), Plenum, New York, pp. 195–248.

7. Miki, T., Bottaro, D. P., Fleming, T. P., Smith, C. L., Burgess, W. H., Chan, A. M., and Aaronson, S. A. (1992) Determination of ligand-binding specificity by alternative splicing: two distinct growth factor receptors encoded by a single gene. *Proc. Natl. Acad. Sci. USA* **89,** 246–250.

8. Werner, S., Peters, K. G., Longaker, M. T., Fuller-Pace, F., Banda, M., and Williams, L. T. (1992) Large induction of keratinocyte growth factor expression in the dermis during wound healing. *Proc. Natl. Acad. Sci. USA* **89,** 6896–6900.

9. Marchese, C., Chedid, M., Dirsch, O. R., Csaky, K. G., Santanelli, F., Latini, C., LaRochelle, W. J., Torrisi, M. R., and Aaronson, S. A. (1995) Modulation of keratinocyte growth factor and its receptor in re-epithelialising human skin. *J. Exp. Med.* **182,** 1369–1376.

10. Ueno, H., Colbert, H., Escobedo, J. A., and Williams, L. T. (1991) Inhibition of PDGF β-receptor by co-expression of a truncated receptor. *Science* **252,** 844–848.

11. Honegger, A. M., Schmidt, A., Ullrich, A., and Schlessinger, J. (1990) Evidence for epidermal growth factor (EGF)-induced intermolecular autophosphorylation of the EGF receptors in living cells. *Mol. Cell Biol.* **10,** 4035–4044.

12. Kashles, O., Yarden, Y., Fischer, R., Ullrich, A., and Schlessinger, J. (1991) A dominant negative mutation suppresses the function of normal epidermal growth factor receptors by heterodimerisation. *Mol. Cell Biol.* **11,** 1454–1463.

13. Mathieu, M., Chatelain, E., Ornitz, D., Bresnick, J., Mason, I., Kiefer, P., and Dickson, C. (1995) Receptor binding and mitogenic properties of mouse fibroblast growth factor 3: modulation of response by heparin. *J. Biol. Chem.* **41,** 24,197–24,203.

14. Yamasaki, M., Miyake, A., Tagashira, S., and Itoh, N. (1996) Structure and expression of the rat mRNA encoding a novel member of the fibroblast growth factor family. *J. Biol. Chem.* **271,** 15,918–15,921.

15. Werner, S., Smola, H., Liao, X., Longaker, M. T., Krieg, T., Hofschneider, P. H., and Williams, L. T. (1994) The function of KGF in epithelial morphogenesis and wound re-epithelialisation. *Science* **266,** 819–822.

16. Guo, L., Degenstein, L., and Fuchs, E. (1996) Keratinocyte growth factor is required for hair development but not for wound healing. *Genes Dev.* **10,** 165–175.

17. Beer, H. D., Florence, C., Dammeier, J., McGuire, L., Werner, S., and Duan, D. R. (1997) Mouse fibroblast growth factor 10: cDNA cloning, protein characterization, and regulation of mRNA expression. *Oncogene* **15,** 2211–2218.

18. Barrandon, Y. and Green, H. (1987) Cell migration is essential for sustained growth of keratinocyte colonies: the roles of transforming growth factor-α and epidermal growth factor. *Cell* **50,** 1131–1137.

19. Schultz, G. S., White, M., Mitchell, R., Brown, G., Lynch, J., Twardzik, D. R., and Todaro, G. J. (1987) Epithelial wound healing enhanced by transforming growth factor-α and vaccinia growth factor. *Science* **235,** 350–352.

20. Mann, G. B., Fowler, K. J., Gabriel, A., Nice, E. C., Williams, R. L., and Dunn, A. R. (1993) Mice with a null mutation of the TGFα gene have abnormal skin architecture, wavy hair, and curly whiskers and often develop corneal inflammation. *Cell* **73,** 249–261.

21. Luetteke, N. C., Qiu, T. H., Peiffer, R. L., Oliver, P., Smithies, O., and Lee, D. C. (1993) TGFα deficiency results in hair follicle and eye abnormalities in targeted and waved-1 mice. *Cell* **73,** 263–278.

22. Marikovsky, M., Breuing, K., Liu, P. Y., Eriksson, E., Higashiyama, S., Farber, P., Abraham, J., and Klagsbrun, M. (1993) Appearance of heparin-binding EGF-like growth factor in wound fluid as a response to injury. *Proc. Natl. Acad. Sci. USA* **90,** 3889–3893.

23. Sibilia, M. and Wagner, E. F. (1995) Strain-dependent epithelial defects in mice lacking the EGF receptor. *Science* **269,** 234–238.

24. Miettinen, P. J., Berger, J. E., Meneses, J., Phung, Y., Pedersen, R. A., Werb, Z., and Derynck, R. (1995) Epithelial immaturity and multiorgan failure in mice lacking epidermal growth factor receptor. *Nature* **376,** 337–341.

25. Murillas, R., Larcher, F., Conti, C. J., Santos, M., Ullrich, A., and Jorcano, J. L. (1995) Expression of a dominant negative mutant of epidermal growth factor receptor in the epidermis of transgenic mice elicits striking alterations in hair follicle development and skin structure. *EMBO J.* **14,** 5216–5223.

26. Bikfalvi, A., Klein, S., Pintucci, G., and Rifkin, D. B. (1997) Biological roles of fibroblast growth factor-2. *Endocr. Rev.* **18,** 26–45.

27. Ortega, S., Ittmann, M., Tsang, S. H., Ehrlich, M., and Basilico, C. (1998) Neuronal defects and delayed wound healing in mice lacking fibroblast growth factor 2. *Proc. Natl. Acad. Sci. USA* **95,** 5672–5677.

28. Gibran, N. S., Isik, F. F., Heimbach, D. M., and Gordon, D. (1994) Basic fibroblast growth factor in the early human burn wound. *J. Surg. Res.* **56,** 226–234.

29. McGee, G. S., Davidson, J. M., Buckley, A., Sommer, A., Woodward, S. C., Aquino, A. M., Barbour, R., and Demetriou, A. A. (1988) Recombinant basic fibroblast growth factor accelerates wound healing. *J. Surg. Res.* **45,** 145–153.

30. Hebda, P. A., Klingbeil, C. K., Abraham, J. A., and Fiddes, J. C. (1990) Basic fibroblast growth factor stimulation of epidermal wound healing in pigs. *J. Invest. Dermatol.* **95,** 626–631.

31. Tsuboi, R. and Rifkin, D. B. (1990) Recombinant basic fibroblast growth factor stimulates wound healing in healing-impaired db/db mice. *J. Exp. Med.* **172,** 245–251.

32. Broadley, K. N., Aquino, A. M., Woodward, S. C., Buckley-Sturrock, A., Sato, Y., Rifkin, D. B., and Davidson, J. M. (1989) Monospecific antibodies implicate basic fibroblast growth factor in normal wound repair. *Lab. Invest.* **61,** 571–575.

33. Massagué, J. (1990) The transforming growth factor-β family. *Annu. Rev. Cell Biol.* **6,** 597–641.

34. Massague, J. and Wotton, D. (2000) Transcriptional control by the TGF-beta/Smad signaling system. *EMBO J.* **19**, 1745–1754.
35. Roberts, A. B. and Sporn, M. B. (2001) Transforming growth factor-β, in *The Molecular and Cellular Biology of Wound Repair*, 2nd ed. (Clark, R. A. F., ed.), Plenum, New York, pp. 275–308.
36. Levine, J. H., Moses, H. L., Gold, L. I., and Nanney, L. B. (1993) Spatial and temporal patterns of immunoreactive TGF-β1, β2, β3 during excisional wound repair. *Am. J. Pathol.* **143**, 368–380.
37. Frank, S., Madlener, M., and Werner, S. (1996) Transforming growth factors β1, β2, and β3 and their receptors are differentially regulated during normal and impaired wound healing. *J. Biol. Chem.* **271**, 10,188–10,193.
38. Shah, M., Foreman, D. M., and Ferguson, M. W. J. (1994) Neutralising antibody to TGF-β1,2 reduces cutaneous scarring in adult rodents. *J. Cell Sci.* **107**, 1137–1157.
39. Shah, M., Foreman, D. M., and Ferguson, M. W. J. (1995) Neutralisation of TGF-β1 and TGF-β2 or exogenous addition of TGF-β3 to cutaneous rat wounds reduces scarring. *J. Cell Sci.* **108**, 985–1002.
40. Brown, R. L., Ormsby, I., Doetschman, T. C., and Greenhalgh, D. G. (1995) Wound healing in the transforming growth factor-β1-deficient mouse. *Wound Rep. Reg.* **3**, 25–36.
41. Shull, M. M., Ormsby, I., Kier, A. B., Pawlowski, S., Diebold, R. J., Yin, M., Allen, R., Sidman, C., Proetzel, G., Calvin, D., Annunziata, N., and Doetschman, T. (1992) Targeted disruption of the mouse transforming growth factor-β1 gene results in multifocal inflammatory disease. *Nature* **359**, 693–699.
42. Kulkarni, A. B., Huh, C.-G., Becker, D., Geiser, A., Lyght, M., Flanders, K. C., Roberts, A. B., Sporn, M. B., Ward, J. M., and Karlsson, S. (1993) Transforming growth factor β1 null mutation in mice causes excessive inflammatory response and early death. *Proc. Natl. Acad. Sci. USA* **90**, 770–774.
43. Letterio, J. J., Geiser, A. G., Kulkarni, A. B, Roche, N. S., Sporn, M. B., and Roberts, A. B. (1994) Maternal rescue of transforming growth factor-β1 null mice. *Science* **264**, 1936–1938.
44. Greenhalgh, D. G. and Gamelli, R. L. (1987) Is impaired wound healing caused by infection or nutritional depletion? *Surgery* **102**, 306–312.
45. Reed, B. R. and Clark, R. A. (1985) Cutaneous tissue repair: practical implications of current knowledge. II. *J. Am. Acad. Dermatol.* **13**, 919–941.
46. Crowe, M. J., Doetschman, T., and Greenhalgh, D. G. (2000) Delayed wound healing in immunodeficient TGF-beta 1 knockout mice. *J. Invest. Dermatol.* **115**, 3–11.
47. Shah, M., Revis, D., Herrick, S., Baillie, R., Thorgeirson, S., Ferguson, M., and Roberts, A. (1999) Role of elevated plasma transforming growth factor-beta1 levels in wound healing. *Am. J. Pathol.* **154**, 1115–1124.
48. Massague, J. (1998) TGF-beta signal transduction. *Annu. Rev. Biochem.* **67**, 753–791.
49. Derynck, R., Zhang, Y., and Feng, X. H. (1998) Smads: transcriptional activators of TGF-beta responses. *Cell* **95**, 737–740.

50. Ashcroft, G. S. and Roberts, A. B. (2000) Loss of Smad3 modulates wound healing. *Cytokine Growth Factor Rev.* **11,** 125–131.

51. Christian, J. L. and Nakayama, T. (1999) Can't get no SMADisfaction: Smad proteins as positive and negative regulators of TGF-beta family signals. *Bioessays* **21,** 382–390.

52. Weinstein, M., Yang, X., Li, C., Xu, X., Gotay, J., and Deng, C. X. (1998) Failure of egg cylinder elongation and mesoderm induction in mouse embryos lacking the tumor suppressor smad2. *Proc. Natl. Acad. Sci. USA* **95,** 9378–9383.

53. Yang, X., Castilla, L. H., Xu, X., Li, C., Gotay, J., Weinstein, M., Liu, P. P., and Deng, C. X. (1999) Angiogenesis defects and mesenchymal apoptosis in mice lacking SMAD5. *Development* **126,** 1571–1580.

54. Ashcroft, G. S., Yang, X., Glick, A. B., Weinstein, M., Letterio, J. L., Mizel, D. E., Anzano, M., Greenwell-Wild, T., Wahl, S. M., Deng, C., and Roberts, A. B. (1999) Mice lacking Smad3 show accelerated wound healing and an impaired local inflammatory response. *Nat. Cell Biol.* **1,** 260–266.

55. Hocevar, B. A., Brown T. L., and Howe, P. H. (1999) TGF-beta induces fibronectin synthesis through a c-Jun N-terminal kinase-dependent, Smad4-independent pathway. *EMBO J.* **18,** 1345–1356.

56. Matzuk, M. M., Kumar, T. R., Vassalli, A., Bickenbach, J. R., Roop, D. R., Jaenisch, R., and Bradley, A. (1995) Functional analysis of activins during mammalian development. *Nature* **374,** 354–356.

57. Matzuk, M. M., Lu, N., Vogel, H., Sellheyer, K., Roop, D. R., and Bradley, A. (1995) Multiple defects and perinatal death in mice deficient in follistatin. *Nature* **374,** 360–363.

58. Hübner, G., Hu, Q., Smola, H., and Werner, S. (1996) Strong induction of activin expression after injury suggests an important role of activin in wound repair. *Dev. Biol.* **173,** 490–498.

59. Munz, B., Smola, H., Engelhardt, F., Bleuel, K., Brauchle, M., Lein, I., Evans, L. W., Huylebroeck, D., Balling, R., and Werner, S. (1999) Overexpression of activin A in the skin of transgenic mice reveals new activities of activin in epidermal morphogenesis, dermal fibrosis and wound repair. *EMBO J.* **18,** 5205–5215.

60. Lyons, K. M., Pelton, R. W., and Hogan, B. L. (1989) Patterns of expression of murine Vgr-1 and BMP-2a RNA suggest that transforming growth factor-beta-like genes coordinately regulate aspects of embryonic development. *Genes Dev.* **3,** 1657–1668.

61. Blessing, M., Schirmacher, P., and Kaiser, S. (1996) Overexpression of bone morphogenetic protein-6 (BMP-6) in the epidermis of transgenic mice: inhibition or stimulation of proliferation depending on the pattern of transgene expression and formation of psoriatic lesions. *J. Cell Biol.* **135,** 227–239.

62. Kaiser, S., Schirmacher, P., Philipp, A., Protschka, M., Moll, I., Nicol, K., and Blessing, M. (1998) Induction of bone morphogenetic protein-6 in skin wounds: delayed reepitheliazation and scar formation in BMP-6 overexpressing transgenic mice. *J. Invest. Dermatol.* **111,** 1145–1152.

63. Paquet, P. and Pierard, G. E. (1996) Interleukin-6 and the skin. *Int. Arch. Allergy Immunol.* **109,** 308–317.
64. Sato, M., Sawamura, D., Ina, S., Yaguchi, T., Hanada, K., and Hashimoto, I. (1999) In vivo introduction of the interleukin 6 gene into human keratinocytes: induction of epidermal proliferation by the fully spliced form of interleukin 6, but not by the alternatively spliced form. *Arch. Dermatol. Res.* **291,** 400–404.
65. Grossman, R. M., Krueger, J., Yourish, D., Granelli-Piperno, A., Murphy D. P., May, L. T., Kupper, T. S., Sehgal, P. B., and Gottlieb, A. B. (1989) Interleukin 6 is expressed in high levels in psoriatic skin and stimulates proliferation of cultured human keratinocytes. *Proc. Natl. Acad. Sci. USA* **86,** 6367–6371.
66. Gallucci, R. M., Simeonova, P. P., Matheson, J. M., Kommineni, C., Guriel, J. L., Sugawara, T., and Luster, M. I. (2000) Impaired cutaneous wound healing in interleukin-6-deficient and immunosuppressed mice. *FASEB J.* **14,** 2525–2531.
67. Bromberg, J. (2001) Activation of STAT proteins and growth control. *Bioessays* **23,** 161–169.
68. Takeda, K., Noguchi, K., Shi, W., Tanaka, T., Matsumoto, M., Yoshida, N., Kishimoto, T., and Akira, S. (1997) Targeted disruption of the mouse Stat3 gene leads to early embryonic lethality. *Proc. Natl. Acad. Sci. USA* **94,** 3801–3804.
69. Sano, S., Itami, S., Takeda, K., Tarutani, M., Yamaguchi, Y., Miura, H., Yoshikawa, K., Akira, S., and Takeda, J. (1999) Keratinocyte-specific ablation of Stat3 exhibits impaired skin remodeling, but does not affect skin morphogenesis. *EMBO J.* **18,** 4657–4668.
70. Devalaraja, M. N. and Richmond, A. (1999) Multiple chemotactic factors: fine control or redundancy? *Trends Pharmacol. Sci.* **20,** 151–156.
71. Engelhardt, E., Toksoy, A., Goebeler, M., Debus, S., Brocker, E. B., and Gillitzer, R. (1998) Chemokines IL-8, GROalpha, MCP-1, IP-10, and Mig are sequentially and differentially expressed during phase-specific infiltration of leukocyte subsets in human wound healing. *Am. J. Pathol.* **153,** 1849–1860.
72. Luster, A. D., Cardiff, R. D., MacLean, J. A., Crowe, K., and Granstein, R. D. (1998) Delayed wound healing and disorganized neovascularization in transgenic mice expressing the IP-10 chemokine. *Proc. Assoc. Am. Physicians* **110,** 183–196.
73. Fivenson, D. P., Faria, D. T., Nickoloff, B. J., Poverini, P. J., Kunkel, S., Burdick, M., and Streiter, R. M. (1997) Chemokine and inflammatory cytokine changes during chronic wound healing. *Wound Rep. Reg.* **5,** 310–322.
74. Cacalano, G., Lee, J., Kikly, K., Ryan, A. M., Pitts-Meek, S., Hultgren, B., Wood, W. I., and Moore, M. W. (1994) Neutrophil and B cell expansion in mice that lack the murine IL-8 receptor homolog. *Science* **265,** 682–684.
75. Devalaraja, R. M., Nanney, L. B., Qian, Q., Du, J., Yu, Y., Devalaraja, M. N., and Richmond, A. (2000) Delayed wound healing in CXCR2 knockout mice. *J. Invest. Dermatol.* **115,** 234–244.
76. Martin, P. (1997) Wound healing—aiming for perfect skin regeneration. *Science* **276,** 75–81.

77. Liechty, K. W., Kim, H. B., Adzick, N. S., and Crombleholme, T. M. (2000) Fetal wound repair results in scar formation in interleukin-10-deficient mice in a syngeneic murine model of scarless fetal wound repair. *J. Pediatr. Surg.* **35**, 866–872; discussion: 872,873.

78. Eckes, B., Colucci-Guyon, E., Smola, H., Nodder, S., Babinet, C., Krieg, T., and Martin, P. (2000) Impaired wound healing in embryonic and adult mice lacking vimentin. *J. Cell Sci.* **113**, 2455–2462.

79. McCluskey, J. and Martin, P. (1995) Analysis of the tissue movements of embryonic wound healing—DiI studies in the limb bud stage mouse embryo. *Dev. Biol.* **170**, 102–114.

80. Brock, J., McCluskey, J., Baribault, H., and Martin, P. (1996) Perfect wound healing in the keratin 8 deficient mouse embryo. *Cell. Motil. Cytoskel.* **35**, 358–366.

81. Rajewsky, K., Gu, H., Kuhn, R., Betz, U. A., Muller, W., Roes, J., and Schwenk, F. (1996) Conditional gene targeting. *J. Clin. Invest.* **98**, 600–603.

82. Indra, A. K., Warot, X., Brocard, J., Bornert, J. M., Xiao, J. H., Chambon, P., and Metzger, D. (1999) Temporally-controlled site-specific mutagenesis in the basal layer of the epidermis: comparison of the recombinase activity of the tamoxifen- inducible Cre-ER(T) and Cre-ER(T2) recombinases. *Nucleic Acids Res.* **27**, 4324–4327.

83. Vasioukhin, V., Degenstein, L., Wise, B., and Fuchs, E. (1999) The magical touch: genome targeting in epidermal stem cells induced by tamoxifen application to mouse skin. *Proc. Natl. Acad. Sci. USA* **96**, 8551–8556.

84. Wang, X. J., Liefer, K. M., Tsai, S., O'Malley, B. W., and Roop, D. R. (1999) Development of gene-switch transgenic mice that inducibly express transforming growth factor beta1 in the epidermis. *Proc. Natl. Acad. Sci. USA* **96**, 8483–8488.

85. Guo, L., Degenstein, L., Dowling, J., Yu, Q.-C., Wollman, R., Perman, B., and Fuchs, E. (1995) Gene targeting of BPAG1: abnormalities in mechanical strength and cell migration in stratified epithelia and neurologic degeneration. *Cell* **81**, 233–243.

86. Abbott, R. E., Corral, C. J., MacIvor, D. M., Lin, X., Ley, T. J., and Mustoe, T. A. (1998) Augmented inflammatory responses and altered wound healing in cathepsin G-deficient mice. *Arch. Surg.* **133**, 1002–1006.

87. Kaya, G., Rodriguez, I., Jorcano, J. L., Vassalli, P., and Stamenkovic, I. (1997) Selective suppression of CD44 in keratinocytes of mice bearing an antisense CD44 transgene driven by a tissue-specific promoter disrupts hyaluronate metabolism in the skin and impairs keratinocyte proliferation. *Genes Dev.* **11**, 996–1007.

88. Hansen, L. A., Alexander, N., Hogan, M. E., Sundberg, J. P., Dlugosz, A., Threadgill, D. W., Magnuson, T., and Yuspa, S. H. (1997) Genetically null mice reveal a central role for epidermal growth factor receptor in the differentiation of the hair follicle and normal hair development. *Am. J. Pathol.* **150**, 1959–1975.

89. Bugge, T. H., Kombrinck, K. W., Flick, M. J., Daugherty, C. C., Danton, M. J., and Degen, J. L. (1996) Loss of fibrinogen rescues mice from the pleiotropic effects of plasminogen deficiency. *Cell* **87**, 709–719.

90. Bezerra, J. A., Carrick, T. L., Degen, J. L., Witte, D., and Degen, S. J. F. (1998) Biological effects of targeted inactivation of hepatocyte growth factor-like protein in mice. *J. Clin. Invest.* **101,** 1175–1183.

91. Huang, X., Griffiths, M., Wu, J., Farese, R.V. Jr., and Sheppard, D. (2000) Normal development, wound healing, and adenovirus susceptibility in beta5-deficient mice. *Mol. Cell. Biol.* **20,** 755–759.

92. Wojcik, S. M., Bundman, D. S., and Roop, D. R. (2000) Delayed wound healing in keratin 6a knockout mice. *Mol. Cell. Biol.* **20,** 5248–5255.

93. Di Colandrea, T., Wang, L., Wille, J., D'Armiento, J., and Chada, K. K. (1998) Epidermal expression of collagenase delays wound-healing in transgenic mice. *J. Invest. Dermatol.* **111,** 1029–1033.

94. Bullard, K. M., Lund, L., Mudgett, J. S., Mellin, T. N., Hunt, T. K., Murphy, B., Ronan, J., Werb, Z., and Banda, M. J. (1999) Impaired wound contraction in stromelysin-1-deficient mice. *Ann. Surg.* **230,** 260–265.

95. Atit, R. P., Crowe, M. J., Greenhalgh, D. G., Wenstrup, R. J., and Ratner, N. (1999) The Nf1 tumor suppressor regulates mouse skin wound healing, fibroblast proliferation, and collagen deposited by fibroblasts. *J. Invest. Dermatol.* **112,** 835–842.

96. Lee, P. C., Salyapongse, A. N., Bragdon, G. A., Shears, L. L. 2nd, Watkins, S. C., Edington, H. D., and Billiar, T. R. (1999) Impaired wound healing and angiogenesis in eNOS-deficient mice. *Am. J. Physiol.* **277,** H1600–H1608.

97. Yamasaki, K., Edington, H. D., McClosky, C., Tzeng, E., Lizonova, A., Kovesdi, I., Steed, D. L., and Billiar, T. R. (1998) Reversal of impaired wound repair in iNOS-deficient mice by topical adenoviral-mediated iNOS gene transfer. *J. Clin. Invest.* **101,** 967–971.

98. Liaw, L., Birk, D. E., Ballas, C. B., Whitsitt, J. S., Davidson, J. M., and Hogan, B. L. (1998) Altered wound healing in mice lacking a functional osteopontin gene (spp1). *J. Clin. Invest.* **101,** 1468–1478.

99. Dougherty, K. M., Pearson, J. M., Yang, A. Y., Westrick, R. J., Baker, M. S., and Ginsburg, D. (1999) The plasminogen activator inhibitor-2 gene is not required for normal murine development or survival. *Proc. Natl. Acad. Sci. USA* **96,** 686–691.

100. Connolly, A. J., Suh, D. Y., Hunt, T. K., and Coughlin, S. R. (1997) Mice lacking the thrombin receptor, PAR1, have normal skin wound healing. *Am. J. Pathol.* **151,** 1199–1204.

101. Romer, J., Bugge, T. H., Pyke C., Lund, L. R., Flick, M. J., Degen, J. L., and Dano, K. (1996) Impaired wound healing in mice with a disrupted plasminogen gene. *Nat. Med.* **2,** 287–292.

102. Subramaniam, M., Saffarpour, S., Van-de-Water, L., Frenette, P. S., Mayadas, T. N., Hynes, R. O., and Wagner, D. D. (1997) Role of endothelial selectins in wound repair. *Am. J. Pathol.* **150,** 1701–1709.

103. Andersen, B., Weinberg, W. C., Rennekampff, O., et al. (1997) Functions of the POU domain genes Skn-1a/i and Tst-1/Oct-6/SCIP in epidermal differentiation. *Genes Dev.* **11,** 1873–1884.

104. Ashcroft, G. S., Lei, K., Jin, W., Longenecker, G., Kulkarni, A. B., Greenwell-Wild, T., Hale-Donze, H., McGrady, G., Song, X. Y., and Wahl, S. M. (2000) Secretory leukocyte protease inhibitor mediates non-redundant functions necessary for normal wound healing. *Nat. Med.* **6,** 1147–1153.

105. Echtermeyer, F., Streit, M., Wilcox-Adelman, S., Saoncella, S., Denhez, F., Detmar, M., and Goetinck, P. F. (2001) Delayed wound repair and impaired angiogenesis in mice lacking syndecan-4. *J. Clin. Invest.* **107,** R9–R14.

106. Forsberg, E., Hirsch, E., Frohlich, L., Meyer, M., Ekblom, P., Aszodi, A., Werner, S., and Fassler, R. (1996) Skin wounds and severed nerves heal normally in mice lacking tenascin-C. *Proc. Natl. Acad. Sci. USA* **93,** 6594–6599.

107. Peterson, J. J., Rayburn, H. B., Lager, D. J., Raife, T. J., Kealey, G. P., Rosenberg, R. D., and Lentz, S. R. (1999) Expression of thrombomodulin and consequences of thrombomodulin deficiency during healing of cutaneous wounds. *Am. J. Pathol.* **155,** 1569–1575.

108. Raife, T. J, Lager, D. J., Peterson, J. J., Erger, R. A., and Lentz, S. R. (1998) Keratinocyte-specific expression of human thrombomodulin in transgenic mice: effects on epidermal differentiation and cutaneous wound healing. *J. Invest. Med.* **46,** 127–133.

109. Streit, M., Velasco, P., Riccardi, L., Spencer, L., Brown, L.F., Janes, L., Lange-Asschenfeldt, B., Yano, K., Hawighorst, T., Iruela-Arispe, L., and Detmar, M. (2000) Thrombospondin-1 suppresses wound healing and granulation tissue formation in the skin of transgenic mice. *EMBO J.* **19,** 3272–3282.

110. Kyriakides, T. R., Tam, J. W., and Bornstein, P. (1999) Accelerated wound healing in mice with a disruption of the thrombospondin 2 gene. *J. Invest. Dermatol.* **113,** 782–787.

111. Carmeliet, P., Schoonjans, L., Kieckens, L., Ream, B., Degen, J., Bronson, R., De Vos, R., van den Oord, J. J., Collen, D., and Mulligan, R. C. (1994) Physiological consequences of loss of plasminogen activator gene function in mice. *Nature* **368,** 419–424.

112. Bugge, T. H., Flick, M. J., Danton, M. J., Daugherty, C. C., Romer, J., Dano, K., Carmeliet, P., Collen, D., and Degen, J. L. (1996) Urokinase-type plasminogen activator is effective in fibrin clearance in the absence of its receptor or tissue-type plasminogen activator. *Proc. Natl. Acad. Sci. USA* **93,** 5899–5904.

113. Inada, R., Matsuki, M., Yamada, K., Morishima, Y., Shen, S., Kuramoto, N., Yasuno, H., Takahashi, K., Miyachi, Y., and Yamanishi, K. (2000) Facilitated wound healing by activation of the transglutaminase 1 gene. *Am. J. Pathol.* **157,** 1875–1882.

114. Jang, Y. C., Tsou, R., Gibran, N. S., and Isik, F. F. (2000) Vitronectin deficiency is associated with increased wound fibrinolysis and decreased microvascular angiogenesis in mice. *Surgery* **127,** 696–704.

16

Wound Repair in Aging

A Review

May J. Reed, Teruhiko Koike, and Pauli Puolakkainen

1. Introduction

The purpose of this chapter is to review the changes in wound healing that occur in the aged. Unlike pathological conditions such as infection or diabetes as a cause for impaired wound repair, aging may simply reduce the speed at which an individual heals. Thus, a goal of this review is to assess whether aging represents truly impaired or merely slowed wound healing.

This chapter focuses on cutaneous wound healing in response to an acute incisional wound, as after surgery, or an acute excisional wound, as after a punch biopsy. Although the general principles that follow will be relevant for most tissues, there are age-associated alterations in certain organs of the body (e.g., sclerosis of the kidney and large blood vessels) that create unique challenges during wound repair. These changes are generally confounded by diseases (such as diabetes) that are more prevalent with age and are, therefore, beyond the scope of this review. Moreover, this review does not address chronic wounds or pressure wounds, pathological conditions that are accentuated by, but not unique to, aged tissue.

2. Alterations in Aging Skin

Human skin or the epidermis (primarily squamous epithelial cells or keratinocytes), dermis (largely fibroblasts and an extracellular matrix [ECM] of collagens I and III, elastin, and glycosaminoglycans), subcutaneous fat, and associated appendages (hair follicles, sensory receptors, sweat and sebaceous glands). As the largest organ of the body, the skin has a critical role as the

From: *Methods in Molecular Medicine, vol. 78: Wound Healing: Methods and Protocols*
Edited by: Luisa A. DiPietro and Aime L. Burns © Humana Press Inc., Totowa, NJ

protective barrier from environmental insults. As such, it is not surprising that in the absence of injury, changes in the skin with age have primarily cosmetic consequences. However, age does have a detrimental effect on the skin's reserves and subsequent response to injury. Although changes caused by intrinsic aging have been recognized in the skin of elderly individuals for many decades, only recently have these changes been analyzed independently of chronic environmental insults such as sun exposure *(1)*.

To provide a framework for a review of aging and wound healing, this chapter begins with a summary of how age affects the morphology and function of the skin *(2–4)*. As the outermost layer, the epidermis is the first line of defense after tissue injury. The total thickness and the four layers of stratified squamous epithelial cells (keratinocytes) are maintained in aged skin, but the cells become more variable in size, shape, and orientation. In addition, the turnover time, the number of days for keratinocytes in the basal layers of the epidermis to migrate and be shed from the skin surface, increases by 50% in the aged. Other cells in the epidermis such as melanocytes (which provide pigment) and Langerhans cells (which are responsible for the immune response in the epidermis) are also reduced in number. Whereas barrier function against water is maintained in aged skin, there is a significant decrease in the ability of the epidermis to regenerate in response to noxious substances such as ammonia *(5)*.

The dermis of humans and other taut-skin animals is divided into the superficial papillary dermis and the deeper reticular dermis. In aged skin the normal ridges at the epidermal-dermal junction flatten, thereby reducing the contact surface between the epidermis and dermis *(6)*. This loss of surface area results in fewer proliferative epidermal cells in the basal layers and a decrease in the strength of epidermal-dermal adhesion. The generalized atrophy and thinning of the dermis with age is a result of decreases in cell number and changes in the surrounding matrix. The former includes fewer fibroblasts, less vascularization, and a decrease in the population of mast cells and macrophages that function as antigen-presenting cells (APCs) in the dermis (for reviews *see* **refs.** *3* and *7*). Changes in dermal protein content with age include a decrease in collagen, the primary structural protein, as a result of both decreased production and increased degradation *(8–11)*. The physical properties are also altered; whereas collagen in young skin is oriented in ropelike bundles, in aged skin the protein becomes disorganized with randomly oriented bundles that appear to unravel and show variable bundle width. Moreover, in the deeper dermis the fiber density is increased with age owing to a decrease in space between the bundles *(12,13)*. It is controversial as to whether the composition of glycosaminoglycan (e.g., hyaluronic acid and dermatan sulfate) is significantly decreased with age (for review *see* **ref.** *7*). These hydrophilic dermal proteins are referred to as the ground substance of the dermis and provide an optimal

microenvironment for cell adhesion and migration. Glycosaminoglycans also maintain skin turgor, and alterations in this class of dermal proteins in the aged may contribute to a flaccid appearance of the dermis. Elastin, the protein most responsible for maintaining skin elasticity (also termed *recoil*), is a large, highly stable protein with minimal turnover with age. Although elastin content does not decrease significantly (and may actually increase) in the aged, there is a greater prevalence of fibers with a disordered morphology resulting in a loss of cutaneous elasticity. The morphological changes are myriad: there are defects termed *lacunae* and cysts in the elastin fibers; the candelabra-like organization of elastin at the epidermal-dermal junction disappears; and the fibers appear granular, fragmented, and about to disintegrate into fibrils (*12*).

In summary, the decreases in cell number and the discussed changes in the matrix result in the thinning and wrinkles that are so characteristic of aged skin. Accompanying functional changes include compromised vascular responses to stress (e.g., excessive cold or heat) as a result of a diminished dermal microcirculation (*14*). In addition, alterations in skin appendages in the aged result in slowed growth of the hair and nails; decreased secretions from the sweat and sebaceous glands; and diminished sensation to light touch, pressure, and pain.

It has recently been appreciated that most of the undesirable changes in aged skin are the result of chronic environmental damage, in particular long-term ultraviolet (UV) (sun) exposure, superimposed on intrinsic aging. This photoaging process creates a low-grade inflammatory response characterized by amorphosis of elastic fibers, activated dermal fibroblasts, and stimulation of the microvasculature in the form of telangiectasias. Fisher et al. (*1*) have shown that exposure to UV irradiation leads to sustained elevations of matrix metalloproteinases (MMPs), such as collagenase-1, gelatinase B, and stromelysin-1, the primary enzymes that control matrix turnover. As a consequence, repeated exposure to UV irradiation degrades collagen and other skin proteins, resulting in a significantly negative impact on the composition of the ECM. Thus, whereas excess MMP activity was previously attributed to an intrinsic dysregulation of metalloproteinases with aging, it is now generally accepted that UV activation of MMPs contributes significantly to the detrimental changes that occur in aged skin (*4*).

3. Models of Wound Repair in Aging

The study of wound repair in aged humans, in the absence of comorbidities, remains a significant challenge. In addition to a high prevalence of diseases that are more common in the aged, such as diabetes and vascular disease, elderly individuals present with variations in nutritional status and exposure to drugs (both prescription and over the counter) that can affect wound repair

(for reviews, *see* **refs. *15–17***). Relevant nutritional deficiencies that are more common in the aged include vitamin C and zinc. Many medications prescribed to the elderly, such as corticosteroids and anticoagulants/antiplatelet agents, can interfere with healing. Over-the-counter medications and high doses of vitamins, in particular vitamin E, can adversely affect the clotting cascade, thereby altering tissue repair. As already noted, the aged demonstrate large variations in exposure to solar damage. Moreover, it is well known that differences among individuals in a given cohort increase with age. Even in a population that is matched for comorbidities and environmental insults, individuals will have inherent differences in the rate at which their skin will age *(18)*. This is especially the case for studies of the "old-old" (those over 85 yr of age), who are much more difficult to study than "young-old" (65–74 yr) and "middle-old" (75–84 yr) humans.

In contrast to humans, laboratory animals have identical genetic backgrounds and controlled environmental exposures. Thus, they age at similar rates and provide useful models for the study of wound repair in aging. Most of the animals have loose skin (with the exception of pigs) and, therefore, do not closely mimic the taut skin of humans. Moreover, whereas mice develop atrophy of the skin with age, rats do not and some strains of rats exhibit thickened skin. In spite of these limitations, studies of mice, rats, and rabbits have yielded important, and largely reproducible, information on general changes in wound healing that occur with age (for review *see* **ref. *7***). Published models have included 22- to 40-mo-old mice and rats and 48- to 60-mo-old rabbits *(19–23)*. The age at which an animal is defined as aged is dependent on the strain (hybrids often live longer) and environmental factors such as diet (caloric-restricted mice and rats live longer). One accepted guideline is that an animal is definitively "aged" at the point in its life-span that 50% of its age-matched cohort has expired.

In addition to studies in vivo, there are numerous in vitro models for the examination of changes in wound repair that are relevant to aging. These include wound explants from the aforementioned aged animals as well as dermal fibroblasts and keratinocytes from aged human donors *(24,25)*. Cells aged in vitro, via serial passage in culture, provide additional information on cellular changes relevant to aging *(26,27)*. Explants and cells in culture, in contrast to live animals, provide a more feasible method of examining specific cellular functions that are relevant to wound repair such as proliferation, migration, and biosynthesis. These methods are discussed in other chapters of this volume.

4. Alterations in Wound Healing in the Aged

4.1. General

The first published observation of altered wound healing with age can be traced to the reports of DuNouy *(28)*, who assessed healing in soldiers of

different age groups (20–40 yr) during World War I. However, the type of wound, infectious complications, and the overall young age of the patients diminished the validity of his conclusions. Halasz *(29)* reported an increase in the incidence of wound dehiscence with age in 3000 patients having undergone duodenal surgery. Again, concurrent morbidity and infectious complications were not recorded. More recently, the majority of studies have found a delay in healing, but less scarring, in the wounds of aged animals and humans relative to their young counterparts *(19,20,22,23,30,31)*.

Wound healing is generally divided into an early inflammatory phase, a middle phase of proliferation/granulation tissue formation, and a final phase of remodeling (for review *see* **ref. 32**). Whereas **Subheading 4.2.** reviews the effect of age on wound repair in light of those phases, this section reviews general principles of cell and tissue behavior.

Examination of the mechanisms of altered wound repair in aging have found decreases in cell proliferation and migration, deficits in matrix secretion, and a paucity of mitogenic growth factors. Each of the cellular components (keratinocytes, fibroblasts, and endothelial cells) show reduced proliferation in the wounds of aged animals. Early studies demonstrated decreased weight of granulation tissue or delayed appearance of cellular invasion in wounds from older animals *(33,34)*. More recent studies have measured proliferation (using specific markers such as incorporation of the DNA analog bromodeoxyuridine) to specifically document less proliferation of fibroblasts and endothelial cells in the wounds of aged animals relative to young controls *(20,30)*.

Generalized changes in matrix deposition in the wounds of aged animals have also been noted. Viljanto's *(35)* group reported that with increasing age there was a concomitant decrease in the amount of hydroxyproline (a biochemical measure of collagen content/production) incorporated into cellulose sponges within human wound sites. Sussman *(36)* noted thicker wounds associated with greater breaking strength in young rats as compared with old animals. These studies suggested that connective-tissue deposition, especially collagen I, was reduced in the wounds of the aged; more recent data support these findings *(19,20)*.

Fibronectin is a large extracellular protein that has also been examined in aging and wound repair. It functions to regulate inflammation and cell adhesion by providing a provisional matrix, along with hyaluronan and collagen III, during the early phases of wound healing *(37)*. Although aged cells have been associated with an increase in fibronectin synthesis in culture *(38)*, studies of aged tissues and wounds from aged animals have shown a decrease in fibronectin expression in association with reduced levels of collagen *(39,40)*.

Wound healing requires the invasion and migration of cells into the area of injury. As such, the proteolysis of the ECM is requisite for proper repair.

This process is regulated by MMPs that are secreted largely by keratinocytes and fibroblasts. Synthesis and activation of MMPs are controlled by several mechanisms including growth factor stimulation, exposure to the ECM, and changes in pH *(41)*. Among MMPs, the expression of collagenases (MMP-1, MMP-13) stromelysins (MMP-3), and gelatinases (MMP-2, MMP-9) have been reported during wound healing *(42–44)*. Whereas the collagenases degrade intact collagen, the gelatinases break down collagen that has been previously denatured (gelatin). The membrane-type MMPs (MT-MMPs) are not only responsible for the activation of MMP-2 at cell surfaces; recent data have demonstrated collagenase activity from cell-surface MT-MMP during migration into collagen *(45,46)*. In early wound repair, MMP-1 enables keratinocytes to migrate between dermal collagen and the fibrin clot *(42,43,47–49)*. During granulation tissue formation, all the MMPs assist the movement of fibroblasts into crosslinked fibrin and the newly deposited ECM. Angiogenesis, the formation of new vessels from preexisting vasculature, occurs during this time and vascularizes the newly formed granulation tissue. Angiogenesis is also dependent on MMP activity to permit the invasion of microvascular endothelial cells into the structural matrix *(50,51)*.

The activity of MMPs, although necessary, must be tightly controlled. Indeed, an excess of proteolytic activity can destroy the support matrix necessary for cell migration and tissue repair. Long-standing observations have associated nonhealing wounds with excessive proteolytic activity *(52)*. In this context, it is not surprising that slowed healing in the aged has been attributed, in part, to increases in the expression of MMPs and decreases in their natural inhibitors, the tissue inhibitors of metalloproteinases (TIMPs) *(53–57)*. Recently, it has become clear that the changes in proteolytic activity with age are not invariant but are cell and tissue specific. For example, whereas dermal keratinocytes and microvascular endothelial cells show a deficit in MMP-1 synthesis with aging, dermal fibroblasts from aged donors show an excess of MMP-1 secretion *(24,25)*. Moreover, studies of transgenic mice demonstrate that both deficits and excesses in MMP activity can inhibit the healing of acute wounds *(58,59)*. Taken together these data highlight the importance of an optimal level of controlled proteolysis for efficient repair of aged tissues.

Growth factors such as platelet-derived growth factor (PDGF), basic fibroblast growth factor (bFGF), transforming growth factor-β (TGF-β), and vascular endothelial growth factor (VEGF) are expressed in tissues during wound healing *(60–64)*. Although their precise spatial and temporal distribution varies with the model examined, it is generally accepted that these factors perform critical regulatory functions during wound healing. Functional roles assigned to these factors include, but are not limited to, cell proliferation, migration, biosynthesis, and control of the secretion of MMPs and TIMPs. The multifunctional roles assigned to these factors is most notable with TGF-β1; this factor is a chemoattractant to fibroblasts, enhances their deposition of collagen and fibronectin, and decreases the synthesis of MMP-1 at the same time it increases TIMP-1 by these same cells (61,65). With increased age, decreased circulating and tissue levels of most of these factors have been reported and are thought to contribute to altered healing in aging (21,66). Whether the decrease in availability is accompanied by a lack of response to exogenous replacement of these growth factors is controversial. There are numerous reports of deficient growth factor responses, attributed largely to defective receptors, in aged cells and tissues (67–71). However, there are many studies demonstrating that aged cells and tissues are able to respond to stimulation with these same factors (19–21,31,72). For example, dermal fibroblasts from aged donors show a deficit in biosynthesis of collagen and collagen gel contraction, but a similar biosynthetic and contractile response to young donors on stimulation with TGF-β1 (72). TGF-β1 applied to dermal wounds accelerated the healing of wounds in aged rats (19,20). Exogenous replacement of estrogen and VEGF has also been shown to reverse impairments in tissue repair and vascularization (21,31). Indeed, a recent study has demonstrated that topical replacement of estrogen in the skin of elderly females can indirectly enhance expression of TGF-β1 in the wound, thereby accelerating healing (31). Observations such as these underscore the complexity of attempting to analyze the effect of any single growth factor on tissue repair in the aged.

4.2. Phases of Wound Healing

Wound healing has traditionally been divided into three phases: inflammatory, granulation tissue formation/proliferative, and remodeling (32). The division is arbitrary and the phases overlap. However, this classification serves to highlight different components of a very complex process; in this section we present additional aspects of altered wound repair in aging utilizing the guidelines provided by this division.

4.2.1. Inflammatory Phase

After injury, the initial inflammatory phase of wound repair is characterized by formation of a fibrin clot, activation of platelets with subsequent release of platelet-derived factors, and an influx of macrophages followed closely by lymphocytes. The activation of circulating and resident cell populations results in the release of soluble mediators such as tumor necrosis factor-α (TNF-α), interleukins, nitric oxide (NO), and growth factors. In addition, epithelial closure (epithelialization) and wound contraction begin in this early stage.

There is a consensus that the inflammatory response is altered with age. However, whether this response is increased or decreased depends on the aspect of inflammation that is examined (for review *see* **ref. 7**). Older studies have shown that aging increases the aggregation of platelets and the adhesion of endothelial cells to monocytes *(73–75)*, changes that could enhance the initial stages of the inflammatory response. Moreover, aged mononuclear cells have been shown to produce increased amounts of the inflammatory mediators interleukin-6 (IL-6) and TNF-α in response to stress *(76)*. By contrast, aged cells release less of the potent vasoactive messenger NO *(21)*. Old skin clearly shows a decrease in the number and function of APCs such as Langerhans cells and mast cells, thereby leading to impaired cell-mediated immunity in stimulated tissues. With age there is a delay in the appearance of monocytes and macrophages during wound repair *(40)*. Age decreases neutrophil respiratory burst activity and the capacity for glucose utilization in lymphocytes and macrophages *(77,78)*. Danon et al. *(79)* demonstrated a functional decline in macrophages during wound healing in aged mice. In their study the application of peritoneal macrophages from young mice to the cutaneous wounds of the aged mice accelerated the repair to rates comparable with those of young animals. Although the number of lymphocytes in the circulation is unchanged, there is a defect in activation and a subsequent delay in the appearance of immunoreactive cells in inflamed tissues in aged humans *(80,81)*.

In summary, the inflammatory phase of wound healing in the aged is associated with an increase in platelet aggregation and endothelial-monocyte adhesion. With the exception of NO, the release of inflammatory mediators is maintained and may be increased. However, the number and function of macrophages and lymphocytes in aged skin is reduced, and their appearance in wounds is delayed.

Epithelialization is critical for wound closure and is dependent on both proliferation and migration. Animal studies have demonstrated that the rate of reepithelialization in the palatal mucosa of aged rats *(82)* and in partial-thickness wounds in old mice is decreased *(83)*. In humans, Grove and colleagues *(5,84)* showed delayed epithelialization and epithelial turnover in an older cohort 65–75 yr of age; as expected, there was significant variability among the aged individuals. Holt et al. *(85)* found a more rapid rate of reepithelialization of superficial split-thickness wounds in subjects ages 18–55 yr as compared with a group of patients over age 65. Recently it has been noted that in addition to reduced proliferation, keratinocytes from aged donors demonstrate significantly slowed migration on type I collagen *(25)*. Thus, under the stress of a wound, both the proliferation and migration of keratinocytes are decreased in aged skin.

4.2.2. Proliferative Phase

The granulation tissue formation or proliferative phase involves nearly every cell type in the skin. Fibroblasts from the surrounding dermis migrate into the injured site and are responsible for contraction, proliferation, and deposition of ECM. Keratinocytes continue the process of reepithelialization. Dermal microvascular endothelial cells, in conjunction with supporting cells such as fibroblasts, enhance blood flow via the process of angiogenesis.

Fibroblasts migrate into the wound area in response to growth factors and signals from the provisional matrix (fibrin and fibronectin) approx 2–4 d after injury. Their major role is the synthesis of an ECM comprising primarily collagen. Whereas fibroblasts deposit type III collagen as part of the provisional matrix early in wound repair, it is their subsequent secretion of type I collagen that provides a structural support for healing. This biosynthetic function is compromised in the wounds of aged persons and may be owing, in part, to a lack of TGF-β1. In addition to secretion of ECM, fibroblasts are the major cell type responsible for wound contraction. Older experimental studies in rabbits, rats, and dogs indicate that in older as compared with younger animals the time before initiation of wound contraction is lengthened, the rate of contraction is lower, and the ultimate degree of contraction is less (for review *see* **ref. 7**). In general, the changes in fibroblast function during wound repair in aging are as follows: proliferation is decreased, migration is often slowed, the capacity to synthesize growth factors (such as TGF-β1 and VEGF) declines, and the response to exogenous growth factors is often preserved *(19,21,24,66,86)*.

Capillaries in the skin comprise microvascular endothelial cells. In the basal state there are fewer capillaries in aged skin *(4)*. Delayed angiogenesis, the formation of new capillaries from existing capillaries, is thought to contribute to slowed wound healing in aging. Holm-Pedersen (*see* **refs. 33,34,** and **87**) was among the first to report that the rate of capillary growth in wounded tissues was decreased in older animals. This decline in neovascularization has been attributed to both decreased endothelial cell proliferation and migration. Other age-related defects in endothelial cell behavior include increased adhesion to leukocytes, enhanced response to TNF-α, and greater IL-1 production *(7,74,75)*. Several studies have specifically examined delayed angiogenesis in aged animals and have found, as expected, reduced levels of angiogenic factors such as TGF-β1 and VEGF *(21,65)*. Replacement of these deficient factors increased angiogenesis *(21,86)*. The extrapolation to enhanced wound repair as a direct result of increased neovascularization (as opposed to the numerous other changes induced by the application of these angiogenic factors) remains to be proven.

4.2.3. Remodeling Phase

The remodeling phase involves continued proliferation of fibroblasts and deposition of newly synthesized matrix (termed *fibroplasia*), completed neovascularization, and formation of mature scar. Collagen (primarily type I) is produced and remodeled throughout this phase, which can last as long as 1 to 2 yr.

Wounds in the aged produce less scarring as compared with young subjects *(31)*. Furthermore, hyperproliferative wound-healing disorders such as keloids and hypertrophic scars are rare in the older population. This is a result, at least in part, of reduced levels of TGF-β in the wounds of the aged. As noted previously, TGF-β is known to enhance net collagen deposition both by increasing its synthesis and by decreasing its degradation. The latter is a result of the effect of TGF-β1 on increasing the secretion of TIMP at the same time it inhibits the production of the primary collagenase, MMP-1 *(65,88)*. In fact, in an experimental study, the use of neutralizing TGF-β antibody was able to prevent excessive scar formation in adult wounds *(89)*. Consistent with these data, Ashcroft et al. *(31)* have shown that treatment with topical estrogen accelerated healing, owing to increased expression of TGF-β1, but resulted in decreased scar quality.

There is a lack of controlled studies of the mechanical properties of healing wounds in the aged. The tensile strength of a wound reflects the organization of the remodeling process and is related to the wound's thickness. By contrast, breaking strength is purely a measure of the ability of a wound to resist disruption. In the past, uncontrolled observations of human postsurgical wounds have noted an increased rate of wound disruption with age, but there was no accounting for concurrent morbidity *(90)*. Animal studies are difficult to interpret because of differences in skin thickness among rodents (whereas mice develop a thinner skin with age, certain strains of rats do not), variability in the definition of mechanical disruption, confounding by other interventions, and small numbers. It is now accepted that wounds in the healthy aged have adequate tensile strength despite an intrinsic decrease in the rate of collagen synthesis relative to the young. Indeed, normal human skin maintains extensibility to the seventh decade; this is in contrast to elasticity, which decreases from an earlier age *(91)*. In both the young and aged, it is important to remember that the tensile strength of a healed wound will never be more than 80% of that of normal, uninjured skin.

In summary, in the absence of comorbidities, there is no conclusive evidence that the mechanical properties of healed wounds in the aged differ significantly from those of the young, but there are no data on very old humans.

5. Clinical Aspects of Wound Healing in the Aged

5.1. Relevance

This chapter has reviewed the healing of acute wounds in the aged. Although significant changes do occur, the clinical impact of aging on wound healing in this scenario is minimal in comparison to the detrimental effects of age on the healing of chronic wounds such as pressure ulcers and ulcers associated with venous hypertension, diabetes, and vascular insufficiency. Thus, the ultimate goal of studies of wound repair in aging is not to alter the course of acute wounds, but to provide information that will contribute to the treatment of chronic wounds in the aged.

5.2. Clinical Issues

Diseases that affect wound healing are more prevalent in the elderly and have a greater adverse effect on healing than in young adults. Thus, concomitant medical problems should be treated vigorously to allow for maximum healing. Moreover, a careful review of medications that can impact wound repair must be performed. The recent increased use among older persons of herbs and over-the-counter products that can affect the clotting cascade (vitamin E, gingko), the absorption of other nutrients, calcium, and the skin itself must be taken into account. Nutritional status also impacts the healing of wounds in the aged (*16*). When to intervene in this area is of great controversy. It is generally accepted that aggressive nutritional intervention and repletion of vitamins and minerals is of value in those who have clear biochemical parameters of deficiency such as hypoalbuminemia or lymphopenia. However, there is no consensus on how to detect an inadequate nutritional state or mineral deficiency in those with normal laboratory values. The latter are usually serum samples; thus, standard assays would fail to detect deficiencies that are present at the tissue level of wound repair.

5.3. Prospects for the Future

The past decade has witnessed a tremendous number of studies that focused on the local or systemic application of mitogenic growth factors as a method to accelerate wound repair in aged animals and other models of altered healing. The factors examined included TGF-β1, bFGF, and PDGF as well as many others and were largely shown to be of benefit in animal models (*21,61,62,93*). Since aged animals demonstrate an approx 40% delay in wound healing relative to their young counterparts (*20*), it is estimated that to be clinically relevant and cost-effective, the acceleration in healing induced by a growth factor should be at least 20–30%. Unfortunately, with the exception of the data on topical use of estrogen (*[31]*; for review *see* **ref. 94**) and PDGF in certain chronic wounds

(92), recent studies on the use of single growth factors in humans have been largely disappointing. Whether a combination of growth factors should be used to enhance wound healing in the aged as a prophylactic or therapeutic measure remains to be evaluated by extensive randomized studies. Thus, our current knowledge does not support their routine use.

In addition to the use of mitogenic factors and hormones that directly affect the behavior of cells in the wound, there is great interest in mechanical means to alter the cellular and extracellular environment of wound repair in the aged *(94)*. Interventions include skin substitutes, grafts, alteration of the matrix with artificial matrices or enzymatic digestion, placement of electrical fields to encourage cell recruitment, devices to change the wound's temperature or ambient oxygen content, and vacuum pumps to minimize the retention of wound fluid. Whether one examines studies of growth factors, hormones, or mechanical devices, it is clear that for any given intervention there may be a subgroup of patients who would benefit even if a study shows no significant effect on a larger scale. This is especially true for more chronic wounds such as pressure ulcers and those that result from diabetes and vascular disease.

In the future, continued advances in molecular biology will undoubtedly lead to additional novel therapies to accelerate wound repair. Studies of the molecular biology of aging are yielding new insights into aging in vivo in skin and other tissues. Initial experiments utilized cells aged in culture (by serial passage) and demonstrated that somatic cells, such as dermal fibroblasts, have a finite ability to undergo cell division. This process was termed *replicative* or *cellular senescence* and provided the foundation for advances in the cell biology of aging *(95)*. Although a causal relationship between cellular senescence and organismic aging in vivo has not been established, recent data indicate that senescent cells could negatively impact aging skin and subsequent wound healing in the aged. Dimri et al. *(96)* have shown that there is an increase in the number of cells that express SA-β-galactosidase, a marker of senescence, in both the dermis and epidermis of aged human skin. Keratinocytes and fibroblasts aged in vitro, by serial passage in culture, and those derived from aged human donors show similar age-related declines in proliferation and migration as well as dysregulation of matrix synthesis and proteolysis *(24–27,97)*.

In addition, there is great interest in the role of telomeres in cellular aging in vitro and in vivo *(98)*. The telomere is the structure at the ends of chromosomes that progressively shortens as cells divide. When the chromosomes of a cell decrease to a certain length as a result of this process, the cell can no longer undergo cell division and becomes senescent. The shortening of telomeres is prevented by the synthetic activities of the ribonucleoprotein enzyme telomerase. Whereas normal human fibroblasts and endothelial cells progressively lose their proliferative capacity in culture, those transfected with

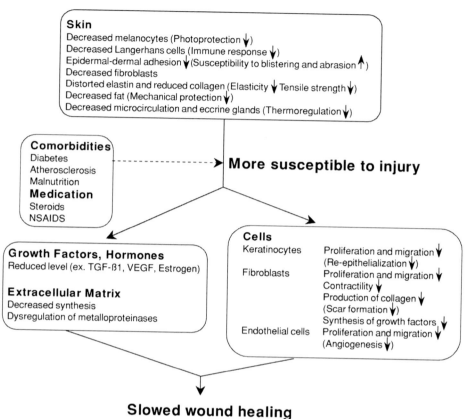

Skin
Decreased melanocytes (Photoprotection ↓)
Decreased Langerhans cells (Immune response ↓)
Epidermal-dermal adhesion ↓ (Susceptibility to blistering and abrasion ↑)
Decreased fibroblasts
Distorted elastin and reduced collagen (Elasticity ↓ Tensile strength ↓)
Decreased fat (Mechanical protection ↓)
Decreased microcirculation and eccrine glands (Thermoregulation ↓)

Comorbidities
Diabetes
Atherosclerosis
Malnutrition
Medication
Steroids
NSAIDS

More susceptible to injury

Growth Factors, Hormones
Reduced level (ex. TGF-ß1, VEGF, Estrogen)

Extracellular Matrix
Decreased synthesis
Dysregulation of metalloproteinases

Cells
Keratinocytes — Proliferation and migration ↓ (Re-epithelialization ↓)
Fibroblasts — Proliferation and migration ↓
Contractility ↓
Production of collagen ↓ (Scar formation ↓)
Synthesis of growth factors ↓
Endothelial cells — Proliferation and migration ↓ (Angiogenesis ↓)

Slowed wound healing

Fig. 1. Drawing illustrates interacting factors that contribute to slowed wound healing in the aged. Solid lines represent components that are intrinsic to aging and largely unavoidable. The dashed line represents risk factors that are not part of normal aging, but are more prevalent in the aged.

telomerase retain their capacity to divide *(98–100)*. In telomerase-deficient mice, progressive telomere shortening occurs after four to six generations of breeding of homozygous-deficient mice. These mice subsequently become sterile, show decreased life expectancy, and demonstrate deficits in wound healing *(101)*. Although skin cells have a minimal requirement for replication in the uninjured state, telomerase-transfected cells have the potential to enhance the proliferation of aged tissues during wound repair *(102)*.

In addition to advances in gene therapy, there is great interest in the use of stem cells for targeted delivery into injured tissues *(103–104)*. It is now accepted that stem cells exist in the marrow and other organs of adult humans, thereby greatly expanding the therapeutic possibilities in even the oldest individuals. In the future, gene therapy, stem cells, and other interventions to maintain a young phenotype in aged tissues will result in the development of novel treatments for wounds in the aged.

6. Conclusion

Aging has adverse effects on wound healing (*see* **Fig. 1**). The effects are related to delayed epithelialization, diminished contraction, slowed angiogenesis, and decreased collagen deposition. However, there are neither new events nor an absence of expected events. Therefore, the healing response is ultimately adequate, albeit delayed. We conclude from this review that wound healing in the aged is simply slowed rather than impaired.

Acknowledgments

We wish to thank Margaret Hamner for her assistance with the manuscript. This work was supported by the Paul Beeson Physician Scholars Program, National Institutes of Health (RO1AG15837 and T32AG00057), American Heart Association, Helsinki University Central Hospital Research Fund, and Japan Foundation for Aging and Health.

References

1. Fisher, G. J., Wang, Z., Datta, S. C., Varani, J., Kang, S., and Voorhees, J. J. (1997) Pathophysiology of premature skin aging induced by ultraviolet light. *N. Engl. J. Med.* **347,** 1419–1428.
2. Frenske, N. A. and Lober, C. W. (1986) Structural and functional changes of normal aging skin. *J. Am. Acad. Dermatol.* **15,** 571–585.
3. Jacobson, R. G. and Flowers, F. P. (1996) Skin changes with aging and disease. *Wound Rep. Reg.* **4,** 311–315.
4. Gilchrest, B. A. (1998) Aging of the skin, in *Principles of Geriatric Medicine and Gerontology* (Hazzard, W. R., Blass, H. P., Ettinger, W. H., Halter, J. B., and Ouslander, J. G., eds.), McGraw-Hill, New York, pp. 573–590.
5. Grove, G. L. (1982) Age-related differences in healing of superficial skin wounds in humans. *Arch. Dermatol. Res.* **272,** 381–385.
6. Kurban, R. S. and Bhavan, J. (1990) Histologic changes in skin associated with aging. *J. Dermatol. Surg. Oncol.* **16,** 908–914.
7. Ashcroft, G. S., Horan, M. A., and Ferguson, M. W. J. (1995) The effects of ageing on cutaneous wound healing in mammals. *J. Anat.* **187,** 1–26.
8. Shuster, S., Black, M. M., and McVitie, E. (1975) The influence of age and sex on skin thickness, skin collagen and density. *Br. J. Dermatol.* **93,** 639–643.
9. Johnson, B. D., Page, R. C., Narayanan, A. S., and Pieters, H. P. (1986) Effects of donor age on protein and collagen synthesis in vitro by human diploid fibroblasts. *Lab. Invest.* **55,** 490–496.

10. West, M. D., Pereira-Smith, O. M., and Smith, J. S (1989) Replicative senescence of human skin fibroblasts correlates with a loss of regulation and overexpression of collagenase activity. *Exp. Cell. Res.* **184,** 138–147.

11. Mays, P. K., McAnulty, R. J., Campa, J. S., and Lauent, G. J. (1991) Age-related changes in collagen synthesis and degradation in rat tissues. *Biochem. J.* **276,** 301–313.

12. Lavker, R. M., Zheng, P., and Dong, G. (1987) Aged skin: a study by light, transmission electron, and scanning electron microscopy. *J. Invest. Dermatol.* **88,** 44–51.

13. Lovell, C. R., Smolenski K. A., Duance, V. C., Light, N. D., Young, S., and Tyson, M. (1987) Type I and III collagen content and fiber distribution in normal human skin during ageing. *J. Dermatol.* **117,** 419–428.

14. Marin, J. (1995) Age-related changes in vascular responses: a review. *Mech. Ageing Dev.* **79,** 71–114.

15. Van de Kerkhof, P. C., Van Bergen, B., Spruijt, K., and Kuiper, J. P. (1994) Age-related changes in wound healing. *Clin. Exp. Dermatol.* **16,** 369–374.

16. Thomas, D. R. (1997) The role of nutrition in prevention and healing of pressure ulcers. *Clin. Geriatr. Med.* **13,** 497–511.

17. Ernst, E. (2000) Adverse effects of herbal drugs in dermatology. *Br. J. Dermatol.* **143,** 923–929.

18. Williams, M. E. (1998) Approach to managing the elderly patient, in *Principles of Geriatric Medicine and Gerontology* (Blass, H. P., Ettinger, W. H., Halter, J. B., Hazzard, W. R., and Ouslander, J. G., eds.), McGraw-Hill, New York, pp. 249–253.

19. Beck, L. S., DeGuzman, L., Lee, W. P., Xu, Y., Siegel, M. W., and Amento, E. P. (1993) One systemic administration of transforming growth factor-$\beta 1$ reverses age- or glucocorticoid-impaired wound healing. *J. Clin. Invest.* **92,** 2841–2849.

20. Puolakkainen, P. A., Reed, M. J., Gombotz, W. R., Twardzik, D. R., Abrass, I. B., and Sage, E. H. (1995) Acceleration of wound healing in rats by topical application of transforming growth factor-$\beta 1$. *Wound Rep. Reg.* **3,** 330–339.

21. Rivard, A., Fabre, J., Silver, M., Chen, D., Murohara, T., Kearney, M., Magner, M., Asahara, T., and Isner, J. (1999) Age-dependent impairment of angiogenesis. *Circulation* **99,** 111–120.

22. Swift, M. E., Hynda, K. K., and DiPietro, L. A. (1999) Impaired wound repair and delayed angiogenesis in aged mice. *Lab. Invest.* **79,** 1479–1487.

23. Wu, L., Xia, Y., Roth, S. I., Gruskin, E., and Mustoe, T. A. (1999) Transforming growth factor-$\beta 1$ fails to stimulate wound healing and impairs its signal transduction in an aged ischemic ulcer model. *Am. J. Pathol.* **154,** 301–309.

24. Reed, M. J., Ferara, N., and Vernon, R. B. (2001) Impaired migration, integrin function, and actin cytoskeletal organization in dermal fibroblasts from a subset of aged human donors. *Mech. Age. Dev.* **122,** 1203–1220.

25. Xia, Y. P., Zhao, Y., Tyrone, J. W., Chen, A., and Mustoe, T. A. (2001) Differential activation of migration by hypoxia in keratinocytes isolated from donors of

increasing age: implications for chronic wounds in the elderly. *J. Invest. Dermatol.* **116,** 50–56.

26. Schneider, E. L. and Mitsui, Y. (1976) The relationship between in vitro cellular aging and in vivo human age. *Proc. Natl. Acad. Sci. USA* **73,** 3584–3588.
27. Takeda, K., Gasiewska, A., and Peterkofsky, B. (1992) Similar, but not identical, modulation of expression of extracellular matrix components during in vitro and in vivo aging of human skin fibroblasts. *J. Cell. Physiol.* **153,** 450–459.
28. DuNouy, P. (1916) The relation between the age of the patient, the area of the wound, and the index of cicatrisation. *J. Exp. Med.* **xxiv,** 461–470.
29. Halasz, N. A. (1968) Dehiscence of laparotomy wounds. *Am. J. Surg.* **116,** 210–214.
30. Reed, M. J., Penn, P. E., Li, Y., Birnbaum, R., Vernon, R. B., Johnson, T. S., Pendergrass, W. R., Sage, E. H., Abrass, I. B., and Wolf, N. S. (1996) Enhanced cell proliferation and biosynthesis mediate improved wound repair in refed, caloric-restricted mice. *Mech. Age. Dev.* **89,** 21–43.
31. Ashcroft, G., Dodsworth, J., van Boxtel, E., Tarnuzzer, R. W., Horan, M. A., Schultz, G. S., and Ferguson, M. W. J. (1997) Estrogen accelerates cutaneous wound healing associated with an increase in TGF-beta 1 levels. *Nat. Med.* **3,** 1209–1215.
32. Singer, A. J. and Clark, R. A. (1999) Mechanisms of disease: cutaneous wound healing. *N. Engl. J. Med.* **341,** 738–746.
33. Holm-Pedersen, P., Nilsson, K., and Branemark, P. I. (1973) The microvascular system of healing wounds in young and old rats. *Adv. Microcirc.* **5,** 80–106.
34. Yamaura, H. and Matsuzawa, T. (1980) Decrease in capillary growth during aging. *Exp. Gerontol.* **15,** 145–150.
35. Viljanto, J. (1969) A sponge implantation method for testing connective tissue regeneration in surgical patients. *Acta. Chir. Scand.* **135,** 297–300.
36. Sussman, M. D. (1973) Aging of connective tissue and physical properties of healing wounds in young and old rats. *Am. J. Physiol.* **224,** 1167–1171.
37. Grinnell, F., Billingham, R. E., and Burgess, L. (1981) Distribution of fibronectin during wound healing in vivo. *J. Invest. Dermatol.* **76,** 181–189.
38. Kumazaki, T., Kobayashi, M., and Mitsui, Y. (1993) Enhanced expression of fibronectin during in vivo cellular aging of human vascular endothelial cells and skin fibroblasts. *Exp. Cell. Res.* **205,** 396–402.
39. Vitellaro-Zuccarello, L., Garbelli, R., and Rossi, V. D. P. (1992) Immunocytochemical localization of collagen types I, III, IV and fibronectin in the human dermis. *Cell Tissue Res.* **268,** 505–511.
40. Ashcroft, G. S., Horan, M. A., and Ferguson, M. W. (1998) Aging alters the inflammatory and endothelial cell adhesion molecule profiles during human cutaneous wound healing. *Lab. Invest.* **78,** 47–58.
41. Nagasi, H. and Woessner, J. F. (1999) Matrix metalloproteinases. *J. Biol. Chem.* **274,** 21,491–21,494.
42. Porras-Reyes, B. H., Blair, H. C., Jeffrey, J. J., and Mustoe, T. A. (1991) Collagenase production at the border of granulation tissue in healing wound: macrophage and mesechymal collagenase production in vivo. *Connect. Tissue Res.* **27,** 63–71.

43. Saarialho-Kere, U., Kovacs, S., Pentland, A., Olerud, J., Welgus, H., and Parks, W. (1993) Cell-matrix interactions modulate interstitial collagenase expression by human keratinocytes actively involved in wound healing. *J. Clin. Invest.* **92,** 2858–2866.

44. Salo, T., Sorsa, T., Lauhio, A., Konttinen, Y. T., Ainamo, A., Kjeldson, L., Borregaard, N., Ranta, H., and Lahdevirta, J. (1994) Expression of matrix metalloproteinase-2 and -9 during early human wound healing. *Lab. Invest.* **70,** 176–182.

45. Okada, A., Tomasetto, C., Lutz, Y., Bellocq, J., Rio, M., and Basset, P. (1997) Expression of matrix metalloproteinases during rat skin wound healing: evidence that membrane type-1 matrix metalloproteinase is a stromal activator of pro-gelatinase A. *J. Cell. Biol.* **137,** 67–77.

46. Hotary, K., Allen, E., Punturieri, A., Yana, I., and Weiss, S. J. (2000) Regulation of cell invasion and morphogenesis in a three-dimensional type I collagen matrix by membrane-type matrix metalloproteinases 1, 2, and 3. *J. Cell. Biol.* **149,** 1309–1323.

47. Inoue, M., Kratz, G., Haegerstrand, A., and Stahle-Backdahl, M. (1995) Collagenase expression is rapidly induced in wound-edge keratinocytes after injury in human skin, persists during healing, and stops at re-epithelialisation. *J. Invest. Dermatol.* **104,** 479–483.

48. Planus, E., Galiacy, S., Matthay, M., Laurent, V., Gavrilovic, J., Murphy, G., Clerici, C., Isabey, D., Lafuma, C., and d'Ortho, M. P.(1999) Role of collagenase in mediating in vitro alveolar epithelial wound repair. *J. Cell. Sci.* **112,** 243–252.

49. Pilcher, B., Dumin, J., Dudbeck, B., Krane, S., Welgus, H., and Parks, W. (1997) The activity of collagenase-1 is required for keratinocyte migration on a type I collagen matrix. *J. Cell. Biol.* **137,** 1445–1457.

50. Cornelius, L., Nehring, L., Roby, J., Parks, W., and Welgus, H. (1995) Human dermal microvascular endothelial cells produce matrix metalloproteinases in response to angiogenic factors and migration. *J. Invest. Dermatol.* **105,** 170–176.

51. Reed, M. J., Corsa, A., Kudravi, S., McCormick, R., and Arthur, W. T. (2000) A deficit in collagenase activity contributes to impaired migration of aged microvascular endothelial cells. *J. Cell. Biochem.* **77,** 116–126.

52. Wysocki, A. B., Staiano-Coico, L., and Grinnell, F. (1993) Wound fluid from chronic leg ulcers contains elevated levels of metalloproteinases MMP-2 and MMP-9. *J. Invest. Dermatol.* **101,** 64–68.

53. Millis, A., McCue, H., Kumar, S., and Baglio, C. (1992) Differential expression of metalloproteinase and TIMP-1 gene expression during replicative senescence. *Exp. Geront.* **27,** 425–428.

54. Zeng,, G. and Millis, A. (1994) Expression of 72-kDa gelatinase and TIMP-2 in early and late passage human fibroblasts. *Exp. Cell. Res.* **213,** 148–155.

55. Zeng, G. and Millis, A. (1996) Differential regulation of collagenase and stromelysin mRNA in late passage cultures of human fibroblasts. *Exp. Cell. Res.* **222,** 250–256.

56. Ashcroft, G., Herrick, S., Tarnuzzer, R., Horan, M., Schultz, G., and Ferguson, M. (1997) Human ageing impairs injury-induced in vivo expression of tissue

inhibitor of matrix metalloproteinases (TIMP)-1 and -2 proteins and mRNA. *J. Pathol.* **183**, 169–176.

57. Ashcroft, G., Horan, M., Herrick, S., Tarnusser, R., Schultz, G., and Ferguson, M. (1997) Age-related differences in the temporal and spatial regulation of matrix metalloproteinases (MMPs) in normal skin and acute cutaneous wounds of healthy humans. *Cell Tissue Res.* **290**, 581–591.

58. Bullard, K. M., Lund, L., Medgett, J. S., Mellin, T. N., Hunt, T. K., Murphy, B., Ronan, J., Werb, Z., and Banda, M. J. (1999) Impaired wound contraction in stromelysin-1-deficient mice. *Ann. Surg.* **230**, 260–265.

59. DiColandrea, T., Wang, L., Wille, J., D'Armiento, J., and Chada, K. K. (1998) Epidermal expression of collagenase delays wound-healing in transgenic mice. *J. Invest. Dermatol.* **111**, 1029–1033.

60. Antoniades, H. N., Galanopoulos, T., Neville-Golden, J., Kiritsy, C. P., and Lynch, S. E. (1991) Injury induces in vivo expression of platelet-derived growth factor (PDGF) and PDGF receptor mRNAs in skin epithelial cells and PDGF mRNA in connective tissue fibroblasts. *Proc. Natl. Acad. Sci. USA* **88**, 565–569.

61. Roberts, A. B., Sporn, M. B., Assoian, R. K., Smith, J. M., Roche, N. S., Wakefield, L. M., Heine, U. I., Liotta, L. A., Falanga, V., Kehrl, J. H., and Fauci, A. S. (1986) Transforming growth factor type-beta: rapid induction of fibrosis and angiogenesis in vivo and stimulation of collagen formation in vitro. *Proc. Natl. Acad. Sci. USA* **83**, 4167–4171.

62. Broadley, K. N., Aquino, A. M., Woodward, S. C., et al. (1989) Monospecific antibodies implicate bFGF in normal wound repair. *Lab. Invest.* **5**, 571–575.

63. Pierce, G. F., Tarpley, J., Yangihara, D., Mustoe, T. A., Fox, G. M., and Thomason, A. (1992) PDGF-BB, TGF-beta 1, and basic FGF in dermal wound healing: neovessel and matrix formation and cessation of repair. *Am. J. Pathol.* **140**, 1375–1388.

64. Brown, L. F., Yeo, K. T., Berse, B., et al. (1992) Expression of vascular permeability factor (vascular endothelial growth factor) by epidermal keratinocytes during wound healing. *J. Exp. Med.* **176**, 1375–1379.

65. Edwards, D. R., Murphy, G., Reynolds, J. J., Whitham, S. E., Docherty, A. J. P., Angel, P., and Heath, J. K. (1987) Transforming growth factor beta modulates the expression of collagenase and metalloproteinase inhibitor. *EMBO J.* **6**, 1899–1904.

66. Reed, M. J., Corsa, A., Penn, P., Pendergrass, W., Sage, E. H., and Abrass, I. B. (1998) Neovascularization of sponge implants in aged mice: delayed angiogenesis is coincident with decreased levels of TGF-β1 and type I collagen. *Am. J. Pathol.* **152**, 113–123.

67. Stanulis-Praeger, B. M. and Gilchrest, B. A. (1986) Growth factor responsiveness declines during adulthood for human skin-derived cells. *Mech. Ageing Dev.* **35**, 185–198.

68. Matsuda, T., Okamura, K., Sato, Y., Morimoto, A., Ono, M., Kohno, K., and Kuwano, M. (1992) Decreased response to epidermal growth factor during cellular

senescence in cultured human microvascular endothelial cells. *J. Cell. Physiol.* **150**, 510–516.

69. Phillips, P. D., Kaji, K., and Cristofalo, V. J. (1984) Progressive loss of the proliferative response of senescing W1-38 cells to platelet-derived growth factor, epidermal growth factor, insulin, transferrin and dexamethasone. *J. Gerontol.* **39**, 11–17.

70. Garfinkel, S., Hu, X., Prudovsky, I. A., McMahon, G. A., Kapnik, E. M., McDowell, S. D., and Maciag, T. (1996) FGF-1-dependent proliferative and migratory responses are impaired in senescent human umbilical vein endothelial cells and correlate with the inability to signal tyrosine phosphorylation of fibroblast growth factor receptor-1 substrates. *J. Cell. Biol.* **134**, 783–791.

71. Shiraha, H., Gupta, K., Drabik, K., and Wells, A. (2000) Aging fibroblasts present reduced epidermal growth factor (EGF) responsiveness due to preferential loss of EGF receptors. *J. Biol. Chem.* **275**, 19,343–19,351.

72. Reed, M. J., Vernon, R. B., Abrass, I. B., and Sage, E. H. (1994) TGF-β1 induces the expression of type 1 collagen and SPARC, and enhances contraction of collagen gels, by fibroblasts from young and aged donors. *J. Cell. Physiol.* **158**, 169–179.

73. Grigorova-Borsos, A. M., Bara, L., Grochuklski, A., et al. (1988) Aging and diabetes increasing the aggregating potency of rat skin collagen towards normal platelets. *Thromb. Haemost.* **60**, 75–78.

74. Molenaar, R., Visser, W. J., Verkerk, A., Koster, J. F., and Jongkind, J. F. (1989) Peroxidative stress and in vitro ageing of endothelial cells increases the monocyte-endothelial cell adherence in a human in vitro system. *Arteriosclerosis* **76**, 193–202.

75. Maier, J. A. M., Statuto, M., and Ragnotti, G. (1993) Senescence stimulates U937-endothelial cell interactions. *Exp. Cell. Res.* **208**, 270–274.

76. Fagiolo, U., Cossarizza, A., Santacaterina, S., et al. (1992) Aging and cellular defence mechanisms. *Ann. NY Acad. Sci.* **663**, 490–493.

77. Lipschitz, D. A. and Udupa, K. B. (1986) Influence of aging and protein deficiency on neutrophil function. *J. Gerontol.* **4**, 690–694.

78. Costa Rosa, L. F. B. P., Almeida, A. F., Safi, D. A., and Curi, R. (1993) Metabolic and functional changes in lymphocytes and macrophages as induced by ageing. *Physiol. Behav.* **53**, 651–656.

79. Danon, D., Kowatch, M. A., and Roth, G. S. (1989) Promotion of wound repair in old mice by local injection of macrophages. *Proc. Natl. Acad. Sci. USA* **86**, 2018–2020.

80. Song, L., Ho Kim, Y., Chopra, R. J., et al. (1993) Age-related effects in T-cell activation and proliferation. *Exp. Gerontol.* **28**, 313–321.

81. Gilhar, A., Aizen, E., Pillar, T., and Eidelman, S. (1992) Response of aged versus young skin to intradermal administration of interferon gamma. *J. Am. Acad. Dermatol.* **27**, 710–716.

82. Butcher, E. O. and Klingsberg, J. (1963) Age, gonadectomy and wound healing in palatal mucosa of the rat. *Oral Surg.* **16**, 482–492.

83. Cox, D., Kunz, S., Cerletti, N., McMaster, G. K., and Burk, R. R. (1992) Wound healing in aged animals: effects of locally applied TGF-beta 2 in different model systems, in *Angiogenesis—Key Principles* (Steiner, R., Weisz, P. B., and Langer, R., eds.), Birkhauser Basel, pp. 287–295.

84. Grove, G. L. and Kligman, A. M. (1983) Age-associated changes in epidermal cell renewal. *Gerontology* **38,** 137–142.

85. Holt, D. R., Kirk, S. J., Regan, M. C., Hurson, M., Lindblad, W. J., and Barbul, A. (1992) Effect of age on wound healing in healthy human beings. *Surgery* **112,** 293–297.

86. Arthur, W. T., Vernon, R. B., Sage, E. H., and Reed, M. J. (1998) Growth factors reverse the impaired sprouting of microvessels from aged mice. *Microvasc. Res.* **55,** 260–270.

87. Holm-Pedersen, P. and Zederfelt, B. (1971) Granulation tissue formation in subcutaneously implanted cellulose sponges in young and old rats. *Scand. J. Plast. Reconstr. Surg.* **5,** 13–16.

88. Edwards, D. R., Leco, K. J., Beaudry, P. P., Atadja, P. W., Veillette, C., and Riabowol, K. T. (1996) Differential effects of transforming growth factor-beta 1 on the expression of matrix metalloproteinases and tissue inhibitors of metalloproteinases in young and old human fibroblasts. *Exp. Gerontol.* **31,** 207–223.

89. Shah, M., Foreman, D. M., and Ferguson, M. W. J. (1992) Control of scarring in adult wounds by neutralizing antibody to transforming growth factor. *Lancet* **339,** 213, 214.

90. Mendoza, C. B. and Postlethwait, R. W. (1970) Incidence of wound disruption following operation. *Arch. Surg.* **101,** 396–398.

91. Escoffier, C., Rigal, J., Rochefort, A., Vasselet, R., Leveque, J. L., and Agache P. G. (1989) Age-related mechanical properties of human skin: an in vivo study. *J. Invest. Dermatol.* **93,** 353–357.

92. Rees, R. S., Robson, M. C. Smiell, J. M., Perry, B. H., and the Pressure Ulcer Study Group (1999) Becaplermin gel in the treatment of pressure ulcers. *Wound Rep. Reg.* **7,** 141–147.

93. Mustoe, T. A., Pierce, G. F., Thomasen, A., Gramates, P., Sporn, M. B., and Deuel, T. F. (1987) Accelerated healing of incisional wounds in rats induced by transforming growth factor-beta. *Science* **237,** 1333–1336.

94. Bello, Y. M. and Phillips, T. J. (2000) Recent advances in wound healing. *JAMA* **283,** 716–718.

95. Hayflick, L. (1965) The limited in vitro lifetime of human diploid cell strains. *Exp. Cell. Res.* **37,** 614–636.

96. Dimri, G. P., Lee, X., Basile, G., Acosta, M., Scott, G., Roskelley, C., Medrano E. E., Linskens, M., Rubeli, I., Pereira-Smith, O., Peacocke, M., and Campisi, J. (1995) A biomarker that identifies senescent human cells in culture and in aging skin in vivo. *Proc. Natl. Acad. Sci. USA* **92,** 9363–9367.

97. Albini, A., Pontz, B., Pulz, M., Allavena, G., Mensing, H., and Muller, P. (1988) Decline of fibroblast chemotaxis with age of donor and cell passage number. *Collagen Rel. Res.* **1,** 23–37.

98. Bodnar, A. G., Ouellette, M., Frolkis, M., Holt, S. E., Chiu, C., Morin, G. B., Harley, C. B., Shay, J. W., Lichtsteiner, S., and Wright, W. E. (1998) Extension of life-span by introduction of telomerase into normal human cells. *Science* **279,** 349–352.
99. Vaziri, H. and Benchimol, S. (1998) Reconstruction of telomerase activity in normal cells leads to elongation of teleomeres and extended replicative life span. *Curr. Biol.* **8,** 279–282.
100. Yang, J., Chang, E., Cherry, A. M., Bangs, C. D., Oei, Y., Bodnar, A., Bronstein, A., Chiu, C. P., and Herron, G. S. (1999) Human endothelial cell life extension by telomerase expression. *J. Biol. Chem.* **274,** 26,141–26,148.
101. Rudolph, K. L., Chang, S., Lee, H.-W., Blasco, M., Gottlieb, G. J., Greider, C., and Depinho, R. A. (1999) Longevity, stress response, and cancer in aging telomerase-deficient mice. *Cell* **96,** 701–712.
102. Fossel, M. (1998) Telomerase and the aging cell. *JAMA* **279,** 1732–1735.
103. Davidson, J. M., Krieg, T., and Eming, S. A. (2000) Particle-mediated gene therapy of wounds. *Wound Rep. Reg.* **8,** 452–459.
104. Kuhnle, I. and Gradell, M. A. (2002) The therapeutic potential of stem cells from adults. *BMJ* **325,** 372–376.

I

EXPERIMENTAL MODELS OF WOUND HEALING

C. HUMAN WOUND HEALING MODELS

17

Specimen Collection and Analysis

Burn Wounds

Areta Kowal-Vern and Barbara A. Latenser

1. Introduction

The incidence of fire deaths in the United States has decreased from 2.5/100,000 population in 1983 to 1.7/100,000 in 1993 *(1)*. In the last century, tremendous strides have occurred in the acute resuscitation of burns, permitting burn clinicians and researchers to concentrate on improving functional outcomes for burn survivors *(2)*. Animal-based laboratory research has contributed to our knowledge of the pathophysiology and microvascular changes in burns *(3)*, and burn wounds have figured prominently in wound-healing studies. One of the difficulties with human burn wound studies, however, has been the uncontrolled circumstance under which a patient acquires the burn wound: What was the temperature? What was the timing? What was the depth or extent?

In contrast to a laboratory burn model, each human burn patient presents with a unique combination of depths of injury, and in some cases with smoke inhalation. Various burn depth studies, utilizing Doppler ultrasound, infrared thermography, and immunofluorescence have not been useful clinically *(4–6)*. The burn surgeon must still rely on his or her clinical assessment of the patient on presentation and during excision and debridement. Although histological evaluations are reliable, they require time and multiple samples to provide an accurate assessment of the total patient. Wound-healing research takes advantage of this modality since tissue is usually available for study once the burn eschar has been excised in preparation for grafting.

From: *Methods in Molecular Medicine, vol. 78: Wound Healing: Methods and Protocols*
Edited by: Luisa A. DiPietro and Aime L. Burns © Humana Press Inc., Totowa, NJ

Table 1
Wound Depth

Parameter	First degree	Second degree	Third degree
Depth	Superficial	Partial thickness	Full thickness
Injured skin layers	Epidermis	Epidermis/partial dermis	Epidermis/dermis
Appearance	Erythema/redness	Erythema/blisters	Whitish/charred/leathery
Sensation	Sensitive/patient withdraws to touch	Extreme pain	Insensate/no feeling

The purpose of this chapter is to assist the researcher in obtaining the appropriate human burn skin samples for intended projects. Three areas are discussed: the phases of burn wound healing *(7–11)*, burn wound specimen collection including controls, and the immunohistochemical protocol utilized. The immunohistochemical method offers a good source of information about cellular infiltrates, since they are an important reference for the study of biological modifiers.

1.1. Normal Skin

As the largest organ in the body, skin is vital for temperature control, cosmetic appearance, and protection against infection and desiccation. It consists of a regenerating outer layer known as the epidermis *(12)*, which consists of the keratinocytes, the major source for the production of cytokines; melanocytes, which are responsible for the pigment; and dendritic histiocytes, which transmit antigenic signals to lymphocytes. In addition, the epidermis is the origin of the sebaceous glands, and adnexa such as hair follicles and sweat glands, which descend into the dermis below. The dermis contains the lymph, blood vessels, pigment, collagen fibers, fibroblasts, perivascular mast cells, dendrocytes, and nerves.

1.2. A Burn

Unlike experiments in a laboratory setting, human burns occur under uncontrolled circumstances and are usually assessed visually and surgically as to depth by the burn surgeon. The postburn response is dynamic with an initial accumulation of cellular infiltrates that generate a transition from the inflammatory phase to the proliferative phase of granulation tissue. Finally, maturation and remodeling ceases 9–12 mo later. The criteria for assessing the depth of injury are provided in **Table 1**. Less common are fourth-degree burns that extend to fascia, and fifth-degree burns that extend to bone.

Burned tissue is destroyed and histologically resembles a pink coagulum of proteins and chemicals that get invaded by neutrophils within 20–30 min, as these cells begin the cleanup and remodeling process (**Fig. 1A**). Even a small burn can initiate a systemic reaction that abates as the dead tissue is removed and an environment conducive to skin regeneration is established. Within 2–4 h after the burn injury, distinct zones of tissue appear. Although the actual burn may last only a few seconds, the destructive inflammatory process set off by the thermal injury may last much longer. This is the reason for the recommendation to cool the burn as soon as possible to stop the burning process. In partial-thickness or second-degree burns, especially if some of the dermis has been preserved, the skin regenerates in pearly white islands as the keratinocytes and adnexal lining cells migrate upward. In deep second and third degree burns, the burned area, or zone of necrosis, is surrounded by the zones of stasis and and erythema, which consist of viable tissue fluctuating between survival and destruction (ranging from 1 to 4 mm in width), and extending from the surface to the tissue underneath the burned area (**Fig. 1C**). Under normal circumstances, part of this area will die, increasing the area injured initially. As regeneration occurs, the epidermis blazes a path forward beneath the dead skin (eschar) (**Fig. 1C**), fortified by the increased cellular infiltration by macrophages and lymphocytes (**Fig. 1D**).

2. Materials

1. Biopsy punches, 5 to 6 mm.
2. Processing/embedding cassettes.
3. Liquid nitrogen.
4. Scalpel.
5. 0.05% Aqueous poly-L-lysine.
6. Xylene.
7. Absolute alcohol.
8. Ethanol; 0.1 mL of concentrated acid in 50 mL of 100% EtOH.
9. Trypsin:
    a. Buffer: Tris (hydroxymethyl) aminomethane base (6 g) and deionized water (900 mL). Add 1 N HCl to obtain pH 7.6. Add deionized water to make 1 L. Store at 4°C.
    b. Solution: Add 50 mg of pancreatic trypsin (T-8128; Sigma, St. Louis, MO) and 50 mg of dihydrate CaCl to 50 mL of Tris buffer, pH 7.6.
10. Ficin: Mix 10 μL of ficin (F-4125; Sigma) with 3 mL of phosphate-buffered saline (PBS).
11. Pepsin: Add one packet of Dako pepsin (cat. no. S3002; Dako, Carpenteria, CA) to 200 mL of deionized water. When dissolved, add 50 mL of 1 N HCl. Store at –20°C.
12. PBS, 10X concentration: monobasic sodium phosphate, monohydrates (50 g); dibasic sodium phosphate, anhydrous (240 g); NaCl (280 g); Tween-20 (4 mL);

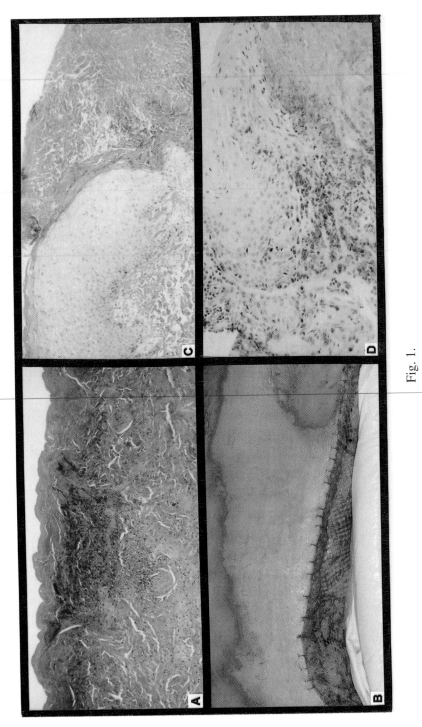

Fig. 1.

and deionized water, to make 4 L. Dilute 1:10 with water to make a working solution.

13. 1% Albumin-saline (PBS-BSA): Bovine serum albumin (BSA), fraction V (1 g), Tween-20 (0.1 mL), and PBS (100 mL). Mix and add, as preservative, sodium azide (50 mg).

14. Streptavidin–horseradish peroxidase (HPP) kits (Kirkegaard-Perry; cat. no. 71-00-18 [mouse, primary]; cat. no. 71-00-19 [rabbit primary]). Each kit contains blocking serum, biotinylated secondary antibody, and streptavidin-HRP conjugate.

15. Diaminobenzidine substrate:
    a. Buffer: Ammonium acetate (3.85 g) and deionized water (900 mL). Add 10% citric acid to obtain pH 5.5. Add water to make 1 L. Store at 4°C.
    b. Substrate solution: Prepare just before using. Add two tablets (10 mg each) of DAB (D-5905; Sigma) for each 50 mL of buffer at room temperature. Allow to dissolve, filter, and add 90 µL of 3% H_2O_2 (H-6520; Sigma) per 50 mL. After use, pour into a bottle containing hypochlorite solution. Treat for 24 h and then dispose via sink. **Hazardous material:** Avoid contact with skin and clothes.

16. Antibodies against immunohistochemical markers are obtained from Dako:
    a. Anti-CD20 (L26) for B-cells.
    b. Anti-CD68 (PG-19) for macrophages.
    c. Anti-CD8 (C8/144B) for cytotoxic T-cells.
    d. Anti-OPD4 (OPD4) for helper T-cells.

17. Harris-type hematoxylin: Solution (nonmercuric) from Newcomer Supply (cat. no. 1201).

Fig. 1. *(facing page)* (**A**) Representative histological section of partial-thickness (2°) burned skin with destruction of epidermal and papillary dermal layers on d 9 postinjury. The tissue surface is nonviable and consists of coagulative necrosis. The acute and chronic cellular infiltrate is part of the inflammatory process that is approaching the surface from the reticular dermis, which is viable (H&E; ×200). (**B**) Photograph of patient with 3° (full-thickness) burn on d 8 after injury. The head and left arm are to the right and the feet are to the left. On the bottom of the patient's side, there is good healing of a meshed skin autograft that has been stapled to the area, once the burned skin was removed or debrided. The white and yellow shiny leathery skin is a full-thickness burn in this area, which is well demarcated from the normal viable tissue by the transitional "zone of stasis," extending into the reddened "zone of erythema," which is part of the local inflammatory response to the injury. (**C**) Representative histological section of burned skin at 28 d postinjury depicting a regenerating epidermis on the left, undermining and removing necrotic skin to provide new surface for injured area. One can appreciate a mononuclear infiltrate at the advancing edge of the newly formed epidermis (H&E, ×200). (**D**) Immunoperoxidase staining with HRP is strongly positive for CD68, which identifies the cells as macrophages (×400).

18. Acid alcohol: 1% HCl in 70% ethanol.
19. 0.1% Ammonia water.
20. Accumount (Stephens, Kalamazoo, MI).

3. Methods
3.1. Specimen Collection
3.1.1. Burn Wound Specimens

Obtain biopsies of burned and unburned skin from patients at the time of debridement and eschar excision, prior to grafting. Skin samples are best obtained from the extremities or torso because these areas provide a good dermal layer for manipulation. Normal skin should not be taken from the face or genital area, to avoid cosmetic complications.

The specimen obtained from the excised burned skin should include the margin between the burned and unburned skin (or zone of stasis and the normal skin). Unburned control skin specimens can be obtained from an area within 5 mm of the zone of stasis; second- and third-degree burn samples are obtained from the area contiguous to the zone of stasis. Small pieces of skin that include the margin between the burned and unburned skin can be removed with a 5- to 6-mm punch biopsy. This biopsy should be deep, extending into the adipose tissue to get a good representative section of the tissue in question. This size of punch biopsy will provide adequate tissue for study and requires only two to three stitches to close the gap created. In addition, it is frequently removed during grafting as part of the eschar.

To get maximum usage out of this skin, the specimen is sectioned perpendicular to the zone of stasis margin to include both types of skin for processing. For comparison studies of normal vs burned skin, each section is further subdivided.

3.1.2. Infected Wound

The burn wound has no innate protection from the environment, so antimicrobial dressings are employed to decrease the rapid colonization of the wound by bacteria, yeast, and/or fungus. Prophylactic antibiotics are not usually administered systemically. However, dressings such as silver sulfadiazine, mafenide acetate, iodine, and Vaseline or Acticoat™, to name a few, are often used. In spite of these measures, the wound may become infected rather than just colonized, and microbial culture may be necessary to make a distinction between the two. Obtaining quantitative cultures per gram of tissue has helped burn surgeons decide between excision and grafting of the area. Thus, if the culture is reported as having 10^5 bacterial count/g of tissue, the wound is

Table 2
Transport and Preservation Medium for Burn Wound Tissue[a]

Procedure	Fresh; no preservative	Fresh; saline	10% Formalin	2.5% Glutaraldehyde	Snap-freezing
DNA and RNA studies	+	+	−	−	+
Western Blot	+	+	−	−	+
ELISA	+	+	−	−	+
Karyotype	+	+	−	−	−
Histology	−	−	+	+	+/−
Immunohistochemistry	−	−	+	+	+/−
In situ hybridization	+	+	+	+	−
Electron microscopy	−	−	−	+	−

[a]Preservation modalities mainly used are formalin, glutaraldehyde, and snap-freezing. ELISA, enzyme-linked immunosorbent assay.

infected and must be treated with antibiotics prior to grafting. On the other hand, a 10^3 bacterial count/g of tissue would be more indicative of only colonization, and, therefore, it would be safe to proceed with the grafting. The recommended culture for microbiological determination of burn wound infection is actually a quantitative culture of burn wound tissue. Swabs are not informative. In obtaining burn tissue for microbial culture, the recommended 1-g sample (postage stamp size) should be removed from the wound edge abutting the normal skin.

3.1.3. Obtaining Specimens

After institutional review board (IRB) approval (*see* **Notes 1–3**), arrangements are made with the surgeon for skin pickup during or after surgery. The researcher should check the operative schedule in the morning to determine whether specimens will be available. Although the researcher may need only a specific piece of skin for the current project, here is an opportunity to maximize the usefulness of the skin sample and establish a skin library or archive by paraffin embedding, plastic embedding, or snap-freezing samples in liquid nitrogen. Tissue transport and storage requirements depend on the experiments planned (**Table 2**) (*see* **Notes 4–10**).

If a thin, ribbon-like section of skin is excised, it should be spread out and rolled on the tips of a forceps, then placed standing in a paraffin-embedding cassette or snap-frozen. Thicker excised skin is cut into 1- to 1.5-cm-wide cross-sections and placed sideways with the cross-section lying flat in the cassette or snap-frozen. In deeper third-degree burns, adipose tissue is present

18

Suction Blister Model of Wound Healing

Vesa Koivukangas and Aarne Oikarinen

1. Introduction

The suction blister model was originally developed for the separation of viable epidermis from dermis by Kiistala *(1)*. Since its development, its use has been expanded and applied to several other applications. One new application assesses the collagen synthesis rate in the human skin in vivo by using the suction blister fluid collected in an assay of collagen propeptides *(2)*. This method is sensitive and can detect changes in collagen synthesis owing to various diseases and topical or systemic therapies. Other applications of the suction blister technique include measurements of pharmacological agents or their derivatives from interstitial fluid, and assays of various enzymes, cytokines, and so on *(3–7)*. Additionally, the suction blister technique has even been used to treat vitiligo by collecting living melanocytes from blister roofs from healthy skin and injecting these into blister cavities induced in diseased skin.

Since the suction blister technique separates epidermis from dermis within the basement membrane *(8)*, this model can also be used to study reepithelization and skin barrier regeneration of superficial wounds of a standard size. The level of separation of epidermis from dermis occurs above type IV collagen, since this collagen remains completely in the blister floor after blistering *(9)*. By contrast, some laminins such as laminin 5 can be found variably in the blister floor and in basal cells of the detached epidermis, indicating that the separation occurs just below the basal cells above the lamina densa layer of basement membrane *(10,11)*.

Epidermal cell proliferation begins at the edge of the wound and the dermal appendages. A few hours after the onset of proliferation, cells start to

From: *Methods in Molecular Medicine, vol. 78: Wound Healing: Methods and Protocols*
Edited by: Luisa A. DiPietro and Aime L. Burns © Humana Press Inc., Totowa, NJ

migrate on the partially intact basement membrane. Simultaneously, the strictly coordinated synthesis of basement membrane components occurs *(10,11)*. The changes in the cytoskeleton and the cell-to-cell and cell-to-matrix connections enable the migration. The process is controlled via cytokines originating from epidermal cells, platelets, fibroblasts, and wound leukocytes.

Reepithelialization can be followed noninvasively by measuring water evaporation from the blister area. One of the main purposes of the epidermis is to restrict water evaporation from the body. Initially water evaporation from a blister wound is 15- to 20-fold compared with basis evaporation from intact skin. When epidermal healing proceeds, water evaporation decreases. This enables noninvasive follow-up of wound healing by measuring the decrease in evaporation (i.e., the restoration of epidermal barrier function). Epithelization can also be followed up by taking skin samples from healing blisters and by studying the samples with appropriate techniques.

Inflammation is an essential part of the healing process. The features of inflammation are increased blood flow in the affected area, leukocyte recruitment, and initiation of regenerative processes. Inflammation is controlled via neuropeptides (e.g., substance P and calcitonin gene-related peptide), prostaglandins, histamine, and various cytokines. The increased blood flow in the blister wound is the result of vasodilatation. The measurement of the level of local inflammation is not straightforward since the phenomenon itself is complex. The level of blood flow in the inflamed area is one reliable parameter. Blood flow can be measured noninvasively using a laser-Doppler flowmeter.

2. Materials

1. Commercially available disposable suction blister devices (Dermovac blistering device; Mucel Co., Nummela, Finland). These are manufactured of butene-styrene, single packed and gamma sterilized. The device contains five holes 6 mm in diameter. The inner diameter of the whole device is 40 mm and the outer diameter, 50 mm. The device is transparent, which makes it easy to observe the blister induction during blistering. It contains a 30-cm rubber tube, which can be connected to a vacuum pump (*see* **Note 1** and **Fig. 1**).
2. A commercially available vacuum pump of the kind generally used in operating rooms. The vacuum pump should be able to generate a vacuum of about 40–70 kPa.
3. Evaporimeter EP1 (Servomed, Stockholm, Sweden). The instrument records the air humidity in an open cylinder probe 12 mm in diameter. The values are given as grams of water evaporation per square meter times hours.
4. Laser-Doppler flowmeter (Periflux Pf 1; Perimed KB, Stockholm, Sweden), for measuring blood flow. The equipment has a multifiber probe 5 mm in diameter. The laser beam penetrates about 1 mm into the tissue. The output signal is relative and shows the number and speed of the blood cells moving in the target area.

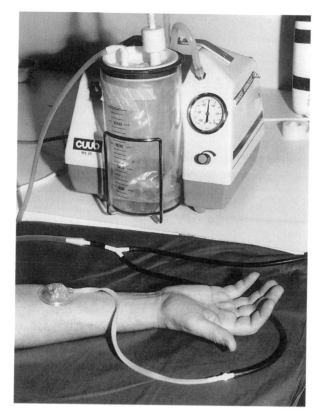

Fig. 1. The suction blister device is attached to the arm and connected to the vacuum pump.

5. Electric lamp (60 W), for warming.
6. Mantoux syringe, to collect blister fluid.
7. 10% Buffered formalin, for fixing tissue samples.

3. Methods

3.1. Suction Blister Induction

1. Suction blisters can be induced on the body, arms, and legs. We have not induced them in the head or facial skin. Make sure that the skin is clean, and remove any hair (*see* **Notes 2** and **3**).
2. Connect the suction blister device to a vacuum pump, and place the device tightly on the skin while turning on the vacuum. The vacuum should be increased to about 50 kPa, so that the device sticks tightly to the skin. Thereafter, it is not necessary to hold the device manually (*see* **Note 4**).

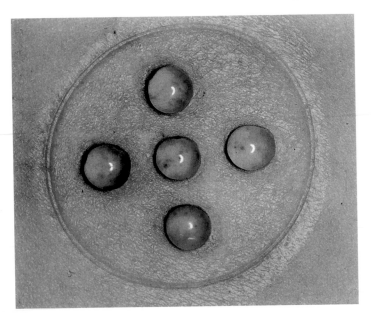

Fig. 2. Fully developed suction blisters.

3. To induce blisters, warming of the skin is essential. Place the lamp about 30 cm above the blistering area. It is important not to burn the skin, but only warm to it *(12)*.
4. Check the induction of blisters about 30 min after the application of vacuum. At this time point, it is possible to see tiny blisters rising from the holes. Remember, do not stop the vacuum or remove the blistering device when checking blistering. It usually takes about 40–120 min for the blisters to be fully developed (**Fig. 2**). Blistering time is dependent on the vacuum and warming of the skin *(12)* (*see* **Notes 5** and **6**).
5. When the blisters are fully developed, turn off the vacuum and carefully remove the suction blister device, so that the blisters do not break.

3.2. Analyses

When the blisters are fully developed, there are several possible analyses to perform, depending on the study design.

3.2.1. Open Blister

To follow the reepithelization of open wounds, the blister roofs should be removed carefully with scissors and pincers. The blister roofs are composed of living cells, which can be used for cell culturing, mRNA analysis, and so on. Before the blister roofs are removed, it is possible to collect blister fluid from the blisters using a mantoux syringe. From one blister it is possible to get 20–50 µL of blister fluid, which means that five blisters contain up to 250 µL of blister fluid, which can be used to analyze cytokines, enzymes, or collagen propeptides, depending on the questions to be answered.

The recovery of the skin barrier can be followed in open blisters using noninvasive techniques, such as measuring transepidermal water evaporation and blood circulation *(13,14)*. Water evaporation can be measured with an Evaporimeter EP2. The probe is placed on the wound, and three measurements are usually made from each blister. Evaporation from healthy skin is also measured. Water evaporation is usually <10 g/(m²• h) in healthy skin. In the blister base immediately after blister induction, water evaporation is about 90–110 g/(m²• h), while after 2 d the value is about 50–80 g/(m²• h) and after 4 d is about 20–40 g/(m²• h) *(14)*. Blood flow can be measured with a laser-Doppler flowmeter from healing blister bases. The values are usually highest in healing blister wounds at 2–4 d after blister induction *(13)*.

3.2.2. Intact Blister

In intact blisters, wound healing can only be studied by excising whole blisters under local anesthesia for analysis. This model is suitable for studying the healing of wounds in conditions in which there is no bacteria or scab over the wound. The intact blisters can be studied for up to 5 d by protecting the blisters with foam plastic rings until the biopsies are taken. From similarly protected intact blisters, it is also possible to collect blister fluid to investigate the induction and regulation of various cytokines, enzymes, and so forth during reepithelization in vivo.

Healing of 6-mm blisters is complete within 6–10 d. Healing can be followed up by excising whole blisters under local anesthesia for histological and immunohistochemical analysis. Before taking an excisional skin biopsy, the skin should be cleaned routinely as before minor operations, and the blister area should be carefully anesthesized with lidocaine-adrenaline. The excisional skin sample containing the whole blister area is then taken with a disposable knife and pincers, avoiding damage to the blister area. The sample can then be divided into two parts. One part is snap-frozen and processed for analysis. The other part can be fixed and embedded into paraffin. If one does not wish to take too many excisional skin samples, it is best to take the skin sample at 4 days after blister induction. At that time point, the blister wound is partially covered by new epidermis. From skin samples numerous parameters can then be analyzed.

4. Notes

1. Earlier, plastic suction cups with variable sizes and variable numbers of holes were used *(1)*. It is still possible to make individual plastic cups of the desired

size and number of holes. Hole size can vary in self-made devices from 3 to 10 mm. The total diameter of the cup can be from 20 to 50 mm.

2. The methodology outlined here can be used to study in vivo reepithelialization of superficial wounds of a standard size, in which healing occurs along the partially restored basement membrane. The disposable suction blister device is highly suitable for human studies, but it can also be used in animals, such as pigs or rats, after the hair has been removed. For mouse studies the device may be too large, but it could be experimentally applied to the dorsal skin.

3. This technique has some drawbacks: it takes about 40–120 min to induce blisters, and there are hyperpigmented spots in the blister bases for up to several months after blistering. However, no scars will remain, if skin biopsies are not taken from the blisters. The method is not applicable to facial skin, scalp, fingers, palms, feet, toes, mouth, or genitalia. We have not used this method in young children, even though it could be used, since it is only minimally invasive and practically painless.

4. Note that it is possible to induce several blisters at the same time using several devices. We have often used four devices connected to the same vacuum pump at the same time to induce blisters in abdominal skin.

5. If no blisters are induced within 2 h, there may be several reasons. The vacuum pump may not be functioning properly, making it unable to generate a vacuum of about 40–50 kPa. The device may not be attached tightly owing to hair, cream, or something else on the skin surface. In some skin diseases, such as lesional skin of psoriasis, ichthyosis, and eczema, blisters may be impossible to induce. In addition, the warming of the skin may not be sufficient. The skin should be warmed with an electric lamp (but only warmed, *not* burned!).

6. Sometimes there are technical defects in the blister device. If this appears to be the case, the investigator should try using another one.

References

1. Kiistala, U. (1968) Suction blister device for separating viable epidermis from dermis. *J. Invest. Dermatol.* **50,** 129–137.
2. Oikarinen, A., Autio, P., Kiistala, U., Risteli, L., and Risteli, J. (1992) A new method to measure type I and III collagen synthesis in human skin in vivo: demonstration of decreased collagen synthesis after topical glucocorticoid treatment. *J. Invest. Dermatol.* **98,** 220–225.
3. Ingemansson-Nordqvist, B., Kiistala, U., and Rorsman, H. (1967) Culture of adult human epidermal cells obtained from roofs of suction blisters. *Acta Dermatol. Venereol.* **47,** 237–240.
4. Averbeck, D., Averbeck, S., Blais, J., Moysan, A., Hüppe, G., Morliére, P., Prognon, P., Vigny, P., and Dubertret, L. (1989) Suction blister fluid: its use for pharmacodynamic and toxicological studies of drugs and metabolites in vivo in human skin after topical or systemic administration, in *Models in Dermatology*, vol. 4 (Maibach, H. I. and Lowe, N. J., eds.), Karger, Basel, pp. 5–11.

5. Benfeldt, E., Serup, J., and Menné, T. (1999) Microdialysis vs. suction blister technique for in vivo sampling of pharmacokinetics in the human dermis. *Acta Dermatol. Venereol.* **79,** 338–342.

6. Oikarinen, A., Kylmäniemi, M., Autio-Harmainen, H., Autio, P., and Salo, T. (1993) Demonstration of 72-kDa and 92-kDa forms of type IV collagenase in human skin: variable expression in various blistering diseases, induction during re-epithelialization and decrease by topical glucocorticoids. *J. Invest. Dermatol.* **101,** 205–210.

7. Kylmäniemi, M., Autio, P., and Oikarinen, A. (1994) Interleukin 1alfa (IL-1alfa) in human skin *in vivo*. Lack of correlation to markers of collagen metabolism. *Acta Dermatol. Venereol.* **74,** 364–367.

8. Kiistala, U. and Mustakallio, K. K. (1967) Dermo-epidermal separation with suction: electron microscopic and histochemical study of initial events of blistering on human skin. *J. Invest. Dermatol.* **48,** 466–477.

9. Oikarinen, A., Savolainen, E.-R., Tryggvason, K., Foidart, J.-M., and Kiistala, U. (1982) Basement membrane components and galactosylhydroxylysyl glucosyltransferase in suction blisters of human skin. *Br. J. Dermatol.* **106,** 257–266.

10. Kainulainen, T., Häkkinen, L., Hamidi, S., Larjava, K., Kallioinen, M., Peltonen J., Salo, T., Larjava, H., and Oikarinen, A. (1998) Laminin-5 expression is independent of the injury and microenvironment during re-epithelialization of wounds. *J. Histochem. Cytochem.* **46,** 353–360.

11. Leivo, T., Kiistala, U., Vesterinen, M., Owaribe, K., Burgeson, R. E., Virtanen, I., and Oikarinen, A. (2000) Re-epithelialization rate and protein expression in suction-induced wound model: comparison between intact blisters, open wounds and calcipotrial-pretreated open wounds. *Br. J. Dermatol.* **142,** 991–1002.

12. Kiistala, U. (1972) Dermal-epidermal separation II. External factors in suction blister formation with special reference to the effects of temperature. *Ann. Clin. Res.* **4,** 236–246.

13. Koivukangas, V., Annala, A.-P., Salmela, P. I., and Oikarinen, A. (1999) Delayed restoration of epidermal barrier function after suction blister injury in patients with diabetes mellitus. *Diabet. Med.* **16,** 563–567.

14. Koivukangas, V. and Oikarinen, A. (1998) Effects of PUVA and UVB treatment on restoration of epidermal barrier function and vascular response after suction blister injury in human skin in vivo. *Photodermatol. Photoimmunol. Photomed.* **14,** 119–124.

19

Implantable Wound Healing Models and the Determination of Subcutaneous Collagen Deposition in Expanded Polytetrafluoroethylene Implants

Lars Nannestad Jorgensen, Søren Munk Madsen, and Finn Gottrup

1. Introduction

Implantable wound-healing models are made of artificial materials and are designed to monitor a systemic or local effect on the wound-healing response induced by a pathological condition or treatment. An ideal implantable model should accurately reproduce a wound, allow multiple assessments, have high exportability with little variability, be easy to apply, be minimally invasive and safe, be functional in more than one species, and be cost-effective. Unfortunately, none of the models fulfill all these criteria. In both animals and humans, these models have mostly been implanted in the sc tissue, and the models may be divided into nondynamic deposition types (the expanded polytetrafluoroethylene [ePTFE], the wire mesh chamber, and the polyvinyl alcohol [PVA] sponge) and dynamic categories (the viscose cellulose sponge model and microdialysis). In this chapter, we briefly review these different models with a focus on the ePTFE model and the determination of collagen deposition levels in the model as assessed by the amount of hydroxyproline detected by high-performance liquid chromatography (HPLC).

1.1. Dynamic Models

1.1.1. Viscose Cellulose Sponge Model (Cellstick®)

The viscose cellulose sponge model is essentially a small wound drain constructed from a gas-permeable silicone tube (15-cm length, 0.18-cm id, and

From: *Methods in Molecular Medicine, vol. 78: Wound Healing: Methods and Protocols*
Edited by: Luisa A. DiPietro and Aime L. Burns © Humana Press Inc., Totowa, NJ

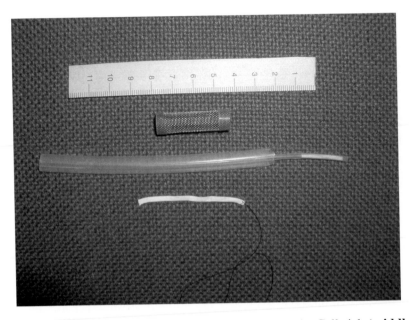

Fig. 1. Hunt-Schilling wire mesh chamber model (**top**), the Cellstick (**middle**), and ePTFE tube model (**bottom**). Scale is in centimeters.

0.25-cm od) containing a 0.13 × 2.0 cm viscose cellulose sponge (Cellomeda OY, Turku, Finland) (**Fig. 1**) *(1)*. Because of a constant leak of fluid through the tube, this model is suitable for the analysis of wound fluid composition during the inflammatory state of the wound. The model is used for studies during the first 3 d after wounding. The sponge matrix entraps a cellular infiltrate that may be analyzed by cytology, histology, or enzyme histochemistry. An early wound maturity profile is obtained from differential counts of the inflammatory cells in the sponge matrix and calculation of their mutual ratios during the first 3 d after wounding. This has been shown to correlate with late tensile strength of surgical wounds in guinea pigs *(2)*. The advantages of this model are easy access to early wound fluid analyses and the potential for studies of the inflammatory response in wound healing. However, the calculations of the wound maturity profile are complicated, and only a few centers have worked with the model so far.

1.1.2. Microdialysis

In microdialysis, probes with an od of 0.2 mm are inserted into the environment of a wound. Semipermeable membranes are used that permit passage of small compounds with a molecular mass of up to 2000 Daltons. Fluid is constantly delivered through the dialysis catheter by a pump. The concentra-

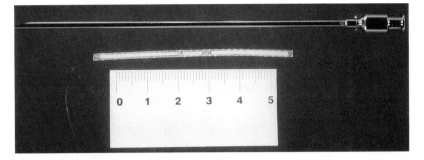

Fig. 2. PVA sponge model and insertion cannula. Scale is in centimeters.

tions of compounds in the sampled fluid mirror the concentration in the interstitial fluid of the wound. If the flow rate is high, the exchange fraction across the membrane will be low. High exchange rates are obtained by low flow rates, but the volumes obtained for analysis are often too small for analysis. However, the extracted fraction may be calculated experimentally from mathematical models *(3)*. The concentration of pharmaceutical compounds within various tissues in humans, (e.g., antibiotics in a wound) may be determined by microdialysis *(4)*. This method measures the free diffusible and often active fraction of a drug and has a high spatial and temporal resolution. Disadvantages are low sample volumes and the requirement of high-sensitivity analyses along with frequent calibration.

1.2. Nondynamic Models

1.2.1. Hunt-Schilling Wire Mesh Chamber Model

The advantages of the Hunt-Shilling model (**Fig. 1**) include easy access to wound fluid and granulation tissue that gradually fill up the cylinder chamber. Multiple samples may be taken for up to 4 wk after wounding *(5)*. The model allows the injection of a test substance into the model chamber. A disadvantage is that the model is not minimally invasive and requires a long implantation time to obtain sufficient amounts of granulation tissue.

1.2.2. PVA Sponge Model

The PVA sponge model consists of three PVA sponges placed inside a perforated, silicone 5.7-cm tube with an od of 0.2 cm (**Fig. 2**). The underlying principle of this model is less encapsulation owing to less tissue adhesion to the outer casing of silicone material *(6)*. The advantages of this model include easy handling and a high suitability for studies of both histology and early

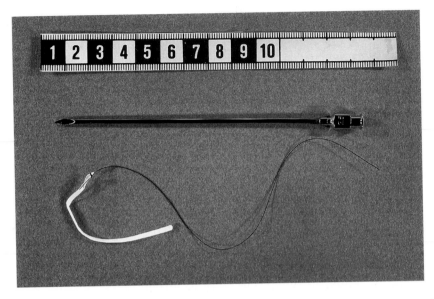

Fig. 3. ePTFE tube model mounted on a suture and insertion cannula. Scale is in centimeters.

wound healing. Drawbacks are relative low collagen deposition and higher variability compared to the ePTFE model *(7)*.

1.2.3. ePTFE Model

The ePTFE model is a tubing with a 1.2-mm id, a 0.6-mm wall thickness, and a 90- to 120-μm pore size formerly known as Impra® (**Figs. 1** and **3**). The deposition levels of collagen (as expressed by hydroxyproline), total protein, and DNA (cellularity) may be determined in this model *(8)*. Histological examination of deposited material in the ePTFE material shows granulation tissue with a normal composition of inflammatory cells; fibroblasts; macrophages; ingrowth of capillaries; and extracellular matrix components such as collagen, elastin, and glycosaminoglycans. The large pore size used results in a high yield of collagen that is higher than for Goretex materials *(9)*. Many groups have used the model for studies of various clinical conditions such as malnutrition, hypovolemia *(10)*, preoperative illness *(11)*, major surgery *(12)*, chemotherapy, use of corticosteroids *(9)*, and smoking *(13)*. These conditions are associated with a diminished deposition of collagen. Accelerated deposition of collagen has been found after optimized tissue perfusion and oxygenation *(10)* and diet supplementation with arginine *(14)*.

The model shows some variability in the measurement of the deposition levels of hydroxyproline, reaching variation coefficients of 15% (within ePTFE) and 23% (between ePTFE). Most of this variation is a biological phenomenon owing to inhomogeneous deposition of granulation tissue along the ePTFE tube *(15)*.

2. Materials

2.1. Preparation and Sterilization of ePTFE Tubes

1. High-porosity tubing (product code: OEM-012-01; International Polymer Engineering, Tempe, AZ). This has a 1.2-mm id, a 0.6-mm wall thickness, and a 90- to 120-μm pore size.
2. 3-0 Nylon suture.
3. Scalpel.
4. Nonpowder surgical gloves.
5. Autoclave.

2.2. Implantation and Removal of ePTFE Tubes

All materials listed must be sterile.
1. 1% Mepivacaine (20 mL) (Carbocain®, AstraZeneca, Södertälje, Sweden).
2. One 20-mL syringe and cannula for sc infiltration anesthesia.
3. Large cannula (13-cm length, 25-mm od).
4. Transparent surgical dressing (e.g., Tegaderm®; 3M Health Care, St. Paul, MN).
5. Chlorhexidine and sterile swabs.
6. Scissors and forceps.
7. Nonpowder surgical gloves.
8. Surgical adhesive aperture drape.

2.3. Delipidization and Drying of Removed ePTFE Tubes

1. Glass vials, 4 mL with polyethylene screw caps (e.g., Sun).
2. Acetone and diethyl ether (analytical grade).

2.4. Measurement of Dried ePTFE Tubes

1. Caliper ruler with 0.1-mm working tolerance.
2. Microbalance with 1-μg working tolerance.

2.5. Hydrolysis

1. Pyrex glass tubes (6 × 50 mm) (Corning).
2. Large vials, 40 mL with Mininert valve caps (Brown, Wertheim, Germany), referred to as *reaction vials* in **Subheading 3.5.**
3. Three-way valve connected to a vacuum pump (end pressure of approx 1 torr) and to nitrogen (1 bar pressure, flow rate of 1 L/min).

  4. Concentrated HCl (analytical grade).
  5. Phenol.

2.6. Determination of Amino Acids

  1. HPLC system with column heater and UV absorbance monitor.
  2. Column packed with silica-bonded C18 (e.g., Hypersil BDS C18, particle size 3 μm, column length and diameter 150 × 4.6 mm; Thermo Quest, Runcorn, Chesire, UK).
  3. Redrying reagent: A mixture of ethanol, water, and triethylamine (analytical grade) in a volume ratio of 2:2:1 (*see* **Note 1**).
  4. Phenylisothiocyanate (PITC) reagent: A mixture of ethanol, water, triethylamine (analytical grade), and phenylisothiocyanate (sequanal grade; Pierce, Rockford, IL) in a volume ratio of 7:1:1:1 (*see* **Note 1**).
  5. Eluent A: One liter of 0.1 M sodium phosphate buffer. Add 560 μL of triethylamine and 200 μL of a 1 mg/mL solution of EDTA disodium salt. Adjust the pH to 5.70, and add 6 vol of acetonitrile (HPLC gradient grade) to 94 vol of the phosphate buffer with additives.
  6. Eluent B: acetonitrile:water (60:40 [v/v]) to which is added 200 μL of a 1 mg/mL solution of EDTA disodium salt per liter.
  7. Amino Acid Standard H (Pierce).
  8. L-4-Hydroxyproline (Merck, Darmstadt, Germany).
  9. δ-Hydroxylysine (Sigma, St. Louis, MO).
  10. L-Citrulline or 3-methoxy-DL-tyrosine (Sigma): 2.25 mM solution in 0.1 M HCl.
  11. Sample diluent: 5 mM sodium phosphate buffer, pH 7.4, containing 5% (v/v) acetonitrile.
  12. 0.1 M HCl.

3. Methods
3.1. Preparation and Sterilization of ePTFE Tubes

  1. Wear gloves and work on a clean table.
  2. Cut the ePTFE material into pieces 4–10 cm long (*see* **Note 2**).
  3. Tie a 3-0 nylon suture to one end of the ePTFE tube after perforating the material with the suture approx 2 to 3 mm from the end. Leave at least a 16-cm length of suture from the ePTFE (**Fig. 3**).
  4. Double-pack the ePTFE tubes in sterilization pouches containing the appropriate number to be used for each subject.
  5. Sterilize at 120°C for 20 min.

3.2. Implantation and Removal of ePTFE Tubes

  1. Disinfect the skin twice on the dorso-lateral part of the upper arm of the subject. Fasten an adhesive aperture drape over the skin.

2. Infiltrate the skin and sc tissue with mepivacaine leaving more anesthetic at the sites planned for entry and exit of the large cannula. Wait at least 5 min before proceeding.

3. Perforate the skin with the large cannula in the distal part of the sterile area. Taking care not to hit the muscular fascia or the skin, guide the cannula proximally in the sc tissue. Direct the cannula out through the skin 10 cm proximal to the site of entry, thus creating an sc tunnel (*see* **Note 3**).

4. With 5 mL of air from a syringe, force out any plug of skin trapped in the syringe.

5. Insert the suture through the distal end of the cannula and pull it through the proximal end until 1 cm of the tube is visible outside the cannula (*see* **Note 4**).

6. Slowly pull out the syringe while controlling the position of the ePTFE implant by keeping the nylon suture tight. Leave 1 cm of the tube protruding through the skin at the proximal site. Remove the syringe from the distal site. Shorten the suture by cutting it 4 cm from the knot on the ePTFE implant, and cover the perforation with an absorbable swab (*see* **Note 5**).

7. Cover the external part of the ePTFE implant and the suture with Tegaderm.

8. The duration of implantation is 7–10 d. Remove the tubes by pulling on the external part of the ePTFE implant using forceps. Anesthesia is not necessary.

3.3. Delipidization and Drying of Removed ePTFE Tubes

1. Engrave glass vials with a code number for identification of the individual section of ePTFE tube. Fill each vial with 3 mL of acetone, close with a polyethylene screw cap, and place at 4°C for a minimum of 1 h (*see* **Note 6**).

2. Divide the ePTFE tubes into sections, cut perpendicularly to the long axis. For the number of sections refer to the planned analyses. Determination of hydroxyproline, hydroxylysine and proline requires an approx 10-mm length of ePTFE tube.

3. Place the section of ePTFE tube in a vial with 3 to 4 mL of cool acetone (*see* **Note 7**).

4. After standing the vial for a minimum of 24 h, decant off the acetone by turning the vial over a beaker (*see* **Note 8**). Fill the vial with 3 mL of fresh acetone, vortex, and place at 4°C for 24 h with occasional shaking.

5. Repeat **Step 4** twice, so that tube samples have been treated with a total of three changes of acetone.

6. Decant off the acetone and replace with 3 to 4 mL of acetone : diethyl ether (1 : 1), and stand the vials at 4°C for 24 h with occasional shaking.

7. Decant off the mixture of acetone and diethyl ether, and aspirate the remaining solvent. Partially fill the vials with pure diethyl ether, and stand at ambient temperature for 24 h in a ventilated hood with occasional shaking.

8. Decant off the diethyl ether and quickly aspirate the remaining ether with a hand-operated pipet. Leave the vials uncapped in the fume hood overnight for evaporation of most of the diethyl ether.

9. Loosely place the caps on the vials. Remove remaining traces of solvents and water by standing the vials in a vacuum desiccator with silica gel or in a freeze dryer run to a chamber pressure of 0.2 torr. Store the completely dried samples in their vials in a vacuum desiccator with silica gel until determination of amino acids. They may be stored up to 3 mo.

3.4. Measurement of Dried ePTFE Tubes

1. Engrave the Pyrex 50-mm glase tubes 6 × with sample identification, heat the tubes in a gas flame heat, and then cool in a desiccator before use.
2. Spike each ePTFE tube section with a thin cannula, hold close to the jaws of a slide caliper, and measure its length with a 0.1-mm working tolerance (*see* **Note 9**).
3. Place each ePTFE tube section on a clean objective slide and divide into four pieces. Tare weigh each Pyrex glass tube on a microbalance and then weigh it with the ePTFE tube pieces immediately after these have been transferred to it with a 1-μg working tolerance.

3.5. Hydrolysis (see Note 10)

1. Place the Pyrex glass tubes with their contents in the reaction vial. Place 500 μL of concentrated HCl and a 1-mm^3 crystal of phenol in the bottom of the reaction vial outside the Pyrex glass tubes and cap the vial (*see* **Note 11**).
2. Connect the connecting piece of the valve cap to one branch of a three-way valve. Connect the other branches to a vacuum and nitrogen, respectively. Evacuate the reaction vial for 10 s, and then fill with nitrogen gas for 10 s. Do this evacuation/flush cycle two more times, and close the valve after a final 10 s evacuation.
3. Place the reaction vial in an oven at 114°C for 24 h.
4. Remove the Pyrex tubes from the reaction vial.
5. Remove remnants from condensation in the tubes by standing in a vacuum oven with silica gel at 45°C for 6 h.

3.6. Determination of Amino Acids (see Note 12)

1. Redissolve the dry residues from the hydrolysates in 240 μL of 0.1 *M* HCl. Close the Pyrex tubes with Parafilm and stand at 4°C for 6 h with occasional vortex mixing for complete dissolution.
2. Centrifuge the hydrolysates at 4000*g* for 10 min.
3. Pipet triplicate 12-μL aliquots and triplicate 60 μL aliquots from the supernatant of each hydrolysate into polypropylene autosampler tubes, and add 20 μL of the 2.25 μ*M* solution of 3-methoxy-DL-tyrosine or L-citrulline.
4. Completely dry the polypropylene autosampler tubes by standing them in a vacuum oven with silica gel at 45°C overnight or longer.
5. Dissolve the samples in 25 μL of redrying reagent and redry completely, preferably by placing in a high-vacuum chamber.

6. React the samples with 25 µL of PITC reagent by standing them at room temperature for 10 min and then at 45°C for 10 min, and dry completely.
7. Redissolve the resulting mixture of phenylthiocarbamyl derivatives from the amino acids in 200 µL of 5 mM phosphate buffer containing acetonitrile. Dissolved derivative samples are stable for 12 h at room temperature.
8. Analyze the samples by HPLC, monitoring the UV absorbance of the eluate from the column at 254 nm. The gradient profile is as follows: starting composition is 100% eluent A, 1.00 mL/min, linear increase of eluent B to 40% after 13 min, then increasing eluent B to 100% to be reached at 14.5 min, flow increasing from 1.00 mL/min to 1.30 mL/min; hold for 4 min, and over 5 min return to starting conditions.
9. Calibrate the instrument from the results by referring to equal analysis and calculation of standards prepared from the Amino Acid Standard H, L-4-hydroxyproline, and δ-hydroxylysine.
10. Calculate the amount of relevant amino acids, in particular hydroxyproline, from the mean value of the results from triplicate aliquots, and give in micrograms per millimeter and per milligram of ePTFE tube. The gross result should be the average of the results from two ePTFE tubes that have been implanted parallel to each other in the same individual.

4. Notes

1. It is convenient to prepare 10 mL of the redrying reagent at a time and aliquot it into 400-µL Eppendorf tubes that are stable at –18°C for 6 mo. The PITC reagent must be prepared immediately before use. PITC comes in 1-mL ampoules. After breaking an ampoule, the contents can be pipeted into a 4-mL vial, which is then flushed with nitrogen, capped with no oxygen coming in, and stored at –18°C for 1 mo.
2. The length of the ePTFE implant depends on the number of different analyses to be performed. At least 1 cm from each piece of implant left outside the sc tissue cannot be used for analysis.
3. Compressing the skin with forceps just proximal to the planned exit site will ease perforation of the skin with the cannula.
4. Take care and pull in the direction of the cannula so as not to cut the suture on the large syringe. Do not pull more than 1 cm of ePTFE tube out of the syringe.
5. Slight oozing from one of the puncture sites is normal. Occasionally, more intense venous bleeding may take place. For hemostasis it will suffice to compress the area for several minutes.
6. If a mechanical refrigerator is used, it should be protected against ignition of vapors inside it.
7. The vials with tubes can be stored at 4°C for up to 3 mo. Alternatively, the sections of ePTFE tube can be placed in labeled cryotubes and stored at –18°C or colder for years.

272 *Jorgensen et al.*

8. Delipidization of the ePTFE tube samples is done with lipophilic, organic solvents, of which acetone and diethyl ether are among the less toxic, but the fire hazard must be considered and the procedures must be carried out in a ventilated hood.

9. The amount of material in each ePTFE tube sample can be determined by measuring of its length or its weight. Both strategies have shortcomings. Measurement of length may be inaccurate owing to slight curvature of some tube sections, bias-cut ends, uneven distribution of ingrown tissue along the tube, and some contraction of the model after ingrowth of granulation tissue. Weighing gives the gross weight of the ePTFE tube and its contents of tissue.

10. The proposed hydrolysis procedure is a gas-phase reaction, involving exposure to hydrogen chloride. Liquid-phase hydrolysis (adding HCl directly to the sample) can also be performed but may result in less complete hydrolysis.

11. Wear eye protection and work in a ventilated hood.

12. HPLC based on PITC derivatization of the amino acids *(16)* is suitable for analysis of hydrolysates from ePTFE tube samples. The volume and number of hydrolysate aliquots taken for analysis depends on the intensity of tissue regeneration while the ePTFE tubes were in place. Taking both low and high volumes ensures that both low levels of hydroxyproline and hydroxylysine and the much higher levels of proline and other amino acids can be accurately determined.

References

1. Viljanto, J. (1991) Assessment of wound healing speed in man, in *Clinical and Experimental Approaches to Dermal and Epidermal Repair: Normal and Chronic Wounds* (Barbul, A., ed.), Wiley-Liss, New York, pp. 279–290.

2. Savunen, T. J. A. and Viljanto, J. A. (1992) Prediction of wound tensile strength: an experimental study. *Br. J. Surg.* **79,** 401–403.

3. Bungay, P. M., Morrison, P. F., and Dedrick, R. L. (1990) Steady-state theory for quantitative microdialysis of solutes and water in vivo and in vitro. *Life Sci.* **46,** 105–119.

4. Lorentzen, H., Kallehave, F., Kolmos, H. J., Knigge, U., Bülow, J., and Gottrup, F. (1996) Gentamicin concentrations in human subcutaneous tissue. *Antimicrob. Agents Chemother.* **40,** 1785–1789.

5. Hunt, T. K., Twomey, P., Zederfeldt, B., and Dunphy, J. E. (1967) Respiratory gas tensions and pH in healing wounds. *Am. J. Surg.* **46,** 702–710.

6. Diegelmann, R. F., Lindblad, W. J., and Cohen, I. K. (1986) A subcutaneous implant for wound healing studies in humans. *J. Surg. Res.* **40,** 229–237.

7. Jorgensen, L. N., Olsen, L., Kallehave, F., Karlsmark, T., Diegelmann, R. F., Cohen, I. K., and Gottrup, F. (1995) The wound healing process in surgical patients evaluated by the expanded polytetrafluoroethylene and the polyvinyl alcohol sponge: a comparison with special reference to intrapatient variability. *Wound Rep. Reg.* **3,** 527–532.

8. Goodson, W. H. and Hunt, T. K. (1982) Development of a new miniature method for the study of wound healing in human subject. *J. Surg. Res.* **33,** 394–401.

9. Wicke, C., Halliday, B. J., Scheuenstuhl, H., Foree, E. F., and Hunt, T. K. (1995) Examination of expanded polytetrafluoroethylene wound healing models. *Wound Rep. Reg.* **3,** 284–291.

10. Hartmann, M., Jonsson, K., and Zederfeldt, B. (1992) Importance of dehydration in anastomotic and subcutaneous wound healing: an experimental study in rats. *Eur. J. Surg.* **158,** 79–82.

11. Goodson, W. H., Lopez Sarmiento, A., Jensen, J. A., West, J., Granja Mena, L., and Chavez Estrella, J. (1988) The influence of a brief preoperative illness on postoperative healing. *Ann. Surg.* **205,** 250–255.

12. Jorgensen, L. N., Kallehave, F., Karlsmark, T., and Gottrup, F. (1996) Less collagen accumulation after major surgery. *Br. J. Surg.* **83,** 1591–1594.

13. Jorgensen, L. N., Kallehave, F., Christensen, E., Siana, J. E., and Gottrup, F. (1998) Less collagen production in smokers. *Surgery* **123,** 450–455.

14. Windsor, J. A., Knight, G. S., and Hill, G. L. (1988) Wound healing response in surgical patients: recent food intake is more important than nutritional status. *Br. J. Surg.* **75,** 135–137.

15. Jorgensen, L. N., Sorensen, L. T., Kallehave, F., Schulze, S., and Gottrup, F. (2001) Increased collagen deposition in an uncomplicated surgical wound compared to a minimal subcutaneous test wound. *Wound Rep. Regen.* **9,** 194–199.

16. Bidlingmeyer, B. A., Tarvin, T. L., and Cohen, S. A. (1986) Amino acid analysis of submicrogram hydrolyzate samples, in *Methods in Protein Sequence Analysis* (Walsh, K. A., ed.), Humana, Clifton, NJ, pp. 229–245.

I

EXPERIMENTAL MODELS OF WOUND HEALING

D. IN VITRO MODELS

20

The Fibroblast-Populated Collagen Lattice

A Model of Fibroblast Collagen Interactions in Repair

H. Paul Ehrlich

1. Introduction

The healing of dermal defects requires the replacement and integration of a new connective-tissue matrix at the repair site. The deposition and organization of that new connective-tissue matrix entails the interaction between fibroblasts and collagen. A better understanding of those interactions may lead to a more rapid closure of wounds and will reduce the frequency of abnormal scarring. An approach to better understand that process is through in vitro models. One such model is the fibroblast-populated collagen lattice (FPCL), introduced by Bell and colleagues *(1)*.

The introduction of cultured fibroblasts into a three-dimensional (3D) collagen matrix leads to the eventual, dynamic reduction in size of that matrix, caused by the reorganization and translocation of randomly orientated collagen fibrils. The degree of organization of the collagen matrix is quantified by the measured reduction in area size of the FPCL over time. With the degree and rate at which an FPCL becomes smaller, the greater the FPCL contraction and the more reorganization of collagen occurs. The FPCL also facilitates the study of fibroblast biology within a 3D matrix. The morphology and physiology of cells residing within the collagen matrix differ from those same cells growing as a monolayer in a tissue culture dish. Morphologically, fibroblasts in monolayer are flattened, have a spindle shape, and demonstrate a prominent ruffling lamellipodia at their leading edge. Those same cells residing within a collagen matrix are greatly elongated, with a cylindrical shape and have prominent, fine, elongated filopodia at their bipolar edges (*see* **Fig. 1**). Bio-

From: *Methods in Molecular Medicine, vol. 78: Wound Healing: Methods and Protocols*
Edited by: Luisa A. DiPietro and Aime L. Burns © Humana Press Inc., Totowa, NJ

A

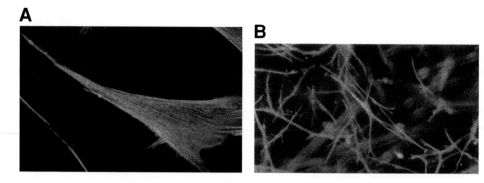

B

Fig. 1. Human dermal fibroblasts cultured on glass and within collagen. **(A)** Fibroblast on glass that has been fixed and stained with rhodamine phalloidin showing prominent lamellipodia at its leading edge (magnification: ×400). **(B)** Fibroblasts in an FPCL 24 h after casting that were viewed with a stereomicroscope equipped with fluorescence optics. Note the randomly arranged elongated cells with prominent filopodia at the polar ends of the cells (magnification: ×40).

chemically, fibroblasts in monolayer synthesize a higher level of collagen compared with the same cells maintained in collagen matrix.

1.1. Modifications of Bell's Model

Experimentation over the years has generated numerous modifications of the FPCL from that first introduced by Bell and his colleagues *(1)*. Bell's "dermal equivalent" was a free-floating FPCL that contained 50,000 human dermal fibroblasts in 1.25 mg of native soluble collagen and culture medium supplemented with fetal bovine serum (FBS) per milliliter of lattice. The entire mixture was contained in a bacteriology dish, and FPCL contraction was determined by following the reduction in the diameter of the FPCL over days.

1.1.1. Attached FPCL

Grinnell and Lamke *(2)* modified the skin equivalent model by substituting tissue culture plastic dishes for bacteriology dishes and introduced the attached FPCL model. The tissue culture dish promoted the adherence of the cast FPCL to the surface of the dish and prevented any change in FPCL diameter. However, the attached FPCL produced a change in thickness, which was the measure of lattice contraction. A modified microscope was used to measure the distance between a focus point on the top surface and a point on the bottom surface. The measured difference determined the change in FPCL thickness in attached FPCL. Attached FPCL contraction is through a cellular spreading and elongation mechanism. By contrast, in the free-floating "dermal equivalent" FPCL, the mechanism for contraction involves the reorganization of collagen fibril bundles by fibroblasts after they have elongated and spread. The attached FPCL contraction takes about 6 h to document differences in FPCL, while the free-floating FPCL takes 24 h or longer to document differences in FPCL contraction. With the free-floating FPCL there is a lag period of 6 h before FPCL diameter changes are recognized. During that 6-h lag period, fibroblasts spread and elongate, causing a reduction in the thickness of the lattice, which is the same process of the attached FPCL. Hence, the reduction in lattice thickness of the free-floating FPCL is identical to the process occurring within the attached FPCL. The major differences between the measurements of lattice contraction of the free-floating FPCL compared with the attached FPCL are related to the cellular mechanism responsible for the translocation of collagen fibril bundles by resident fibroblasts and the time of measurement.

1.1.2. Stress-Relaxed FPCL

Another modification of the FPCL contraction model combines both the attached FPCL and free-floating FPCL models. In the stress-relaxed FPCL contraction model, the FPCL is cast in a tissue culture dish, where it remains attached for 4 d *(3)*. At d 4 the FPCL is detached and the released FPCL undergoes a rapid decrease in diameter size, which is completed within 30 min following detachment. In this model, elongated spread fibroblasts residing in the matrix are seen to undergo cell contraction during the contraction of the matrix. Hence, the mechanism for the stress-relaxed FPCL contraction model involves cell contraction.

1.2. Mechanism for FPCL Contraction

All three in vitro models require translocation of collagen fibrils. With the free-floating FPCL model, translocation of collagen fibrils is by elongated cells. With the attached FPCL model, translocation of collagen fibrils is by the spreading of round cells. With the stress-relaxed FPCL model, translocation of collagen fibrils is through a process of cell contraction. In all three models, actin-myosin filament sliding of cytoskeleton microfilaments is involved. All three FPCL contraction models require the translocation of collagen fibrils through the participation of microfilaments. When randomly oriented, collagen fibril bundles are rearranged in parallel arrays; they demonstrate a birefringence pattern by polarized light microscopy. At 24 h after casting, a free-floating FPCL that is undergoing a reduction in diameter, collagen birefringence patterns appear associated with elongated spread fibroblasts. There is no birefringence pattern demonstrated within an attached FPCL, which undergoes a reduction in thickness. Likewise, after 4 d, a stress-relaxed

FPCL that undergoes rapid lattice contraction does not demonstrate a collagen birefringence after lattice contraction.

1.2.1. Myofibroblast and Cell Contraction

The reorientation and reorganization of collagen both in vivo and in vitro requires cell participation. A widely held idea is that a specialized cell, the myofibroblast, is responsible for wound contraction and the reorganization of collagen. The myofibroblast is identified by the presence of the α–smooth muscle isoform of actin within its cytoplasmic stress fibers *(4)*. Myofibroblasts are fibroblasts with prominent α–smooth muscle actin stress fibers that have been identified in open wounds undergoing wound contraction, in scars undergoing scar contracture, and in other contractile fibrotic disease processes such as Dupuytren contracture *(5)*. In vitro myofibroblasts have been identified in monolayer culture, where they represent 5–20% of the cell population. Populations of fibroblasts in culture will spontaneously develop into myofibro-blasts. Myofibroblasts spontaneously appear in areas of high cell density, such as in confluent monolayer cell layers in vitro as well as in granulation tissue in vivo. Histologically, cytoplasmic stress fibers containing α–smooth muscle actin have not been reported within fibroblasts residing in free-floating FPCL. It would appear that myofibroblasts are not a participant in free-floating FPCL contraction. Histologically, in attached FPCL only 3% of the cell population expresses α–smooth muscle actin in cytoplasmic stress fibers *(6)*.

1.2.2. Fibroblasts and Tractional Forces

A proportion of fibroblasts derived from dermis grown in monolayer culture has the capacity to develop cytoplasmic stress fibers, which contain α–smooth muscle actin. Cytoplasmic stress fibers are aggregates of microfilaments composed of actin and myosin II. In general, fibroblast populations that demonstrate fine cytoplasmic microfilaments are associated with cells undergo-ing cell movement. On the other hand, fibroblasts containing cytoplasmic stress fibers are associated with stationary cells. The fibroblasts in FPCL demonstrate both cell populations within distinct locations. When a free-floating FPCL undergoes lattice contraction, the fibroblasts at the periphery of that lattice are at a high cell density, have multiple cell-cell contacts, and show prominent cytoplasmic stress fibers (without expressing α–smooth muscle actin within the stress fibers). Fibroblasts within the central portion of the FPCL are at lower cell density, show few cell-cell contacts, contain fine cytoplasmic microfila-ments, and do not express α–smooth muscle actin. Based on morphological characteristics, fibroblasts at the periphery of the FPCL are stationary cells, whereas fibroblasts residing within the center have the capacity to undergo cell movement. FPCL contraction requires both the translocation of collagen fibrils and their reorientation.

Which cell population, the stationary or locomotive phenotype, has the capacity to translocate collagen fibrils and generate FPCL contraction? The mechanism for the translocation of collagen fibrils by stationary fibroblasts suggests a process of cell contraction. Fibroblast populations with fine cytoplasmic microfilaments would be expected to demonstrate a mechanism for the translocation of collagen fibrils by the cell locomotive process such as cell tractional forces as described by Harris et al. *(7)*. A mechanism involving cell tractional forces would imply the translocation of collagen fibrils over the surface of an elongated fibroblast by a cytoskeletal mechanism related to cell locomotion. Both processes of cell contraction and cell tractional forces require myosin adenosine triphosphatase (ATPase) activity. Optimal myosin ATPase activity is controlled by the phosphorylation state of its associated regulatory myosin light chains. Inhibiting the phosphorylation of the regulatory myosin light chains within fibroblasts residing in FPCL will inhibit free-floating FPCL contraction *(8)*.

The cellular mechanism proposed for free-floating FPCL contraction is through the generation of tractional forces. Harris et al. *(7)* described tractional forces, in which fibroblasts plated on thin silicone films wrinkle that film surface (*see* **Fig. 2**). Wrinkles appear beneath the elongated cells and not under round cells. Hence, cell contraction is not responsible for generating the wrinkles. The generation of tractional forces by fibroblasts is similar to the movement of the tread on a military tank. In the free-floating FPCL contraction, the locomotive forces have a quality like that of a tank tread. Attached collagen fibrils are pulled over the surface of the elongated fibroblasts, generating a reorientation of the collagen fiber bundles. As the microfilaments of the cytoskeleton undergo contraction by myosin-actin sliding, the cell does not contract; rather, the attached collagen fiber sites on the surface of the fibroblasts are pulled over that surface. Fibroblasts need to be elongated in order to produce contractual forces if they are to be effective at translocating collagen fibrils. If the surface of the fibroblast were flexible, the cell would buckle and collagen fibrils would not be moved. Such a cell would undergo cell contraction without realigning attached collagen fibrils. As the collagen fibrils are moved over the surface of the cell, they come in contact with other collagen fibrils. Contacts between collagen fibrils leads to the aggregation of fibrils into thicker, longer collagen fiber bundles.

In free-floating FPCL, there is an early rapid rate of lattice contraction—a log phase of contraction—lasting about 2 d. Fine collagen fibrils are more easily pulled over the fibroblast cell surfaces compared with thicker, more

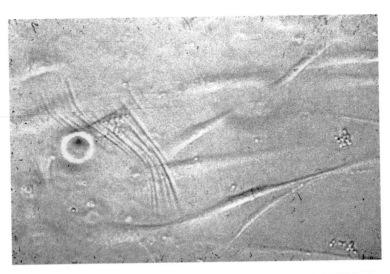

Fig. 2. Fibroblasts wrinkling a fine silicone rubber surface. Human dermal fibroblasts were plated onto a fine silicone rubber surface and maintained in culture for 6 h. At 6 h wrinkles appeared within the silicone surface beneath elongated fibroblasts.

mature collagen fibrils. After that initial log phase of lattice contraction, there is a slower rate of FPCL contraction. Hence, as collagen fibers become thicker and longer, i.e., more organized, they become more difficult for the fibroblasts to translocate. These larger fiber bundles become more stabilized and are less susceptible to being translocated by fibroblast-generated tractional forces. It is proposed that this slowdown in FPCL contraction is a consequence of collagen fiber thickening and elongation. The longer, thicker collagen fibers are less susceptible to translocation through forces generated by resident fibroblasts.

1.3. Summary

The FPCL contraction model has demonstrated that fibroblasts organize collagen through the compaction of collagen fibrils and the generation of organized fiber bundles. Organized collagen fiber bundles within a compacted FPCL demonstrate a birefringence pattern. The more rapidly the FPCL becomes smaller (contracts), the faster the translocation of collagen fibrils by the resident fibroblasts. The degree of FPCL contraction is dependent on the density of packing of the collagen fiber bundles. In vivo wound contraction and scar contracture involve the same process of collagen fibril translocation and the reorganization of the newly deposited collagen. The morphology and physiology of cells residing within the collagen matrix differ from those same cells in monolayer culture, whereby the fibroblasts on a flat surface have a lamellipodia at their leading edge. Like fibroblasts in granulation tissue, cells in FPCL have elongated filopodia that are extended out into the surrounding newly polymerized collagen matrix. The fibroblasts within a 3D collagen lattice form a continuous, linked 3D cell complex that is in contact and interacting with a 3D collagen matrix. Such a complex structure is very different from the flat two-dimensional structure of those same cells on a plastic surface. Morphological differences and numerous biochemical differences between cells in collagen and on plastic support the notion that caution must be applied when extrapolating from in vivo and in vitro experiments.

2. Materials
2.1. Isolation and Purification of Collagen
1. Rat tails for the preparation of collagen solution (*see* **Notes 1–4**).
2. 1 mM HCl.
3. 0.5 M Acetic acid.
4. NaCl.

2.2. Casting Free-Floating FPCL
1. Cells: Cells derived from a variety of tissues have been used to manufacture FPCL *(9,10)* (*see* **Notes 5–12**).
2. Tissue culture medium: A variety of culture media have been used in the manufacture of FPCL. In the original study by Bell and coworkers *(1)*, Medium-199 was used. The most common medium used today is Dulbecco's modified Eagle's medium.
3. FBS (*see* **Notes 13** and **14**).
4. Bacterial culture plates (*see* **Note 15**).
5. CO_2 incubator.
6. Ruler.

3. Methods
3.1. Isolation and Purification of Collagen
1. Collect rat tails and tease the tendons from their sheath by pulling them free with fine-nose pliers.
2. Place the freed tendons from five rat tails in 500 mL of ice-cold 0.5 M acetic acid and stir in the cold for 2 d.
3. Clear the viscous solution by centrifuging for 30 min at 10,000g.
4. Save the clear viscous collagen solution and add 10% (w/v) NaCl.
5. Stir the salt solution in the cold overnight, and collect the insoluble collagen precipitate by centrifuging for 10 min at 10,000g.
6. Resuspend the pellet in 100 mL of ice-cold 0.1 M acetic acid, and dialyze with four changes against 4 L of 1 mM HCl in the cold. Each of the four dialysis changes requires a minimum duration of 6 h.

Table 1
Makeup of FPCL for Different Volumes

Culture dish	Area	Volume (mL)	No. of cells	Collagen[a]	Medium (mL)	Serum[b] (mL)
24-Well	201 mm²	0.5	25,000	625 µg : 0.125 mL	0.325	0.05
35-mm	962 mm²	2.0	100,000	2.5 mg : 0.5 mL	1.3	0.2
60-mm	28 cm²	4.0	200,000	5.0 mg : 1.0 mL	2.6	0.4
100-mm	78.5 cm²	10	500,000	12.5 mg : 2.5 mL	6.5	1.0

[a]Collagen stock solution is 5 mg/mL in 1 mM HCl.
[b]FBS.

7. Freeze the salt-free collagen solution, lyophilize, weigh, and resuspend in ice-cold filter-sterilized 1 mM HCl at 5.0 mg/mL (*see* **Note 16**). Store the collagen solution in a refrigerator until needed.

3.2. Casting Free-Floating FPCL

1. Release the cultured cells from monolayer culture by trypsinization, suspend in culture medium, and count.
2. Mix the appropriate number of cells, tissue culture medium, and serum as outlined in **Table 1**. The tissue culture medium should be a room temperature. The final concentration of FBS in the FPCL will be 10% (v/v). Add the indicated amount of collagen solution, mix rapidly, and pour into the bacterial culture dish (*see* **Note 15**). For the original free-floating FPCL, the optimal cell density was 50,000 cells/mL (*1*). The recipes given in **Table 1** are based on that cell density. Bell (*1*) reported that when lattices were cast with <10,000 human dermal fibroblasts/mL no FPCL contraction occurred. That study found that a moderate density of 50,000 human dermal fibroblasts/mL of lattice produced maximal FPCL contraction (*see* **Fig. 3** and **Notes 17** and **18**).
3. Transfer the tissue culture dish to a 37°C, 5% CO_2/95% air incubator with an H_2O-saturated atmosphere. The gel will polymerize rapidly.
4. Measure the diameter of the FPLC with a ruler at 24-h intervals. Calculate the area using the average of two separate measurements of diameter.

4. Notes

1. An important player in the FPCL contraction model is collagen. The isolation of native collagen from rat tails can be performed using the salt purification method outlined in **Subheading 3.**
2. The concentrations of collagen effect the rate and final degree of FPCL contraction. The greater the concentration of collagen, the lesser the rate and degree of FPCL contraction (*1*). During lattice contraction, fibroblasts compact collagen fibrils, and the initial density of the collagen fibrils within the matrix will influence the degree of compaction of that matrix. With an equal number of

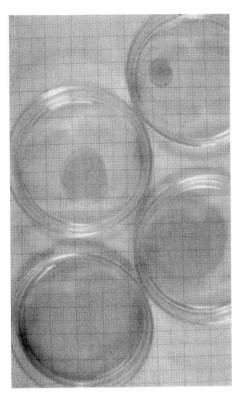

Fig. 3. FPCL undergoing contraction. Four FPCLs prepared with different cell numbers per 2 mL of lattice are shown 24 h after casting. (**Bottom left**) FPCL with 5000 fibroblasts; (**bottom right**) FPCL with 25,000 fibroblasts; (**top left**) FPCL with 50,000 fibroblasts; (**top right**) FPCL with 100,000 fibroblasts.

cells, fewer collagen fibrils will be compacted in smaller volume than a high concentration of collagen fibrils. FPCL containing 1 mg/mL of collagen will contract faster and to a greater degree than at 1.5 mg/mL. At the termination of the log phase of FPCL contraction, a level of equilibrium is reached at which the further translocation of collagen fibrils ceases. The equilibrium is attributed to the size and degree of organization of the collagen fiber bundles of the contracted FPCL. The bulk of the collagen bundles makes it difficult to undergo further modification of the bundles without damaging these structures in such a way as to establish new points for growth.

3. Besides the concentration of collagen, the types of collagen making up the FPCL will influence the rate and final degree of FPCL contraction (*11*). Type I collagen from human dermis, type II collagen from human cartilage; and type III collagen from a benign uterine tumor, a leiomyoma were isolated and purified by salt fractionation. When equal amounts by dry weight of these collagens were cast

into FPCLs with normal human dermal fibroblasts, there were differences in the rate and final degree of FPCL contraction. The type II collagen FPCL showed the slowest rate and least final degree of FPCL contraction compared with other types of collagen. On the other hand, the type III collagen FPCL showed the greatest rate and degree of FPCL contraction compared with other collagens. It is unclear what the mechanism for these differences is. One possibility is that the type III collagen fibrils can be packed closer together compared with the type I or type II collagen fibrils. Another possibility is that fibroblasts have more attachment sites or have a higher affinity for type III collagen. This would facilitate the more rapid translocation of these fibrils over the cell surface. In vivo granulation tissue and hypertrophic scar have a connective-tissue matrix enriched in type III collagen. In vivo granulation tissue undergoes wound contraction and hypertrophic scar undergoes scar contracture. The increased contraction of FPCL in vitro, when enriched in type III collagen, is in agreement with the in vivo situations.

4. The protein structure of collagen can be modified by limited proteolytic digestion, whereby the N- and C-terminal peptides, telopeptides, are removed. The smaller collagen molecules have the capacity to be polymerized and cast into FPCL. Salt-soluble rat tail tendon collagen was treated with pepsin for 18 h in the cold, and modified collagen was purified by salt fractionation. By gel electrophoresis it was shown that the α-chains from the pepsin-treated collagen preparation were smaller and migrated faster than the α-chains from the untreated collagen preparation. FPCLs were cast with equal numbers of human dermal fibroblasts contained in either the pepsin-treated or untreated rat tail tendon collagen preparations. FPCLs made with pepsin-treated collagen contracted slower and to a lesser degree than the FPCL made with the untreated collagen preparation. It is unclear why there is a difference in FPCL contraction between FPCL made with pepsin-treated and untreated collagen preparations. One possibility is that the telopeptides play an important role in optimizing the packing of collagen fibrils *(12)*. With optimal packing of collagen fibrils, the FPCL can be compacted into its minimal volume.

5. Most culture fibroblasts have the capacity to rearrange collagen fibrils leading to FPCL contraction. Other mesenchymal cells, such as blood vessel smooth muscle cells and normal bone cells, will also produce collagen lattice contraction.

6. It has been shown that transformed fibroblasts are poor at FPCL contraction *(13)*. Cell division and DNA synthesis are not essential for FPCL contraction *(1)*. There are a number of differences between transformed fibroblasts and normal fibroblasts, which may explain transformed cell deficiencies at FPCL contraction. Those differences include but are not limited to the expression of integrin, gap junction communications, cytoskeletal machinery, and cell morphology.

7. A measure of cell-collagen interaction capacities can be compared among different cell populations through following FPCL contraction. One example is the human osteosarcoma (HOS) cell line, which lacks the capacity to contract

collagen lattices. It appears that this inability to contract collagen lattices is related to a defect in the expression of a specific integrin. When HOS cells are transfected with the gene for α2 integrin, the transfected cells have the capacity to contract FPCL *(14)*. Hence, the importance of the α2 integrin appears to involve the attachment of the fibroblasts to the collagen *(15)*. That attachment is necessary for the subsequent translocation of the collagen fibrils. The induced expression of the α2 integrin is sufficient to promote cell-collagen interactions. It is implied that HOS cells contain the cytoskeletal machinery necessary to translocate collagen fibrils but cannot integrate that assembly with the collagen fibrils.

8. Cells derived from tissues affected by different diseases have been demonstrated to show alterations in their ability to contract collagen lattices. Fibroblasts derived from the dermis of patients with epidermolysis bullosa dystrophica (EBdr) were studied. Dermal fibroblasts from EBdr patients show impaired FPCL contraction *(16)*. This defect in cell-collagen interactions appears to be linked to the excess accumulation of cAMP. One cause of the increased intracellular accumulation of cAMP is an increased synthesis of prostaglandins. The inclusion of indomethacin, an inhibitor of prostaglandin synthesis, antagonized EBdr fibroblast inhibition of FPCL contraction and restored lattice contraction toward normal. It was suggested that the elevated levels of cAMP inhibit the activity of myosin ATPase, the enzyme that triggers the contraction of microfilaments. In the presence of excess levels of cAMP, myosin light chains are not correctly phosphorylated and actin-myosin filament sliding within microfilaments is inhibited. Hence, the translocation of collagen fibrils over the cell surface does not occur.

9. The modulation of cellular function through electroporesis of proteins has been shown to alter FPCL contraction *(8)*. It was reported that in the presence of high intracellular levels of cAMP, FPCL contraction proceeded normally by the intracellular inoculation of a modified myosin light chain kinase enzyme by electroporesis prior to its incorporation into collagen lattices. The modified myosin light chain kinase enzyme was unaffected by high intracellular levels of cAMP. The treated fibroblasts contracted FPCL at an optimal rate.

10. Cells derived from tissues affected by fibrotic diseases also show differences in the rate and degree of FPCL contraction. One example is the comparison of fibroblasts derived from Dupuytren nodules and cords. Dupuytren disease is a malady characterized by the permanent flexion of fingers caused by a fibrosis within the palmer fascia. Two anatomical components of the fibrotic palmer fascia are the nodules and cords. Histologically, nodules are composed of fibroblasts at high density contained in a moderate concentration of connective tissue. Cords are composed of cells at a low density contained in a dense connective-tissue matrix. FPCLs were cast with fibroblasts derived from normal human dermis, Dupuytren nodules, and Dupuytren cords. The cord-derived FPCL showed the lowest rate and degree of FPCL contraction compared to the other two cell lines. The Dupuytren nodule–derived fibroblasts were equal to the dermal-derived

fibroblasts in the FPCL contraction assay. The reasons for these differences between Dupuytren nodule– and cord-derived fibroblast interactions with collagen are unclear.

11. Crohn disease is an inflammatory disease of the bowel wall. Smooth muscle cells derived from involved and uninvolved bowel from the same patient with Crohn disease undergoing surgery were compared in the FPCL contraction assay. Smooth muscle cells derived from the affected bowel wall of the patient showed a reduced rate and final degree of collagen lattice contraction compared with smooth muscle cells derived from uninvolved bowel wall *(17)*. Hence, resident smooth muscle cells from the chronically inflamed bowel wall of patients with Crohn disease change their phenotype. This change in phenotype is retained when these smooth muscle cells are grown in cell culture.

12. Keratinocytes substituted for fibroblasts, when suspended in collagen lattices, will contract that matrix.

13. The most common type of serum used in the casting of FPCL is FBS. There is some variation in the rate and degree of FPCL contraction related to the lot of FBS used. It is wise to have enough serum from the same lot to complete an experiment. The presence of serum during the manufacture of FPCL is required for FPCL contraction. The concentration of 10% serum appears to be optimal for the promotion of FPCL contraction *(1)*. Serum contains a number of growth factors, which includes transforming growth factor-β (TGF-β) and platelet-derived growth factor (PDGF). It is reported that TGF-β enhances FPCL contraction in the presence of serum *(18)*, whereas PDGF does not *(19)*. However, PDGF in the absence of serum will promote FPCL contraction *(20)*.

14. It was found that substituting dialyzed serum in the casting of FPCL inhibited FPCL contraction *(21)*. Growth factors such as TGF-β and PDGF are nondialyzable polypeptides and are not removed from serum by dialysis. Hence, they were not removed from the serum, yet FPCL contraction did not proceed. Dialyzed serum is devoid of free fatty acids (FFAs). The mechanism of FPCL contraction through the generation of tractional forces will be altered by cell membrane fluidity. Cell membrane fluidity is influenced by the membrane's fatty acid composition. A plasma membrane enriched in the 12 carbon (C-12 laurate)–saturated FFA will demonstrate increased membrane fluidity compared with cell membranes enriched in the 18 carbon (C-18 stereate)–saturated FFA. Shorter FFA substitution of lipids in the cell plasma membrane increases membrane fluidity and more rapid movement of proteins in the plane of the cell membrane. Those plasma membrane proteins can include integrins linked to collagen. The saturated FFA makeup of human fibroblasts was modified prior to their incorporation into FPCL made with dialyzed serum. The laurate (C-12)-treated fibroblasts contracted collagen lattices to 33% of their initial size in 24 h compared to FPCLs in whole serum, which were still 60% of their initial size. FPCLs, which were made with stereate (C-18) treated fibroblasts, and dialyzed serum, contracted to 57% of their initial size in 24 h, which is similar to whole serum. It suggests that stereate inclusion as the major fatty acid in the cell membrane creates a cell membrane

fluidity similar to that of whole serum. The rate of FPCL contraction with laurate (C-12)-treated fibroblasts was almost two times faster compared with the same cells in whole serum or stereate-treated fibroblasts in dialyzed serum. Substituting laurate as the major membrane fatty acid species resulted in an increase in the rate of FPCL contraction, which supports the notion of an association of FPCL contraction with cell membrane fluidly. This further supports the concept of tractional forces being responsible for the translocation of collagen, resulting in FPCL contraction.

15. The best dish for preventing fibroblast adherence to its surface is a bacteriology dish. Tissue culture dishes can be used if the FPCLs are released within 4 h of casting.

16. Since 1 mM HCl has no buffering capacity, and the addition of that collagen solution to culture medium creates no pH change in the medium. Collagen solutions made with acetic acid, which is an excellent buffer, require neutralization by the addition of NaOH, in order to prevent a pH drop in the culture medium, which is detrimental to the cells and impairs collagen polymerization.

17. With experimental tissue culture models, there are concerns about what changes occur by the transfer of fibroblasts from an in vivo environment to an in vitro one. When examining fibroblasts within a collagen matrix, cell density also needs to be considered. As an example, in vitro vanadate has been shown to inhibit high-density FPCL contraction *(22)*. With moderate-density FPCLs, the inclusion of vanadate does not inhibit lattice contraction. Likewise, in vivo, the chronic ingestion of vanadate by rats does not inhibit wound contraction *(23)*. Data generated from in vitro studies need to be viewed with caution when applied to wound contraction and scar contracture problems.

18. The effects of fibroblast density of FPCL on lattice contraction have been investigated *(19)*. By increasing the cell number to 500,000 cells/mL, the initial measurable change in FPCL diameter was reduced to 2 h and the log phase of FPCL contraction was completed by 8 h. By comparison, an FPCL with 50,000 cells requires 4–6 h to show a change in diameter, and the log phase of lattice contraction takes 48 h. The morphology of an 8-h-old FPCL with 50,000 cells/mL showed elongated and spread fibroblasts. High-density FPCL with 500,000 cells/mL at 8 h, the time of termination of further lattice contraction, also showed elongated and spread cells. With moderate-density FPCL no lattice contraction occurred prior to cell elongation, but with high density FPCL no lattice contraction occurred after cell elongation. The difference between high- and moderate-density FPCL contraction is the mechanism involved in translocating collagen fibrils. With free-floating, high-density FPCL, 500,000 cells/mL, the mechanism for lattice contraction is by cell elongation and spreading. With moderate-density FPCL, 50,000 cells/mL, the mechanism of lattice contraction is through the translocation collagen fibrils over elongated fibroblasts through tractional forces. High-density FPCL contraction does produce collagen birefringence. On the other hand, moderate-density contracted FPCL demonstrates collagen birefringence patterns.

References

1. Bell, E., Ivarsson, B., and Merrill, C. (1979) Production of a tissue-like structure by contraction of collagen lattices by human fibroblasts of different proliferative potential in vitro. *Proc. Nat. Acad. Sci. USA* **76,** 1274–1278.
2. Grinnell, F. and Lamke, C. R. (1984) Reorganization of hydrated collagen lattices by human skin fibroblasts. *J. Cell. Sci.* **66,** 51–63.
3. Tomasek, J. J., Haaksma, C. J., Eddy, R. J., and Vaughan, M. B. (1992) Fibroblast contraction occurs on released attention in attached collagen lattices: dependency on an organized exercise skeleton and serum. *Anat. Rec.* **232,** 359–368.
4. Darby, I., Skalli, O., and Gabbiani. (1990) Alpha-smooth muscle actin is transiently expressed by myofibroblasts during experimental wound healing. *Lab. Invest.* **63,** 21–29.
5. Tomasek, J. J., Vaughan, M. B., and Haaksma, C. J. (1999) Cellular structure and biology of Dupuytren's disease. *Hand Clin.* **15,** 21–34.
6. Vaughan, M. B., Howard, E. W., and Tomasek, J. J. (2000) Transforming growth factor-beta1 promotes the morphological and functional differentiation of the myofibroblast. *Exp. Cell. Res.* **257,** 180–189.
7. Harris, A. K., Wild, P., and Stopak, D. (1980) A new wrinkle in the study of cell locomotion. *Science* **280,** 177–179.
8. Ehrlich, H. P., Rockwell, W. B., Cornwell, T. L., and Rajaratnam, J. B. (1991) Demonstration of a direct role for myosin light chain kinase in fibroblast-populated collagen lattice contraction. *J. Cell. Physiol.* **146,** 1–7.
9. Bowman, N., Donahue, H., and Ehrlich, H. P. (1998) Gap junctional intercellular communication contribution to the contraction of rat osteoblast populated collagen lattices. *J. Bone Miner. Res.* **7,** 1700–1713.
10. Graham, M. F., Diegelmann, R. F., Bitar, K. N., and Ehrlich, H. P. (1987) Heparin modulates human intestinal smooth muscle cell proliferation, protein synthesis and lattice contraction. *Gastroenterology* **93,** 801–809.
11. Ehrlich, H. P. (1988) The modulation of contraction of fibroblast populated collagen lattices by types I, II, and III collagen. *Tissue Cell* **20,** 47–50.
12. Woodley, D., Yamauchi, M., Wynn, K. C., Mechanic, G., and Briggaman, R. A. (1991) Collagen telopeptides (cross-linking sites) play a role in collagen gel lattice contraction. *J. Invest. Dermatol.* **97,** 580–585.
13. Buttle, D. J. and Ehrlich, H. P. (1983) Comparative studies of collagen lattice contraction utilizing a normal and transformed cell line. *J. Cell Physiol.* **116,** 159–166.
14. Cooke, M. E., Sakai, T., and Mosher, D. F. (2000) Contraction of collagen matrices mediated by alpha2beta1A and alpha(v)beta3 integrins. *J. Cell. Sci.* **113,** 2375–2383.
15. Schiro, J. A., Chan, B. M., Roswit, W. T., Kassner, P. D., Pentland, A. P., Hemler, M. E., Eisen, A. Z., and Kupper, T. S. (1991) Integrin alpha 2 beta 1 (VLA-2) mediates reorganization and contraction of collagen matrices by human cells. *Cell* **67,** 403–410.

16. Ehrlich, H. P. and White, M. E. (1983) Effect of increased concentrations of PGE levels with EBdr fibroblasts within a populated collagen lattice. *J. Invest. Dermatol.* **81,** 572–575.

17. Ehrlich, H. P., Allison, G. M., Page, M. J., Koltun, W. A., and Graham, M. F. (2000) Increased gelsolin expression and retarded collagen lattice contraction with Crohn's diseased intestinal smooth muscle cells. *J. Cell. Physiol.* **182,** 303–309.

18. Monesano, B. and Orci, L. (1988) Transforming growth factor β stimulates collagen-matrix contraction by fibroblasts. *Proc. Natl. Acad. Sci. USA* **85,** 4894–4897.

19. Ehrlich, H. P. and Rittenberg, T. (2000) Differences in the mechanism for high versus moderate density fibroblast populated collagen lattice contraction. *J. Cell. Physiol.* **185,** 432–439.

20. Han, Y. P., Hughes, M., and Garner, W. L. (2002) rhPDGF-BB and TGFβ mediate contraction of human dermal FPCLs is inhibited by RHO/GTPase inhibitor but does not require Phophatidylinsositol-3 kinase. *Wound Rep. Regen.* **10,** 169–176.

21. Rittenberg, T. and Ehrlich, H. P. (1992) Free fatty acids and dialyzed serum alterations of fibroblast populated collagen lattice contraction. *Tissue Cell* **24,** 243–251.

22. Lin, Y. C. and Grinnell, F. (1995) Treatment of human fibroblasts with vanadate and platelet-derived growth factor in the presence of serum inhibits collagen matrix contraction. *Exp. Cell. Res.* **221,** 73–82.

23. Ehrlich, H. P., Keefer, K. A., Myers, R. I., and Passaniti, A. (1999) Wound contraction, vanadate and myofibroblasts. *Arch. Surg.* **134,** 494–501.

21

A Quantifiable In Vitro Model to Assess Effects of PAI-1 Gene Targeting on Epithelial Cell Motility

Kirwin M. Providence, Lisa Staiano-Coico, and Paul J. Higgins

1. Introduction

Gene "knockout" studies and analysis of physiologically relevant in vitro models have clarified basic mechanisms in the tissue response to injury *(1–5)*. Fundamental to this process is the genetic reprogramming required for conversion of normally sedentary cells to an actively motile, invasive phenotype *(5,6)*. It is difficult, however, to identify important events among the diverse changes associated with the initiation and maintenance of migration or the acquisition of "plasticity" in a specific cell type in the intact animal. Thus, the development of in vitro approaches that closely mimic defined stages in epidermal wound repair facilitates discovery of the critical elements and provides an opportunity to probe the underlying molecular mechanisms.

Several in vitro assays address particular aspects of the wound repair process, such as the Boyden chamber model for evaluation of barrier-dependent or barrier-free motility, and suspension gels of varying matrix composition and rigidity to assess three-dimensional constraints on cellular behavior. Although such systems provide relevant information, the spatial relationship among distinct cohorts of cells that participate in wound repair (i.e., the proliferative, locomoting, and distal quiescent compartments) is not maintained in either the Boyden chamber or in-gel methods. Migration of substrate-anchored epithelial cells into scrape-denuded areas of a previously intact monolayer, by contrast, provides a simple, highly reproducible, spatial, and temporal context in which to dissect mechanisms associated with epithelial wound repair (discussed in **ref. 3**). More important, the proliferating compartment (required to maintain

From: *Methods in Molecular Medicine, vol. 78: Wound Healing: Methods and Protocols*
Edited by: Luisa A. DiPietro and Aime L. Burns © Humana Press Inc., Totowa, NJ

the integrity of the migrating front) and the motile population induced in response to epithelial monolayer trauma are physically distinct and easily accessible for molecular, biochemical, and immunocytochemical analysis *(3)*. A similar functional distribution occurs during wound healing in vivo, indicating that several important aspects of injury repair are recapitulated in the monolayer scrape model *(1,3,4,7,8)*. Indeed, such in vitro modeling approaches combined with molecular genetic manipulations have served to highlight the role of plasminogen activator inhibitor type-1 (PAI-1), the major physiological regulator of plasmin generation, an injury-response gene, and an important modulator of cell-to-substrate adhesion *(9–12)*, in wound-associated cellular migration *(3,13,14)*.

We have developed an in vitro epithelial injury model that reproduces subpopulation-specific cell function similar to that evident during the in vivo wound repair response *(3)*. This chapter describes methods for use of this quantifiable system of trauma resolution to identify cohort-dependent changes in gene expression and assess the effects of gene targeting on epithelial cell motility (using antisense PAI-1 construct delivery as an example).

2. Materials
2.1. Cell Culture and Microscopy

1. An established line of newborn rat epidermal keratinocytes is used in the monolayer denudation injury model *(15)*; primary keratinocyte cultures derived from pup skin produce equivalent results (*see* **Note 1**).
2. Dulbecco's modified Eagle's medium [DMEM]; 1 g of D-glucose/L, from Gibco-BRL or Cellgro) supplemented with 10% (v/v) fetal bovine serum (FBS), L-glutamine (20 mM), streptomycin (1 mg/mL), and penicillin (1000 U/mL) is used in all experiments (*see* **Note 2**).
3. Hank's balanced salt solution (HBSS), pH 7.0 : 1.3 mM CaCl$_2$, 5 mM KCl, 0.3 mM KH$_2$PO$_4$, 0.5 mM MgCl$_2$, 4 mM MgSO$_4$, 0.14 M NaCl, 4 mM NaHCO$_3$, 0.3 mM Na$_2$HPO$_4$, 5.6 mM glucose.
4. Only tissue culture–grade plastic should be used for rat keratinocyte culture (35 × 10 and 100 × 20 mm diameter Corning dishes, cat. no. 430165 and 430167, respectively, provide sufficient cells for wound closure assessments and mRNA/protein analyses, respectively) (*see* **Note 3**).
5. P1000 plastic pipet tips (Continental, San Diego, CA).
6. A Nikon TMS phase-contrast inverted microscope equipped with a ×10 objective is used for all wound repair assessments. In one of the ×15 wide-field oculars an eyepiece grid reticle (10 × 10 mm, partitioned into 0.5- or 1.0-mm squares; Fisher part no. 12-561-RG2 and 12-561-RG3, respectively) is mounted (Fisher, Pittsburgh, PA). A stage micrometer or calibration plate is required to calculate migratory front closure rate (micrometers per hour).

2.2. Northern Blot

1. Purescript RNA isolation kit (Gentra, Minneapolis, MN).
2. RNA denaturation buffer: 1X MOPS buffer, 6.5% formaldehyde, and 50% formamide. 10X MOPS buffer consists of 0.4 M 3-N-morpholino-propanesulfonic acid, pH 7.0; 0.1 M sodium acetate; and 0.01 M EDTA-Na$_2$ (*see* **Note 4**).
3. Agarose/formaldehyde gels: 1.2% agarose; 1.1% formaldehyde; 1X MOPS, pH 8.0.
4. RNA gel-loading buffer: 1 mM EDTA, pH 8.0, 0.25% bromophenol blue, 0.25% xylene cyanol, 50% glycerol.
5. Ethidium bromide (EtBr) (0.5 μg/mL in water).
6. RNA transfer solution (10X SSPE): 1.5 M NaCl, 96 mM NaH$_2$PO$_4$, 10 mM EDTA-Na$_2$.
7. Prehybridization buffer: 50% formamide, 2.8% sodium dodecyl sulfate (SDS), 5.6X Denhardt's solution (10% ficoll, 10% polyvinylpyrrolidine, 10% bovine serum albumin), 5X SSPE, 100 μg/mL of sheared salmon sperm DNA (phenol-chloroform extracted, ethanol precipitated, boiled and rapidly cooled).
8. Hybridization buffer: 50% formamide, 2.2X Denhardt's solution, 5X SSPE, 1% SDS, 100 μg/mL of sheared salmon sperm DNA, 10% dextran sulfate.
9. Northern blot wash buffer: 0.1X SSPE/0.1% SDS.
10. X-ray film or phosphorimager screen.

2.3. Construction of Vector and Transfection of Rat Keratinocytes

1. Vector design: pBluescript containing a full-length rat PAI-1 cDNA is digested with *Eco*RI and *Hind*III to generate a 2.6-kb insert (representing nucleotides –118 to +2572 relative to the start site of transcription). Agarose gel–purified DNA is blunt ended with Klenow fragment/dNTPs using a fill-in reaction. *Not*I linkers are ligated and the fragments digested with *Not*I and purified by agarose gel electrophoresis. Flanked inserts are ligated to *Not*I-digested phosphatase-treated Rc/CMV expression vector DNA and subsequently transformed into competent INVαF′ *Escherichia coli*. Plasmid DNA is isolated from ampicillin-resistant colonies; restriction endonuclease digestion and Southern blot analysis, using a 726-bp *Pst*I/*Apa*I-digested PAI-1 cDNA fragment as a probe, confirms sense (Rc/CMVPAI) and antisense (Rc/CMVIAP) insert orientation (**Fig. 1**). Insert template activity can be assessed in vitro for both constructs using T7 polymerase to initiate PAI-1 antisense and sense transcripts (confirmed by hybridization analysis and coupled STP3 transcription-translation [Novagen]/Western blotting, respectively) (*see* **Note 5**).
2. Qiagen plasmid purification kits.
3. Luria-Bertoni (LB) medium containing 50 μg/mL of ampicillin.
4. Chloramphenicol, in 70% ethanol.
5. TE buffer: 10 mM Tris-HCl, 1 mM EDTA, pH 8.0.
6. For transient transfection, DNA:LipofectAMINE (Gibco) ratios of 2–6 μg of DNA:18 μL of LipofectAMINE are optimal for transfection of 35- and

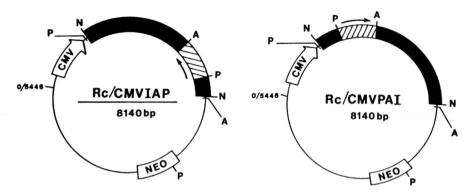

Fig. 1. Schematics of PAI-1 antisense (Rc/CMVIAP) and sense (Rc/CMVPAI) expression vector pair; solid black regions correspond to PAI-1 cDNA. Topography of known restriction sites (P, *Pst*I; N, *Not*I; A, *Apa*I) is used to interpret endonuclease digest patterns. The cross-hatched areas in the cloned cDNA inserts represent the 726-bp *Pst*I-*Apa*I fragment used in Southern blot confirmation of insert orientation (*see* **ref. 16** for details).

100-mm dish cultures, respectively. For solution A, 9 µL of antibiotic- and serum-free DMEM (*see* **Subheading 2.1., item 2**) is combined with 18 µL of LipofectAMINE. Solution B consists of 9 µL of antibiotic- and serum-free DMEM containing 2 or 6 µg of DNA. Solutions A and B are mixed, left at room temperature for 30 min, and 1 or 5 mL of antibiotic- and serum-free DMEM is added (depending on whether transfection is designed for 35- or 100-mm dishes) prior to addition to rat keratinocyte cultures (*see* **Notes 6** and **7**).

2.4. Protein Gel Electrophoresis

1. Cell extraction (sample) buffer: 50 m*M* Tris-HCl, pH 8.0, 1% 2-mercaptoethanol, 2% SDS, 0.01% bromophenol blue, 10% glycerol.
2. Separating gel (1.5-mm-thick gel): 9% acrylamide, 0.24% bisacrylamide, 0.375 *M* Tris-HCl, pH 8.8; 0.1% SDS, 0.03% ammonium persulfate, 0.025% TEMED.
3. Stacking gel: 3% acrylamide, 0.08% bisacrylamide, 0.125 *M* Tris-HCl, pH 6.8, 0.1% SDS, 0.03% ammonium persulfate, 0.05% TEMED.

3. Methods
3.1. Microscopic Measurement of Wound Closure Rate

1. Seed rat keratinocytes at high initial cell densities into serum-containing DMEM (*see* **Note 1**).
2. Immediately after attaining confluency, aspirate the growth medium and wash the monolayers twice with HBSS. Wash volumes are 2 and 5 mL for 35- and 100-mm culture dishes, respectively.

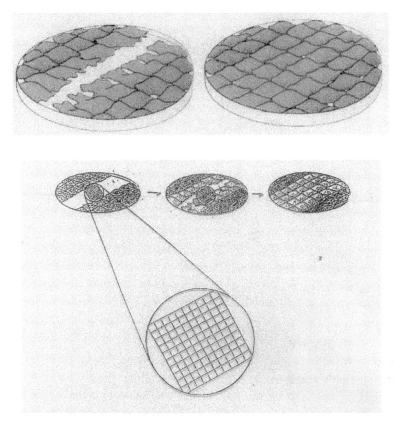

Fig. 2. Rat keratinocytes are grown to confluency and maintained in serum-free DMEM for 3 d to create a contact-inhibited quiescent population. A single scrape wound is created in the monolayer using the narrow end of a P1000 plastic pipet tip initiating migration from the cohort of cells immediately bordering the wound edge (**top left**). In the rat keratinocyte system, this wound is completely resolved within 28–30 h (**top right**) (*see* **Fig. 3**). Immediately after wounding, the size of the injury "bed" is measured by superimposition of the ocular grid over the wound field, and measurements are taken at 20 distinct regions over the length of the scrape site (**bottom left**). At specified intervals over the subsequent 30 h, the size of the "unhealed" region is assessed again over 20 distinct areas as the wound area is resolving (**bottom middle**) and until the injury is completely closed (**bottom right**).

3. Add serum-free DMEM and maintain the cells in this medium for 3 d prior to use; this creates a contact-inhibited quiescent population that approximates the in vivo epidermis.
4. Create wounds in the monolayers by pushing the narrow end of a sterile P1000 plastic pipet tip through the monolayer (**Fig. 2**).

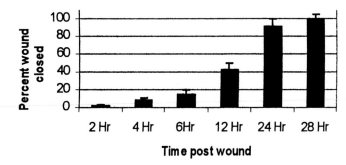

Fig. 3. Kinetics of monolayer wound repair in rat keratinocyte system. Scrape injury to confluent cultures of rat keratinocytes, maintained in serum-free DMEM for 3 d prior to creation of wound with a P1000 pipet tip (*see* **Subheading 3.1.**), initiates a repair response that culminates in complete trauma site "healing" within 28 h. Data plotted are the mean ± SD of measurements from three independent experiments.

5. Place the culture dish on the microscope stage, with one axis of the ocular grid aligned parallel to the long axis of the scrape wound and the stage positioned so that one side of the wound border meets the edge of the first grid square.
6. Measure the size of the "unhealed" wound bed over 20 distinct sites at defined hourly intervals to yield a wound repair profile (**Fig. 3**). The type of pipet tip type is not critical but should be kept constant to obtain reproducible wound widths. The P1000 was selected because it provided a scrape injury that was effectively healed in the rat keratinocyte system (with a wound closure rate of approx 40 µm/h) within 28–30 h (**Fig. 3**) while providing easy microscopic visualization of the entire wound field using a ×10 objective (*see* **Note 8**).

3.2. Cohort-Specific Evaluation of mRNA Abundance

1. Harvest cells immediately adjacent to the wound (termed *edge isolates*) by pushing the wide end of a P1000 pipet tip (i.e., the end opposite that used to create the original scrape injury) along the existing wound tract (*see* **Note 9**). This displaces cells directly at, and 5 mm from, the wound edge; time-lapse microscopy estimates that this procedure recovers the major fraction of the motile cohort.
2. Carefully aspirate the medium and subsequently collect the scrape-released cells by centrifuging at 1400*g*.
3. Wash the remaining monolayers once with serum-free medium.
4. Immediately release the cells located 40 mm from the wound site (i.e., in the intact, uninvolved monolayer region; termed *monolayer isolates*) by scraping and collect by centrifugation.
5. Disrupt the harvested cells in 1.2 mL of Purescript lysis solution.
6. Add 400 µL of DNA-protein precipitation buffer.
7. Incubate on ice for 5 min.

8. After centrifuging for 5 min at 15,000*g*, collect the supernatant.
9. Precipitate the RNA with an equal volume of isopropanol.
10. Harvest by centrifuging at 15,000*g* for 5 min at room temperature.
11. Wash the RNA pellet in 70% ethanol and store in TE buffer.
12. Suspend 10 µg of RNA in denaturation buffer and incubate at 55°C for 15 min.
13. Add a 1/5 vol of RNA gel-loading buffer, place the samples in the agarose gel slots, and separate for 3 h at 70 V in 1X MOPS buffer.
14. Stain the gels for 30 min with EtBr, wash twice for 30 min in water, and photograph to check the integrity of the 28S and 18S ribosomal species.
15. Transfer the RNA from EtBr-stained gels to Nytran maximum strength nylon membranes by capillary action in 10X SSPE for 16 h, and immobilize onto the membrane using a UV Stratalinker on the autolink setting.
16. Incubate the membrane at 42°C for 2 h in prehybridization buffer followed by hybridization with random-primed ^{32}P-labeled cDNA probes (5×10^6 cpm) to PAI-1 (and an appropriate normalization cDNA; e.g., A-50) *(3,15)* in hybridization buffer for 16 h at 42°C. (Probe preparation and labeling procedures are standard and, therefore, not detailed in this chapter.)
17. Wash the membranes three times in wash buffer for 15 min each at 42°C, then an additional three times for 15 min each at 55°C.
18. Expose the blots to Kodak X-OMAT AR-5 film using intensifying screens or place in a Storm Phosphorimager for analysis.
19. Using this combined method of location-specific cell harvest and Northern blot assessment of PAI-1 mRNA abundance, identify the transcripts that are differentially expressed in the migrating cohort (**Fig. 4**).

3.3. Preparation of Transfectant-Grade DNA

Large-scale preparations of plasmid DNA are obtained using Qiagen kits.

1. Inoculate LB medium (10 mL) containing ampicillin with one colony of expression vector–transformed *(16)* E. *coli* bacteria and incubate overnight at 37°C with moderate shaking.
2. Add culture to 500 mL of LB medium containing ampicillin and grow to an OD_{600} of 0.8.
3. Add chloramphenicol to a final concentration of 1 mg/mL for overnight incubation at 37°C with shaking to amplify plasmid copy number and inhibit bacterial replication.
4. Centrifuge the bacteria at 6000*g* for 15 min at 4°C, and process the samples according to the manufacturer's instructions.
5. After precipitation of the purified plasmid, wash the pellet twice with 70% ethanol, air-dry, and resuspend in TE buffer.

3.4. Vector Delivery and Assessment of Function

1. Aspirate the medium in confluent rat keratinocyte cultures and incubate the cells for 5 h with DNA/LipofectAMINE complexes (Rc/CMV empty vector, Rc/CMVIAP, or Rc/CMVPAI) as prepared in **Subheading 2.3., item 1**.

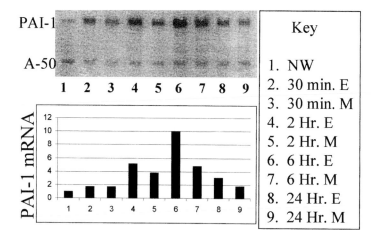

Fig. 4. Wound-induced PAI-1 transcript expression is particularly abundant in the edge cell subpopulation as compared to the monolayer isolates. (**Top**) Representative Northern blot illustrating PAI-1 and A-50 mRNA levels. A-50 is used as a normalization control since its expression does not change as a function of wounding in cultured cells *(3)*. (**Bottom**) PAI-1 mRNA abundance in edge (E) as compared to monolayer (M) isolates at various times (30 min to 24 h) after scrape injury to confluent rat keratinocyte cultures; PAI-1 expression is normalized to the corresponding A-50 transcript signal as assessed with a Storm Phosphorimager. NW, nonwounded control.

2. After transfection, add an equal volume of DMEM/10% FBS medium for an overnight incubation.
3. The next day, aspirate the medium, wash the cultures with HBSS, and incubate the cells in serum-free DMEM for 3 d prior to wounding.
4. Following monolayer scrape injury, assess the extent of trauma closure at defined times by the ocular grid method (*see* **Subheading 3.1.**), and plot the data as a function of time (**Fig. 5**). In any such genetic approach, however, it is necessary to confirm that the introduced constructs affect expression of the targeted protein.
5. Harvest the edge and monolayer isolates (*see* **Subheading 3.2.**), directly lyse the cells in extraction buffer (*see* **Subheading 2.4., item 1**), and separate the constituent proteins on SDS/9% acrylamide gels.
6. After blotting to nylon membranes, confirm the level of PAI-1 expression by standard Western-blotting procedures (detailed in **ref.** *17*) (see inset in **Fig. 5**).
7. Incubate the protein blots with rabbit antibodies to rat PAI-1 (5 µg of IgG/mL), and visualize antigen-antibody complexes with horseradish peroxidase–conjugated secondary antibody and chemiluminescence *(17)*.

4. Notes

1. It is important to maintain initial population input levels of $\geq 10^3$ cells/cm^2 to prevent premature keratinocyte differentiation. Initiation of culture with clonal

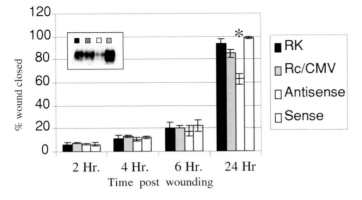

Fig. 5. Genetic modification of PAI-1 protein levels in wound-stimulated rat keratinocyte (RK) migration. RKs were transfected with non-insert-containing expression vector (Rc/CMV) or the PAI-1 antisense (Rc/CMVIAP) or sense (Rc/CMVPAI) constructs. Cells were maintained in serum-free DMEM for 3 d prior to wounding. The extent (percentage) of wound closure (on *y*-axis) for each transfected population was assessed relative to nontransfected (RK) controls. The inset is a representative Western blot depicting PAI-1 protein levels in leading-edge cells harvested at the 24-h time point. The Rc/CMVIAP construct effectively attenuated PAI-1 expression in migrating RKs. The histogram illustrates the mean ± SD of three independent experiments. *Significant statistical difference between PAI-1 antisense-transfected cells and the three other experimental conditions indicating that PAI-1 downregulation markedly impaired directed cell motility.

    seeding densities of rat keratinocytes and primary rat keratinocytes promotes both intraclonal suprabasal maturation and stratification.

2. It is critical that low Ca^2 content "keratinocyte" growth medium (available from several vendors) not be used in the monolayer scrape wound system. Such low Ca^{+2} media generally are not conducive to formation and/or maintenance of close epithelial cell-to-cell contacts, at least to the extent evident in standard Ca^{+2} content growth medium. This can significantly impact the interpretation of outcome since the polarization of function (i.e., migration, proliferation, region-specific gene expression) in the wounded monolayer is likely to be, at least partly, dependent on cell-to-cell communication. The expression of particular genes activated in response to trauma (such as PAI-1), for example, is strongly influenced by distance from the wound edge in vivo as well as in vitro and extent of culture confluency *(3,14)*.

3. The use of glass-surface (regardless of the type) dishes and even glass cover slips is strongly discouraged for wounding studies with rat keratinocytes. Scrape injury of rat keratinocytes maintained on glass results in the elaboration of a migrating front consisting largely of cells with little or no cell-to-cell contact. This is morphologically unlike cells that comprise the migrating tongue in vivo

and is in marked contrast to the migratory response on plastic surfaces on which the cells locomote as a cohesive sheet with only minimal and occasional gaps in neighbor contact.

4. This buffer can be stored for 3 mo at 4°C and should be discarded if yellow; caution must be observed when using formaldehyde and formamide.

5. Details of expression vector construction, determination of insert orientation by restriction site mapping/Southern blotting, and description of the coupled transcription-translation reaction are beyond the scope of this chapter. This information can be found in **ref. *15***.

6. This procedure differs substantially from routine transfection protocols using LipofectAMINE in that relatively small volumes of transfection reagent are used and the level of input DNA is low. The present design is optimal for gene delivery to rat keratinocytes; a transfection efficiency of >80% in rat keratinocytes can be easily obtained with this method.

7. While other liposome formulations have been reported to be maximized for delivery and expression of exogenous genes in epidermal keratinocytes, the system developed here routinely yields the highest transfection efficiencies in primary, established, and transformed newborn rat keratinocyte cultures.

8. The width of the original "wound bed" can vary as a result of pressure differences exerted on the pipet tip. It is critical, therefore, that the wound size be determined by microscopy immediately after scraping and that this value be recorded for each dish in order to properly evaluate closure rates from time zero.

9. It is highly recommended that the tract of the initial scrape injury be traced on the bottom of the culture dish with a marker because this greatly facilitates harvesting of "edge isolates." Cells are best dislodged by placing the culture dish on top of a white sheet of paper and following the marker path with the pipet tip held upside down (i.e., wide end on the wound) and perpendicular to the monolayer surface.

Acknowledgments

This work was supported by grants from the National Institutes of Health (GM57242) and the Department of the Army (DAMD17-98-1-8015, DAMD17-00-1-0124).

References

1. Garlick, J. A. and Taichman, L. B. (1994) Fate of human keratinocytes during reepithelialization in an organotypic culture model. *Lab. Invest.* **70**, 916–924.

2. Romer, J., Lund, L. R., Kriksen, J., Pyke, C., Kristensen, P., and Dano, K. (1996) Impaired wound healing in mice with a disrupted plasminogen gene. *Nat. Med.* **2**, 287–292.

3. Providence, K. M., Kutz, S. M., Staiano-Coico, L., and Higgins, P. J. (2000) PAI-1 gene expression is regionally induced in wounded epithelial cell monolayers and required for injury repair. *J. Cell. Physiol.* **182**, 269–280.

4. Coulombe, P. A. (1997) Towards a molecular definition of keratinocyte activation after acute injury to stratified epithelia. *Biochem. Biophys. Res. Commun.* **236,** 231–238.

5. Sato, Y. and Rifkin, D. B. (1988) Autocrine activities of basic fibroblast growth factor: regulation of endothelial cell movement, plasminogen activator synthesis, and DNA synthesis. *J. Cell Biol.* **107,** 1199–1205.

6. Ando, Y. and Jensen, P.J. (1996) Protein kinase C mediates up-regulation of urokinase and its receptor in migrating keratinocytes of wounded cultures, but urokinase is not required for movement across a substratum *in vitro. J. Cell. Physiol.* **167,** 500–511.

7. Reidy, M., Irwin, C., and Lindner, V. (1995) Migration of arterial wall cells. *Circ. Res.* **78,** 405–414.

8. Zahm, J. M., Kaplan, H., Herard, A. L., Doriot, F., Pierrot, D., Somelette, P., and Puchelle, E. (1997) Cell migration and proliferation during the *in vitro* wound repair of the respiratory epithelium. *Cell Motil. Cytoskel.* **37,** 33–43.

9. Andreasen, P. A., Kjoller, L., Christensen, L., and Duffy, M. J. (1997) The urokinase-type plasminogen activator system in cancer metastasis: a review. *Int. J. Cancer* **72,** 1–22.

10. Blasi, F. (1997) uPA, uPAR, PAI-1: key intersection of proteolytic, adhesive and chemotactic highways? *Immunol. Today* **18,** 415–417.

11. Loskutoff, D. J., Curriden, S. A., Hu, G., and Deng, G. (1999) Regulation of cell adhesion by PAI-1. *APMIS* **107,** 54–61.

12. Stefansson, S. and Lawrence, D. A. (1996) The serpin PAI-1 inhibits cell migration by blocking integrin $\alpha v \beta 5$ binding to vitronectin. *Nature* **383,** 441–443.

13. Bajou, K., Noel, A., Gerard, R. D., Masson, V., Brunner, N., Holst-Hansen, C., Skobe, M., Fusenig, N. E., Carmeliet, P., Collen, D., and Foidart, J. M. (1998) Absence of host plasminogen activator inhibitor 1 prevents cancer invasion and vascularization. *Nat. Med.* **4,** 923–938.

14. Romer, J., Lund, L. R., Eriksen, J., Ralfkiaer, E., Zeheb, R., Gelehrter, T. D., Dano, K., and Kristensen, P. (1991) Differential expression of urokinase-type plasminogen activator and its type-1 inhibitor during healing of mouse skin wounds. *J. Invest. Dermatol.* **97,** 803–811.

15. Boehm, J. R., Kutz, S. M., Sage, E. H., Staiano-Coico, L., and Higgins, P. J. (1999) Growth state-dependent regulation of plasminogen activator inhibitor type-1 gene expression during epithelial cell stimulation by serum and transforming growth factor-$\beta1$. *J. Cell. Physiol.* **181,** 96–106.

16. Higgins, P. J., Ryan, M. P., and Jelley, D. M. (1997) p52[PAI-1] gene expression in butyrate-induced flat revertants of v-*ras*-transformed rat kidney cells: mechanism of induction and involvement in the morphologic response. *Biochem. J.* **321,** 431–437.

17. Li, F., Goncalves, J., Faughnan, K., Steiner, M. G., Pagan-Charry, I., Esposito, D., Chin, B., Providence, K. M., Higgins, P. J., and Staiano-Coico, L. (2000) Targeted inhibition of wound-induced PAI-1 expression alters migration and differentiation in human epidermal keratinocytes. *Exp. Cell Res.* **258,** 245–253.

22

Human Skin Organ Culture

Ingrid Moll

1. Introduction

Reepithelialization is the main process during wound healing that specifically defines the reconstruction of the stratified squamous epithelium. In partial-thickness epidermal wounds, reepithelialization arises from viable epidermal cells at the wound edges as well as from adnexa remaining in the wound bed itself. During the processes involved in epidermal wound healing, keratinocytes undergo a series of behavioral changes including cell migration, proliferation, and differentiation at the wound margins (*1,2*). Migration has been shown to be the first event, which includes the movement of suprabasal cells followed by a mitotic burst (*3,4*). The process of differentiation of the newly formed epidermis starts at a short distance behind the migrating tips, very early before reepithelialization of the whole wound has been completed (*5,6*). These processes are under the influence of chemical attractants, mainly growth factors and extracellular matrix proteins (*7,8*).

These complex processes involved in reepithelialization have mainly been studied in vivo using various animal models (*9*). However, owing to the very different structures of various species and the complex nature of the wounded microenvironment, it is difficult to obtain acceptable, precise data concerning the various stages of reepithelialization for human skin (*10*).

To overcome such difficulties in studying human epidermal wound healing, we have developed a new skin organ culture model, which involves the complete removal of the epidermis from the central portion of a skin disk. The viability and efficiency of such models has been previously demonstrated in various studies investigating complex aspects of cutaneous dendritic cell

From: *Methods in Molecular Medicine, vol. 78: Wound Healing: Methods and Protocols*
Edited by: Luisa A. DiPietro and Aime L. Burns © Humana Press Inc., Totowa, NJ

systems *(11,12)*. We have also used it to investigate both ultraviolet damage within the epidermis *(13)* and keratinocyte transplantation *(14)*. It has also been used to study the expression of basement membrane zone antigens *(15)*.

2. Materials

1. Tissues: Adult human skin samples are used immediately after excision.
2. Dermal biopsy punches, 3- and 6-mm.
3. Falcon culture dish (1 cm in diameter).
4. Medium for cell cultures: Stock medium is Dulbecco's modified Eagle's medium (DMEM) containing 3.7 g/L of $NaHCO_3$, 4.5 g/L of D-glucose, 1.028 g/L of N-acetyl-L-alanyl-L-glutamine, without sodium pyruvate. To prepare medium for cultures, supplement each 100 mL of medium with 0.08 µg of hydrocortisone, 10,000 U of penicillin, 10 mg of streptomycin, and 2 or 5% fetal calf serum (FCS).
5. Dulbecco's phosphate-buffered saline (PBS): without Ca^{2+} or Mg^{2+}.
6. PBS supplemented with 0.1% trypsin and 0.2% EDTA.
7. Acetone.
8. Diaminobenzidine (DAB).
9. Avidin-biotin-peroxidase complex (ABC) (ABC Elite; Vector, Burlingame, CA).
10. H_2O_2.
11. Methanol.
12. Shandon Sequenza apparatus (Shandon-Life Science, Frankfurt/Main, Germany).

3. Methods

3.1. Skin Organ Culture

1. Using a punch subdivide all skin samples into round pieces (diameter: 6 mm). Using a needle fix each sample and remove a punch biopsy (diameter: 3 mm) including the whole epidermis and the papillary dermis from its center (*see* **Notes 1–3**).
2. Place each sample dermis side down on gauze in a culture dish and add DMEM with 2 or 5% FCS. Use approx 1 mL for each dish (**Fig. 1**).
3. Carefully check each skin sample to make sure that the medium is only in contact with the underside of the sample and that the epidermis and the wound bed remain completely exposed to the air.
4. Incubate cultures at 37°C with 10% CO_2 for 3–7 d, depending on the experimental procedure.
5. Change the medium every other day.
6. Transplant freshly isolated or cultured single keratinocytes to the central wound 1 d after establishing the cultures (*see* **Note 4**).

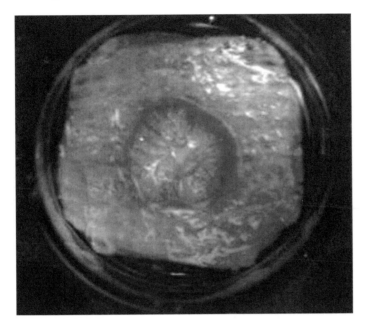

Fig. 1. Skin organ culture model after establishing a central wound.

3.2. Preparation and Transplantation of Isolated Keratinocytes

1. Obtain keratinocytes from the outer root sheath of human hair follicles from freshly plucked anagen hair follicles. Autologous, but also allogenic, keratinocytes can be used.
2. Incubate the follicles in trypsin-PBS solution for 1 h at 37°C.
3. Mechanically separate the cells into solution using sterile pipets.
4. Suspend a total of 1 to 2×10^6 keratinocytes in 5 μL of PBS.
5. Apply one drop (about 200,000 cells) with a micropipet into the center of each wound of the skin organ culture 1 d after its establishment.

3.3. Morphological Evaluation

3.3.1. Hemotoxylin and Eosin Staining

1. Freeze or paraffin embed the skin organ culture specimens and prepare serial sections through each central area (*see* **Note 5**).
2. Stain the sections with hematoxylin and eosin using routine methods. If no part of the central area of the wound lacks an epithelium, even though this might be only one cell layer thick, samples are classified as healed (**Fig. 2**). Samples that fail to show this continuous epithelial cell layer are considered to be unhealed.

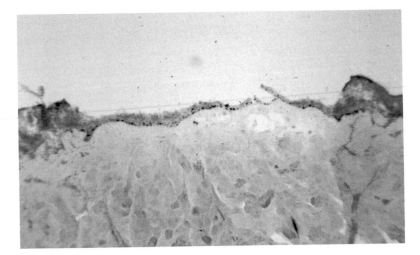

Fig. 2. Frozen section of central wound in a skin organ culture model (7 d). A thin two- to four-cell-layer-thick neoepithelium has developed. Staining was done with antibody MIB I against Ki 67 (Dianova, Hamburg, Germany) to demonstrate the distribution of proliferation (×200).

3.3.2. Immunohistochemical Techniques

For studying the state of differentiation and proliferation, sections are stained immunohistochemically using the primary antibody of interest.

1. Fix frozen or deparaffinized sections in acetone at −20°C for 10 min.
2. For frozen sections, perform indirect immunoperoxidase staining using peroxidase-coupled goat antibodies against mouse or rabbit immunoglobulins (Dako, Hamburg, Germany) as secondary antibodies with DAB and H_2O_2 being employed for the staining reactions.
3. For paraffin sections, apply the ABC:
   a. Deparaffinize and rehydrate the sections.
   b. Block endogenous peroxidase activity using 1% H_2O_2 in methanol for 30 min.
   c. Apply primary antibodies for 1 h at 37°C using a Shandon Sequenza apparatus.
   d. Apply secondary antibodies for 30 min at room temperature using biotin related anti–mouse antibodies (1 : 100; Vector).
   e. Apply ABC Elite reagent for 30 min at room temperature.
   f. Develop the staining reaction using DAB and H_2O_2.

4. Notes

1. All procedures must be done very shortly after excision and under sterile conditions.

2. For one series of experiments, skin of identical localizations and of patients of similar age should be used exclusively; otherwise, differences might be owing to various ages, skin viabilities, and thicknesses.
3. Additionally, sun exposure, application of ointments, or other diagnostic procedures prior to excision should be carefully noted, and the results should be correlated to those additional treatments.
4. No differences between cultured or freshly isolated keratinocytes are obvious within 7 d of culture.
5. Frozen sections are cut 5–7 µm thick, and paraffin section, 3 to 4 µm.

References

1. Palladini, R. D., Takahashi, K., Bravo, N. S., and Coulombe, P. A. (1996) Onset of re-epithelialization after skin injury correlates with a reorganization of keratin filaments in wound edge keratinocytes: defining a potential role for keratin 16. *J. Cell. Biol.* **132,** 381–397.
2. Eisen, A. Z., Holyoke, J. B., and Lobitz, W. C. (1955) Responses of the superficial portion of the human pilosebaceous apparatus to controlled injury. *J. Invest. Dermatol.* **15,** 145–156.
3. Marks, S. and Nishikawa, T. (1973) Active epidermal movement in human skin in vitro. *Br. J. Dermatol.* **88,** 245–248.
4. Garlick, J. A. and Taichman, L. D. (1994) Fate of human keratinocytes during reepithelialization in an organotypic culture model. *Lab. Invest.* **6,** 916–924.
5. Brandner, J. M., Houdek, P., Kief, S., and Moll, I. (1999) Changes of cell junctions during early wound healing. *Arch. Dermatol. Res.* **291,** 134.
6. Moll, I., Houdek, P., Schäfer, S., Nuber, U., and Moll, R. (1999) Diversity of desmosomal proteins in regenerating epidermis: immunohistochemical study using a human skin organ culture model. *Arch. Dermatol. Res.* **291,** 437–446.
7. Moulin, V. (1995) Growth factors in skin wound healing. *Eur. J. Cell Biol.* **68,** 1–7.
8. Martin, P. (1997) Wound healing—aiming for perfect skin regeneration. *Science* **276,** 75–81.
9. Mainsbridge, J. N. and Knapp, A. M. (1987) Changes in keratinocyte maturation during wound healing. *J. Invest. Dermatol.* **89,** 253–263.
10. Oliver, A. M., Kaawach, W., Weiler Mithoff, E., Watt, A., Abramovic, D. R., and Rayner, C. R. (1991) The differentiation and proliferation of newly formed epidermis on wounds treated with cultured epithelial allografts. *Br. J. Dermatol.* **125,** 147–154.
11. Pope, M., Betjes, M. G. H., Hirmand, H., Hoffmann, L., and Steinmann, R. M. (1995) Both dendritic cells and memory T lymphocytes emigrate from organ cultures of human skin and form distinctive dendritic-T-cell conjugates. *J. Invest. Dermatol.* **104,** 11–17.
12. Lukas, M., Stössel, H., Hefel, L., Imamura, S., Fritsch, P., Sepp, N. T., Schuler, G., and Romani, N. (1996) Human cutaneous dendritic cells migrate through dermal

lymphatic vessels in a skin organ culture model. *J. Invest. Dermatol.* **106,** 1293–1299.

13. Bohnert, E., Moll, I., and Jung, E. G. (1993) Formation and quantitation of SBCs in UV-irradiated, short-term primary, and organotypic keratinocyte cultures. *Arch. Dermatol. Res.* **258,** 70.

14. Moll, I., Houdek, P., Schmidt, H., and Moll, R. (1998) Characterization of epidermal wound healing in a human skin organ culture model: acceleration by transplanted keratinocytes. *J. Invest. Dermatol.* **111,** 251–258.

15. Hintner, H., Frisch, P. O., Foidart, J. M., Stingl, G., Schuler, G., and Katz, S. L. (1980) Expression of basement membrane zone antigens at the dermoepidermal junction in organ cultures of human skin. *J. Invest. Dermatol.* 74, 200–204.

23

In Vitro Matrigel Angiogenesis Model

Anna M. Szpaderska and Luisa A. DiPietro

1. Introduction

Angiogenesis, the formation of new blood vessels, is a key process in wound healing. During the angiogenic phase of injured tissue repair, epithelial cells sprout and branch from preexisting vessels, evolving into a network of new capillaries. This formation of vasculature, necessary for normal granulation tissue, is tightly regulated spatially and temporally. Blood capillaries regress in a relatively short time after tissue integrity is restored.

Physiological angiogenesis observed in healing wounds as well as excessive blood vessel proliferation in pathological states have been extensively studied in recent years (1). Advances in in vivo and in vitro assays of angiogenesis have been powerful tools for increasing our understanding of regulation of angiogenesis (2). A convenient model for studying endothelial cell differentiation in vitro is the tube formation assay on Matrigel. Matrigel is a mixture of basement membrane proteins and growth factors secreted by Engelbreth-Holm-Swarm murine sarcoma cells. It consists of laminin, type IV collagen, entactin, nidogen, heparan sulfate proteoglycan, and growth factors including transforming growth factor-β, epidermal growth factor, platelet-derived growth factor, and insulin growth factor-1 (3,4).

When endothelial cells are grown in vitro on Matrigel, these cells organize into capillary-like tubules (5). Within 1 h of plating on the gel, endothelial cells form cords, which develop into a three-dimensional branching network (**Fig. 1**). By mixing test substances with Matrigel prior to gel polymerization or by adding them to endothelial cell suspension, both putative inducers and inhibitors of neovascularization can be studied.

From: *Methods in Molecular Medicine, vol. 78: Wound Healing: Methods and Protocols*
Edited by: Luisa A. DiPietro and Aime L. Burns © Humana Press Inc., Totowa, NJ

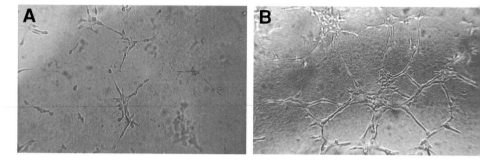

Fig. 1. Morphology of SVEC4-10 cells on Matrigel. Cells were cultured for **(A**
4 h and **(B)** 8 h.

In this chapter, we describe a modification of the in vitro angiogenesis
assay that can be used to assess the relative angiogenic phenotype of wound
tissue.

2. Materials
2.1. Preparation of Conditioned Medium
1. Wound tissue (collect all samples in triplicate).
2. Phosphate-buffered saline (PBS), sterile.
3. Serum-free Dulbecco's modified Eagle's medium (DMEM) containing 4.5 g/L
   of glucose and supplemented with 100 U/mL of penicillin, 100 µg/mL of streptomycin, and 0.25 µg/mL of fungizone.
4. 70% Ethanol solution made with sterile distilled water.
5. Sterile distilled water.
6. Tissue culture plates (100 mm).
7. 12-Well tissue culture plates.
8. Sterile microtubes (1.5 mL).
9. Ultrafree-4 Centrifugal Filter Units with 5000 nominal molecular weight limit
   (NMWL) Membrane (Millipore, Bedford, MA).
10. Gel-loading pipet tips for sample removal from the filter unit.
11. No. 10 scalpels (Becton Dickinson, Hancock, NY).
12. Centrifuge with swinging-bucket or fixed-angle rotor that accommodates 17 ×
    120 mm 15-mL tubes, capable of 7500g.

2.2. Cell Culture

1. SVEC4-10 murine endothelial cell line (American Type Culture Collection,
   Rockville, MD) (*see* **Note 1**).
2. DMEM containing 4.5 g/L of glucose and supplemented with 10% fetal bovine
   serum, 100 U/mL of penicillin, 100 µg/mL of streptomycin, and 0.25 µg/mL
   of fungizone.

3. Trypsin (0.25%)-EDTA (0.1%) solution.
4. Cell culture dishes (100 mm).
5. Sterile tubes (15 mL).

2.3. Preparation of Matrigel

1. Matrigel (Collaborative Biomedical Products, Bedford, MA).
2. Sterile pipet tips chilled to 4°C.
3. 48-Well plates chilled to 4°C.

2.4. Image Analysis and Quantitation

1. Microscope with camera mounted on an ocular tube connector (Leitz DM IL).
2. Charge coupled device (CCD) camera and camera control unit (DEI-750D; Optronics Engineering, Goleta, CA).
3. Color monitor (Sony Trinitron PVM-14N1U; Sony, San Jose, CA).
4. Image acquisition software (Optronics Acquisition; Optronics Engineering).
5. Computer (Gateway 2000, Pentium Pro 333 MHz, 128 Mb RAM).

3. Methods

3.1. Preparation of Conditioned Medium

1. Collect the wound tissue. Place the collected wounds into culture dishes filled with sterile PBS to prevent drying.
2. Mince the wound tissue in a sterile 100-mm tissue culture plate with a scalpel.
3. Transfer the minced wound tissue with the scalpel into the wells of a 12-well plate filled with 1 mL of serum-free DMEM.
4. Incubate the minced tissue in the media in a humidified incubator at 37°C in 5% CO_2 for 24 h.
5. Transfer the conditioned medium with a sterile pipet tip into a microtube.
6. Spin the medium at 10,000g for 5 min at 4°C to pellet the wound tissue.
7. Rinse the Ultrafree-4 centrifugal filter unit with 70% ethanol and with sterile distilled water (*see* **Note 2**).
8. Transfer the supernatant into the Ultrafree-4 centrifugal filter unit (*see* **Note 3**).
9. Concentrate according to the manufacturer's instruction to a final volume of 100 µL.
10. Retrieve the concentrate from the filter units with a gel-loading tip (*see* **Note 4**).

3.2. Angiogenic Assay

1. Grow SVEC4-10 cells to near confluence in DMEM.
2. Thaw Matrigel on ice at 4°C overnight (*see* **Note 5**).
3. Place a 48-well plate on ice.
4. Coat the wells of a 48-well plate with Matrigel (150 µL/well). Use chilled pipet tips (*see* **Note 6**).
5. Place the Matrigel-coated plate in a tissue culture incubator for 30–60 min to polymerize the gel.

6. Collect the cells by trypsin-EDTA treatment. Neutralize the trypsin with DMEM containing 10% serum.
7. Transfer the cells into a 15-mL tube and spin at 700g for 3 min at 4°C.
8. Discard the supernatant.
9. To wash the cells gently, resuspend the pellet in serum-free DMEM and spin the cells at 700g for 3 min at 4°C.
10. Discard the supernatant.
11. Gently resuspend the cells in serum-free DMEM at 1.3×10^5 cells/mL. Keep the cell suspension on ice.
12. Plate 150 μL of cell suspension/well (1.95×10^4 cells/well).
13. Add 100 μL of the wound tissue–conditioned medium to the 150-μL of the cell suspension.
14. Incubate the cells for 6–8 h at 37°C in a 5% CO_2 humidified atmosphere (*see* **Note 7**).

3.3. Analysis and Quantitation of Tube Formation

1. Choose the lowest magnification of the microscope that will include all of the areas to be analyzed (*see* **Note 8**).
2. Adjust the focus so that the image through the ocular as well as the image on the monitor is in focus.
3. Adjust contrast, exposure, and color.
4. Capture the image using software that is associated with the CCD camera and save the image in a TIFF format.
5. Print the images. Count the number of tubes formed in a blinded fashion (*see* **Note 9**).

4. Notes

1. Other endothelial cell lines (e.g., human umbilical vein endothelial cell) can also be used.
2. Ultrafree-4 centrifugal filters are not sterile and they cannot be autoclaved. They can be treated with ethylene oxide, instead of rinsing with 70% ethanol.
3. Take care not to transfer minced wound tissue into the Ultrafree-4 centrifugal filter unit because this will clog the filter membrane. If necessary, after the first centrifugation, transfer the supernatant to a new tube and centrifuge for an additional 5 min.
4. If not used immediately, conditioned media can be stored at –80°C. Quick-freeze the media in 1.5-mL microtubes in a dry ice–ethanol mixture.
5. Keep Matrigel on ice at all times. Matrigel polymerizes at 24–37°C.
6. Do not dilute Matrigel; dilution dramatically reduces tube formation.
7. SVEC4-10 cells will start growing as a monolayer 36–48 h after plating on Matrigel.
8. It is helpful to draw a grid on the bottom of each well on the outside of the plate. Dividing the well into several fields facilitates quantitation.
9. All images should be counted by the same person.

References

1. Folkman, J. (1995) Angiogenesis in cancer, vascular, rheumatiod and other disease. *Nat. Med.* **1,** 27–31.
2. Jain, R. K., Schlenger, K., Hackel, M., and Yuan, F. (1997) Quantitative angiogenesis assays: progress and problems. *Nat. Med.* **3,** 1203–1208.
3. Kleinman, H. K., McGarvey, M. L., Hassel, J. R., Star, V. L., Cannon, F. B., Laurie, G. W., and Martin, G. R. (1986) Basement membrane complexes with biological activity. *Biochemistry* **25,** 312–318.
4. Vukicevic, S., Kleinman, H. K., Luyten, F. P., Roberts, A., Roche, N. S., and Reddi, A. H. (1992) Identification of multiple growth factors in basement membrane matrigel suggest caution in interpretation of cellular activity related to extracellular matrix components. *Exp. Cell Res.* **202,** 1–8.
5. Kubota, Y., Kleinman, H. K., Martin, G. R., and Lawrey, T. J. (1988) Role of laminin and basement membrane in the morphological differentiation of human endothelial cells into capillary-like structures. *J. Cell. Biol.* **107,** 1589–1598.

II

ANALYSIS AND MANIPULATION OF WOUND HEALING

24

Quantification of Wound Angiogenesis

Quentin E. H. Low and Luisa A. DiPietro

1. Introduction

Angiogenesis occurs during embryonic development and in adult tissues *(1)*. In developmental angiogenesis, the primitive vascular network formed during neovasculogenesis matures to form the circulatory system. In the adult animal, physiological angiogenesis occurs in the ovaries during the menstrual cycle and in tissue repair. Pathological angiogenesis is observed in many diseases, including inflammatory diseases, diabetic retinopathy, and cancer *(2,3)*. Because angiogenesis plays such crucial roles in both instances, it is not surprising that this phenomenon is widely studied. Parallel to the numerous studies, there are also a large variety of angiogenic assays described *(4)*.

One key feature in these angiogenic assays is the enumeration of vessels to ascertain the angiogenic response to endogenous or exogenous agents. For vessel quantification, investigators have traditionally counted the number of vessels formed. This approach has been used both for in vitro assays and for measuring the degree of angiogenesis *in situ*. Reagents directed against endothelial cell markers allow for more specific identification of vessels. Surface markers such as von Willebrand factor *(5)*, VE-cadherin *(6–8)*, endothelial cell surface marker-1 *(9)*, and CD31 (PECAM-1) *(10)* have been utilized for endothelial cell detection. In addition, lectins such as *Ulex europaens* agglutinin-1 *(11,12)* have been successfully used to visualize endothelial cells. A more systematic manner of quantification is possible when immunohistochemistry or histological approaches are used in conjunction with image analysis programs. Currently, a wide variety of programs are available, such as Optimas and Image-Pro Plus (Media Cybernetic, Silver Spring, MD), analySIS (Soft Imaging, Lakewood, CO), and NIH Image (National Institutes of Health, Bethesda, MD). These imaging approaches are amenable to both in

From: *Methods in Molecular Medicine, vol. 78: Wound Healing: Methods and Protocols*
Edited by: Luisa A. DiPietro and Aime L. Burns © Humana Press Inc., Totowa, NJ

vitro and in vivo assays of angiogenesis and also have particular advantages for analysis of heterogeneous environments, like that found in wounds.

Tissue repair is a complex biological process, involving many soluble factors, multiple cell types, and a variety of extracellular matrix molecules, and it spans four overlapping stages: hemostasis, inflammation, tissue proliferation, and wound resolution *(13,14)*. Therefore, analysis of wound healing in either normal or diseased conditions relies on determining inflammatory cell influx, angiogenesis, reepithelialization, collagen content, and wound-breaking strength. Together the knowledge obtained from measuring these parameters contributes to a complete picture of normal and impaired repair.

In this chapter, we describe a method for measuring blood vessel density in a model of dermal wound repair. This method utilizes imaging software in distinguishing vessel-specific signals from those of the background and enumeration of vessel-specific areas.

2. Materials
2.1 Animals, Anesthesia, and Euthanasia

1. Five- to 6-wk-old female BALB/c mice (Harlan Sprague Dawley, Indianapolis, IN).
2. Halothane (Halocarbon Laboratories, Riveredge, NJ).
3. Olive oil.
4. Glass desiccant jar.

2.2. Full-Thickness Excisional Wound Model

1. Biopsy punch (3 mm) (Acuderm, Ft. Lauderdale, FL), for creating full-thickness wound.
2. Biopsy punch (5 mm) for isolating wound.

2.3. Sample Collection and Embedding

1. Specimen base mold (Fisher Tissue Path., Fisher Scientific, Pittsburgh, PA).
2. TBS Tissue Freezing Media (Triangle Biomedical Science, Durham, NC).
3. Dry ice or liquid nitrogen.
4. Dissecting tools.

2.4. Tissue Sectioning

1. Cryostat (CM 3000; Leica Microsystems, Deerfield, IL).
2. Superfrost Plus slides (Fisher Scientific).
3. Hematoxylin.

2.5. Immunohistochemistry

1. PAP pen (Kiyota; Research Products, Mount Prospect, IL).
2. Acetone.

3. Methanol.
4. Phosphate-buffered saline (PBS), pH 7.4.
5. 30% H_2O_2.
6. Normal mouse serum (Harlan Bioproducts, Indianapolis, IN).
7. Monoclonal rat anti–mouse CD31 antibody (clone MEC13.3; Pharmingen, San Diego, CA).
8. Biotinylated mouse anti–rat IgG antibody (Jackson Immunoresearch Laboratories, West Grove, PA).
9. Horseradish peroxidase–linked avidin-biotin complex (ABC-HRP) (Vector, Burlingame, CA).
10. Stock solution of diaminobenzidine (25 mg/mL) (DAB) (Kirkegaard and Perry, Gaithersburg, MD).
11. 0.1 M Tris-Cl, pH 7.6.
12. Harris hematoxylin (Sigma, St. Louis, MO).
13. Whatman #1 Qualitative Filter Papers (Whatman, Maidstone, England).
14. 95% and 100% Ethanol.
15. Cytoseal 280 (Stephens Scientific, Kalamazoo, MI).

2.6. Image Analysis (see Note 1)

Equipment used in our setup is given in parentheses.

1. Microscope with camera mounting on the ocular tube connector (Zeiss Axioskop 20 with photo tube; Carl Zeiss, Thornwood, NY).
2. Charge-coupled device (CCD) camera and camera control unit (DEI-750D; Optronics Engineering, Goleta, CA).
3. Color monitor (separate from the computer system) (Sony Trinitron PVM-14N1U; Sony, San Jose, CA).
4. Image analysis software. (we used Scion Image [Scion, Frederick, MD] but NIH Image [National Institutes of Health] can also be used). Scion Image can be downloaded from Scion's Web site at www.scion.com. NIH Image (for Apple Macintosh) can also be used. This program can be obtained from http://rsb.info.nih.gov/nih-image. For Scion Image, an IBM-compatible computer with a Pentium processor with at least 32 Mb of RAM running any of the following operating systems is needed: Windows 95, Windows 98, Windows ME, Windows NT, or Windows 2000. For NIH Image, a color Macintosh with at least 4Mb of RAM operating on System 7.0 or later is needed.
5. Image acquisition software (Optronic Acquisition for Windows 95).
6. Computer system (Gateway 2000, Pentium Pro 333 MHz, 128Mb RAM operating on Windows 95).

3. Methods

3.1. Animals, Anesthesia, and Euthanasia (see Note 2)

1. For anesthesia, mix an 8:24 dilution of halothane in olive oil in a 50-mL conical tube (*see* **Note 3**).

2. Introduce the agent into the lower chamber of a glass desiccant jar, and allow the fumes to saturate the chamber for a few minutes (*see* **Note 4**).
3. Put the mouse into the top chamber and monitor its response to the anesthesia (*see* **Note 5**). Check the animal's response to the anesthesia and proceed with wound tissue isolation as outlined in **Subheading 3.2.**
4. For euthanasia, either a desiccant jar or covered jar can be used. Put some gauze in the bottom of the jar and saturate it with 1 to 2 mL of halothane. Allow sufficient fumes to build up for an overdose.

3.2. Full-Thickness Excisional Wound Model

1. Shave the anesthetized mice on the dorsal side.
2. Lift up the skin longitudinally along the middle of the back of the mouse by grasping it between two fingers below the neck and just above the base of the tail. The skin will naturally form a double layer as it is lifted up and away from the body.
3. Place the mouse on its side so that the folded skin rests on a firm surface (*see* **Note 6**).
4. Using a 3-mm dermal punch, create one full-thickness punch wound on either side of the midline by punching through both layers of skin.
5. Create a total of six 3-mm wounds, three on each side of the folded skin, and space each wound between 0.5 and 1 cm apart from edge to edge.
6. For wound harvest, remove the dorsal skin from the euthanized mouse by making a small incision at the base of the neck and cutting around the collection of wounds, taking care not to damage them.
7. Place the excised skin on a firm surface, and remove the wound and its surrounding tissue by using a 5-mm dermal punch or by cutting around the wound with a scalpel (*see* **Note 7**).

3.3. Tissue Sectioning

1. Prepare 10-μm sections from frozen embedded tissues (*see* **Note 8**).
2. Collect the middle of the wound for analysis.
3. Mount two sections on one slide so that they are parallel to each other within 1–1.5 cm apart.
4. Store the sections at –80°C.

3.4. Immunohistochemistry

1. Allow the frozen slides to come to room temperature and wipe off the condensation on them.
2. Using a PAP pen, draw a circle around the sections to form a hydrophobic barrier.
3. Fix the sections in acetone for 15 min at room temperature (*see* **Note 9**).
4. Wash the slides three times for 5 min each in PBS, pH 7.4.
5. To quench endogenous peroxidase, treat the sections with 0.3% (v/v) H_2O_2 in methanol for 30 min.

6. Wash the slides three times for 5 min each in PBS, pH 7.4.
7. Block nonspecific protein-protein interactions by incubating the sections in a 1 : 10 dilution of normal mouse serum in PBS, pH 7.4, for 30 min (*see* **Note 10**).
8. Prior to incubation with the primary antibody, blot the pool of blocking serum off the slide by tilting it on its side onto paper towels.
9. For endothelial cell detection, incubate the sections in 1.0 µg/mL of MEC 13.3 primary antibody for 30 min.
10. Wash the slides three times for 5 min each in PBS, pH 7.4.
11. Incubate the slides in 13.0 µg/mL of biotinylated mouse anti–rat IgG antibody for another 30 min.
12. Wash the slides three times for 5 min each in PBS, pH 7.4.
13. Incubate the slides in ABC-HRP for 30 min.
14. Wash the slides three times for 5 min each in PBS, pH 7.4.
15. After the final set of washes in PBS, pH 7.4, incubate the slides in DAB for 10 min. The working concentration of DAB is 2% (v/v) in 0.1 M Tris-HCl, pH 7.6. It is activated with 0.1 mL of 0.5% H_2O_2/5 mL of 2% DAB solution (*see* **Note 11**).
16. Wash the slides in distilled water for 10 min.
17. Counterstain the sections by dipping the slides once or twice in Harris hematoxylin (*see* **Note 12**).
18. Rinse the slides under running tap water until the water runs clear.
19. Dehydrate the slides by immersing them twice in 95% ethanol for 1 min followed by two immersions in 100% ethanol.
20. Allow the slides to dry and then mount them with Cytoseal.

3.5. Image Analysis

1. Choose the lowest magnification on the microscope that will include all of the area to be analyzed (*see* **Note 13**).
2. Adjust the focus so that the image through the ocular as well as the image on the monitor is in focus.
3. Move the sample off to the side so that a background (glass only) reading can be taken.
4. Move the sample back into view and adjust other components, such as contrast, exposure, and color correction, until a bright, sharp image is obtained.
5. Capture the image using software that is associated with the CCD camera and save the image in the TIFF format.
6. Open the saved files in NIH Image.
7. Use the Freehand Selection Tool to draw an outline of the entire wound bed (**Fig. 1**).
8. Measure the total area in pixels.
9. Select the Automatic Outlining Tool (wand) and double-click to activate the Look Up Table (LUT). Adjust the LUT tool so that the degree of false coloring matches that of the DAB staining (*see* **Note 14**). Restore the previous selection (from **step 7**) and measure the LUT colored area (**Fig. 2**).

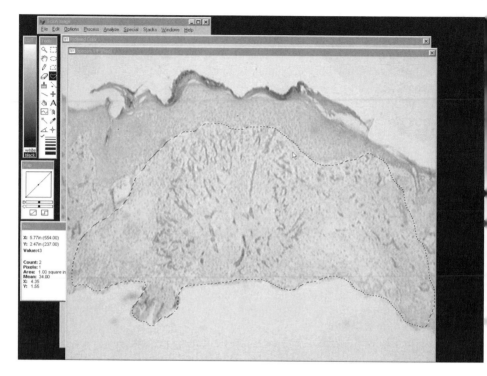

Fig. 1. Freehand selection of wound bed area. The d 5 wound section was captured and converted to TIFF format. The image was opened in Scion Image, and the dermal wound bed was outlined using the Freehand Selection Tool. This area was then measured and the measurement represents the total wound area.

10. Select Show Results in the Analyze tab to get the pixel values for the two areas measured.
11. Measure the CD31-positive area within the wound bed and calculate the percentage of vascularization as follows:

$$\% \text{ Vascularization} = \frac{\text{CD31-positive area}}{\text{Total wound bed area}} \times 100\%$$

4. Notes

1. The mounted camera feeds into the camera control unit and is linked from the camera control unit to the computer via the LPT1 port. Another connection exits between the camera control unit and the Sony monitor via Y/C ports. Because there is only one LPT1 port on the computer, we have installed a data switch so that we are able to toggle between the camera input signal and the signal going out to the printer.

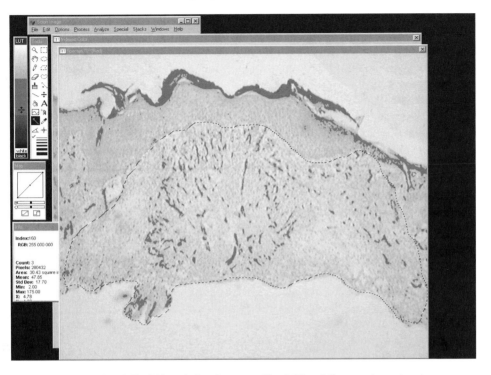

Fig. 2. Analysis of CD31[+] staining in wound bed. The d 5 wound section image was highlighted with Automatic Outlining Tool to falsely color the CD31-stained regions in the wound bed. The intensity of the coloring was adjusted by changing the threshold levels using the LUT. The initial wound selection was restored (dotted lines) and the area measured to determine the area occupied by the false coloring within the defined wound area.

2. Inbred strains are housed in a specific-pathogen-free environment. All animal procedures were approved by the Loyola University Medical Center Institute Animal Care and Use Committee.
3. Other forms of anesthetic agents can also be used, such as phenobarbital, however, we prefer inhalation anesthesia, because this is relatively easy to administer.
4. Instead of pipeting the halothane:olive oil mixture directly into the lower chamber of the desiccant jar, a handful of cotton balls or a wad of gauze can also be saturated with the anesthetic agent and placed in a dish.
5. One 32-mL mixture of halothane and olive oil should be sufficient to anesthetize eight 20- to 25-g mice.

6. We use a hockey puck for our wounding and harvesting procedures. This provides a firm surface to support the mouse while being pliable enough for the punch to embed into the puck, allowing for a complete excision of the wound. Some investigators have found a hard rubber door wedge to be more suitable than a hockey puck.

7. For wound harvesting, a 5-mm biopsy punch could be used. Typically, we cut a 1×1 cm square around the wound. This provides a greater amount of surrounding uninjured skin, making the sample easier to embed and less prone to tearing during preparation of the frozen section.

8. Follow the manufacturer's instructions for optimal temperature and knife angle for creating skin sections. Some wound samples may be more difficult to create because they are more fragile in nature. This is especially true for excisional wound samples isolated from the earlier healing time points (up to 3 d postwounding).

9. Incubations in acetone, H_2O_2/methanol, PBS washes, and hematoxylin counter-staining can be carried out in slide holders or Coplin jars, depending on the number of slides to be immunostained. Incubations with blocking serum, both primary and secondary antibodies, ABC-HRP, and DAB can be performed by pipeting 50–100 µL of a reagent on a slide, within a circle drawn with the PAP pen.

10. All dilutions, unless otherwise, are in PBS, pH 7.4. For ABC-HRP complex, create the complexes at least 30 min before use.

11. The antibodies and ABC-HRP complex are stable at 4°C for 1 wk; however, the DAB solution needs to be made fresh each time. We find that the background from DAB is reduced when the slides are incubated in the dark. DAB is a carcinogen, so handle accordingly and refer to the manufacturer's instructions for deactivation and disposal.

12. Filter the hematoxylin prior to counterstaining. This step helps to eliminate any particulate that may contribute to increased background. Furthermore, a few dips in hematoxylin are sufficient to reveal the wound's architecture. While it is crucial that the level of hematoxylin staining be kept to a lower intensity than normal, it is also important that enough staining is achieved so that the architecture of the wound is still distinguishable. Increased staining time may mask the signal from DAB and result in a lower contrast between the primary DAB signal and those from the hematoxylin and, consequently, the distinction by the imaging software between CD31+ signals and background.

13. Depending on the image analysis setup, one will have to adjust the image size so that the area of interest is within the image field of view. It is also important to be aware of the size variations that exist in your model, because it is crucial that comparison among samples be done at the same magnification. Typically, we perform our measurements under ×25 magnification. Some cameras may have different fields of view, which may affect the area available for analysis.

14. When background intensity is high, the false coloring often includes DAB-positive areas as well as DAB-negative areas. To eliminate false positives, activate the Eraser tool, and click and drag over those areas.

Acknowledgment

This work was supported by National Institutes of Health grants GM 55238 and GM 50875.

References

1. Carmeliet, P. (2000) Mechanisms of angiogenesis and arteriogenesis. *Nat. Med.* **6,** 389–395.
2. Carmeliet, P. and Jain, R. K. (2000) Angiogenesis in cancer and other diseases. *Nature* **407,** 249–257.
3. Folkman, J. and D'Amore, P. A. (1996) Blood vessel formation: what is its molecular basis? *Cell* **87,** 1153–1155.
4. Jain, R. K., Schlenger, K., Hockel, M., and Yuan, F. (1997) Quantitative angiogenesis assays: progress and problems. *Nat. Med.* **3,** 1203–1208.
5. Weidner, N., Semple, J. P., Welch, W. R., and Folkman, J. (1991) Tumor angiogenesis and metastasis—correlation in invasive breast carcinoma. *N. Engl. J. Med.* **324,** 1–8.
6. Kawashima, M. and Kitagawa, M. (1998) An immunohistochemical study of cadherin 5 (VE-cadherin) in vascular endothelial cells in placentas with gestosis. *J. Obstet. Gynaecol. Res.* **24,** 375–384.
7. Martin-Padura, I., De Castellarnau, C., Uccini, S., Pilozzi, E., Natali, P. G., Nicotra, M. R., Ughi, F., Azzolini, C., Dejana, E., and Ruco, L. (1995) Expression of VE (vascular endothelial)-cadherin and other endothelial-specific markers in haemangiomas. *J. Pathol.* **175,** 51–57.
8. Wong, R. K., Baldwin, A. L., and Heimark, R. L. (1999) Cadherin-5 redistribution at sites of TNF-alpha and IFN-gamma-induced permeability in mesenteric venules. *Am. J. Physiol.* **276,** H736–H748.
9. Lassalle, P., Molet, S., Janin, A., Heyden, J. V., Tavernier, J., Fiers, W., Devos, R., and Tonnel, A. B. (1996) ESM-1 is a novel human endothelial cell-specific molecule expressed in lung and regulated by cytokines. *J. Biol. Chem.* **271,** 20,458–20,464.
10. Vanzulli, S., Gazzaniga, S., Braidot, M. F., Vecchi, A., Mantovani, A., and Wainstok de Calmanovici, R. (1997) Detection of endothelial cells by MEC 13.3 monoclonal antibody in mice mammary tumors. *Biocell* **21,** 39–46.
11. Suri, C., McClain, J., Thurston, G., McDonald, D. M., Zhou, H., Oldmixon, E. H., Sato, T. N., and Yancopoulos, G. D. (1998) Increased vascularization in mice overexpressing angiopoietin-1. *Science* **282,** 468–471.
12. Thurston, G., Suri, C., Smith, K., McClain, J., Sato, T. N., Yancopoulos, G. D., and McDonald, D. M. (1999) Leakage-resistant blood vessels in mice transgenically overexpressing angiopoietin-1. *Science* **286,** 2511–2514.
13. Martin, P. (1997) Wound healing—aiming for perfect skin regeneration. *Science* **276,** 75–81.
14. Singer, A. J. and Clark, R. A. (1999) Cutaneous wound healing. *N. Engl. J. Med.* **341,** 738–746.

25

In Vivo Matrigel Migration and Angiogenesis Assays

Katherine M. Malinda

1. Introduction

Angiogenesis, the process of new blood vessels forming from preexisting vessels, is an important feature in developmental processes, wound healing, and pathologic conditions such as cancer and vascular diseases. Owing to the importance of angiogenesis, a relatively simple and rapid in vivo method to determine the angiogenic potential of compounds is desirable to augment in vitro findings.

One such quantitative method is the murine Matrigel plug assay, which can measure both angiogenesis and antiangiogenesis. Matrigel, an extract of the Englebreth-Holm-Swarm tumor composed of basement membrane components, is liquid at 4°C and forms a gel when warmed to 37°C *(1)*. When plated on Matrigel, human umbilical vein endothelial cells undergo differentiation into capillary-like tube structures in vitro *(2,3)*. In vivo, Matrigel is either injected alone or mixed with potential angiogenic compounds and injected subcutaneously into the ventral region of mice, where it solidifies, forming a "Matrigel plug." When known angiogenic factors, such as basic fibroblast growth factor (bFGF), are mixed with the Matrigel and injected, endothelial cells migrate into the plug and form vessels. The level of angiogenesis is typically viewed by embedding and sectioning the plugs in paraffin and staining using Masson's Trichrome, which stains the Matrigel blue and the endothelial cells/vessels red **(Fig. 1)**. These vessels contain erythrocytes, indicating that they form functional capillaries. Additionally, these capillaries stain positively for factor VIII–related antigen *(4,5)*. In unsupplemented Matrigel, few cells invade the plug. Strongly angiogenic compounds result in

From: *Methods in Molecular Medicine, vol. 78: Wound Healing: Methods and Protocols*
Edited by: Luisa A. DiPietro and Aime L. Burns © Humana Press Inc., Totowa, NJ

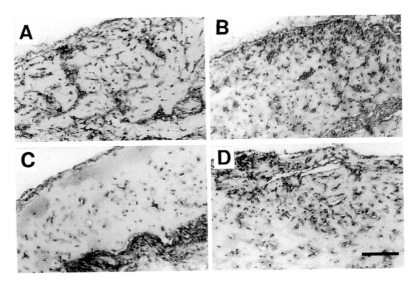

Fig. 1. Sections of Matrigel plugs stained with Masson's trichrome. All sections are oriented with the side underlying the skin at the top of the image. (**A,B**) Representative fields of plugs containing 5 μg/mL of Tβ4. (**C**) Field showing Matrigel alone. (**D**) Representative field of a plug with 10 ng/mL of ECGS (positive control). Sections with Tβ4 contain many more cells than Matrigel alone and have cells with a morphology similar to those in the ECGS control. Bar = 100 μm. With permission from Malinda, K. M., Goldstein, A. L., and Kleinman, H. K. (1997). Thymosin β4 stimulates directional migration of human umbilical vein endothelial cells. *FASEB J.* **11**, 474–481.

yellowish plugs, so initial indications of activity can be made at the time when plugs are removed from the mice.

The assay also can be utilized when putative antiangiogenic compounds are being tested. In this assay, Matrigel is premixed with bFGF (angiogenic compound), and the test substances are then added. Thus, test antiangiogenic substances inhibit the formation of vessels induced by bFGF in the Matrigel plug. In this case, the plugs removed from the mouse are relatively colorless, and when viewed by Masson's trichrome staining should contain few endothelial cells. Because of the strong vascular response to bFGF, it is also possible to measure hemoglobin levels with the Drabkin assay *(4)*.

One important consideration in using either of the above assays is the degree of variability that will be observed. Differences in the mice and in the basement membrane preparations will affect the background levels of blood vessel formation one observes. Age and gender of the mice selected also can result in different results between experiments. Vessel formation in young mice (6 mo old) is reduced as compared to mice 12–24 mo old *(4)*. Additionally, if

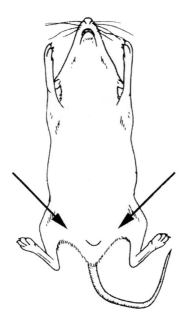

Fig. 2. Diagram of ventral side of a mouse. Arrows show optimal sites for Matrigel injection.

the Matrigel is injected into different sites in the mouse, variability can result. Lower angiogenic response is observed if the material is injected into the dorsal surface of the animal, while one of the best areas in terms of angiogenic response is the ventral surface of the mouse in the groin area close to the ventral midline (**Fig. 2**). Regardless of these potential problems, this assay is one of the best for the rapid screening of potential angiogenic and antiangiogenic compounds.

2. Materials

2.1. General Materials

1. C57Bl/6N female mice. Three or four mice are needed for each test group.
2. Additional cages and supplies, one for each test group.
3. Matrigel (Collaborative Biomedical, Bedford, MA); store at –20°C. Enough will be needed to inject 0.5 or 1 mL per mouse.
4. 6-mL Syringes (Monoject).
5. 25-gauge Needles (Monoject).
6. 14-mL Falcon round-bottomed tubes (#2059) (Becton Dickinson, Rutherford, NJ).
7. 10X Phosphate-buffered saline (PBS) (Biofluids, Rockville, MD) diluted to 1X in sterile, distilled H$_2$O.

8. Endothelial cell growth supplement (bovine brain extract containing acid fibroblast growth factor and bFGF [ECGS]) (Collaborative Biomedical, Becton-Dickinson, Rutherford, NJ): Prepare a 1 mg/mL solution just before use in sterile, distilled H_2O and store unused portion in aliquots at $-20°C$ (loses activity after 1 mo, according to manufacturer). Or for bFGF (Collaborative Biomedical), prepare a 1 mg/mL solution just before use in sterile, distilled H_2O and store unused portion in aliquots at $-20°C$. Final concentration used in experiment is either 10 ng/mL and 100 ng/mL of ECGS or 150 ng/mL of bFGF (concentration of bFGF varies with lot and supplier).
9. Tabletop vortex (Vortex Genie 2; Scientific Industries).
10. Sterile pipet tips.
11. Sterile 5-mL disposable pipets.
12. Scalpel or dissecting scissors.

2.2. Embedding and Quantitation

1. Scintillation vials or specimen vials.
2. 10% Formalin in PBS.
3. Histology service for paraffin embedding, sectioning, and staining with Masson's trichrome stain.
4. Microscope equipped with a video system linked to a computer with NIH Image software (free to the public).
5. Spreadsheet software.

3. Methods

3.1. Screening Putative Angiogenic Compounds

1. Thaw Matrigel on ice overnight at 4°C. At no time should Matrigel be warmed to room temperature during handling.
2. Mix Matrigel on a vortex; place on ice (*see* **Notes 1** and **2**).
3. Pipet equal amounts of Matrigel for each test condition in separate 14-mL tubes on ice. Each mouse injection requires 0.5–1 mL with three or four mice for each condition (*see* **Notes 2** and **3**).
4. Tubes should be included for the positive and negative controls. Negative control is Matrigel alone; positive control contains either 10 and 100 ng/mL of ECGS or 150 ng/mL of bFGF added to Matrigel.
5. Equalize the volumes with cold PBS so that after test substances have been added, all tubes contain Matrigel at equal dilutions (*see* **Note 4**). Mix on the vortex.
6. Load syringes with each solution and inject 0.5 or 1 mL subcutaneously into the ventral area of each mouse (*see* **Fig. 2**; **Notes 5** and **6**).
7. Place the animals of each test group in separate labeled cages.
8. After 7–10 d, sacrifice the animals and remove the Matrigel plugs. Plugs appear as bumps on the ventral side of the animal and are removed using a sharp pair of scissors or a scalpel. Remove the plug with some surrounding tissue for orientation when histology is performed.

3.2. Screening Putative Antiangiogenic Compounds

1. Thaw Matrigel on ice overnight at 4°C.
2. Mix Matrigel on a vortex; place on ice (*see* **Note 1**).
3. Pipet equal amounts of Matrigel for each test condition in separate 14-mL tubes on ice. Each mouse injection requires 0.5–1 mL, three or four mice for each condition (*see* **Notes 2** and **3**).
4. Add 150 ng/mL of bFGF to all tubes except the one used for the negative control containing Matrigel alone.
5. Equalize the volumes with cold PBS so that after putative antiangiogenic ogenic substances have been added, all tubes contain Matrigel at equal dilutions (*see* **Note 4**). Mix on the vortex.
6. Load syringes with each solution and inject 0.5 or 1 mL subcutaneously into the ventral area of each mouse (*see* **Fig. 2**; **Notes 5** and **6**).
7. Place the animals of each test group in separate labeled cages.
8. After 7–10 d, sacrifice the animals and remove the plugs. Plugs appear as bumps on the ventral side of the animal and are removed using a sharp pair of scissors or a scalpel. Remove the plug with some surrounding tissue for orientation when histology is performed.

3.3. Fixation and Quantitation by Microscopy

1. Place the plugs in labeled scintillation or specimen vials filled with 10% formalin. Allow the plugs to fix overnight before embedding in paraffin.
2. Section and stain with Masson's trichrome, which stains the endothelial cells/vessels dark red and the Matrigel blue (*see* **Note 7**).
3. Visually inspect the sections to determine whether the test substance is stimulatory or inhibitory and whether further quantitation is necessary (**Fig. 1**).
4. Capture images at ×10 magnification of the area underlying the skin (*see* **Note 8**).
5. Adjust the image to selectively highlight the gray level corresponding to the endothelial cells/vessels by using the *density slice function* of the software and the light level of the microscope.
6. Use the *measure option* to measure the area occupied by all cells selected by the *density slice function* (*see* **Notes 9** and **10**).
7. Count at least three random fields of the area underlying the skin on each slide.
8. Load the numbers into a spreadsheet and calculate the total area occupied by endothelial cells in the three fields and then average these areas among the three or four replicate mouse plugs.
9. Compare the resulting numbers for statistical significance.

4. Notes

1. Bubbles form when Matrigel is vortexed. Minimize vortexing to keep bubbles to a minimum or injection problems will occur. Also, allowing the tubes to stand on ice for 10 min will reduce the number of bubbles.

2. All reagents should be kept as sterile as possible to prevent infecting the mice.
3. Always use gloves when working with reagents.
4. Keep the dilution of Matrigel to a minimum. If too dilute, it will not gel when injected.
5. Use caution when handling animals. Only approved personnel should handle animals. Contact your animal safety officer for the appropriate safety regulations you must follow. Wear gloves, masks, gowns, hair cover, and boots when appropriate.
6. Inject solutions slowly; a bump should form under the skin. If the skin is punctured during injection, the material will flow out. Allow the Matrigel to gel for about 10 s before removing the needle at the end of the injection; otherwise injected material will leak out.
7. Fixation according to these methods can inactivate epitopes so that immunohistochemical analysis may not work. An alternative is to make frozen sections of the tissue and eliminate the fixation and paraffin steps.
8. An alternative method of quantitating vessel ingrowth is to measure the hemoglobin content using, e.g., a Drabkin reagent 525 kit (Sigma, St. Louis, MO).
9. Selecting only a portion of the image may be required, to avoid counting areas that contain bubbles, cracks, or other artifacts that refract the light and may be picked up by the density slice feature. If this is necessary, use the drawing tool to draw a box, note the size in the "info" window, and draw the same size box on all sections for the entire experiment.
10. Since animals will have different responses to the injected material, it is not unusual to experience variability in the responses of animals to different test substances.

Acknowledgment

This chapter is reprinted from *Methods in Molecular Medicine, Vol. 46: Angiogenesis Protocols*, edited by J. C. Murray, © 2001 Humana Press, Totowa, NJ. It was written while the author was employed at the National Institute of Dental and Craniofacial Research, National Institutes of Health, Bethesda, MD, and was prepared as part of the author's official duties as a US government employee.

References

1. Kleinman, H. K., McGarvey, M. L., Liotta, L. A., Gehron-Robbey, P., Tryggvasson, K., and Martin, G. R. (1982) Isolation and characterization of type IV procollagen, laminin, and heparin sulfate proteoglycan from the EHS sarcoma. *Biochemistry* **24,** 6188–6193.
2. Kubota, Y., Kleinman, H. K., Martin, G. R., and Lawley, T. J. (1988) Role of laminin and basement membrane in the morphological differentiation of human endothelial cells into capillary-like structures. *J. Cell Biol.* **107,** 1589–1598.

3. Grant, D. S., Kinsella, J. L., Fridman, R., Auerbach, R., Piasecki, B. A., Yamada, Y., Zain, M., and Kleinman, H. K. (1992) Interaction of endothelial cells with a laminin A chain peptide (SIKVAV) in vitro and induction of angiogenic behavior in vivo. *J. Cell Physiol.* **153,** 614–625.

4. Passaniti, A., Taylor, R. M., Pili, R., Guo, Y., Long, P. V., Haney, J. A., Pauly, R. R., Grant, D. G., and Martin, G. R. (1992) A simple, quantitative method for assessing angiogenesis and antiangiogenic agents using reconstituted basement membrane, heparin, and fibroblast growth factor. *Lab. Invest.* **67,** 519–528.

5. Kibbey, M. C., Corcoran, M. L., Wahl, L. M., and Kleinman, H. K. (1994) Laminin SIKVAV peptide-induced angiogenesis in vivo is potentiated by neutrophils. *J. Cell Physiol.* **160,** 185–193.

26

Endothelial Cell Migration Assay

A Quantitative Assay for Prediction of In Vivo Biology

Mark W. Lingen

1. Introduction

Angiogenesis, the growth of new blood vessels from preexisting ones, is one of the essential phenotypes of tumor formation and is also important in a number of normal physiological processes including growth and development *(1)*, wound healing *(2)*, and reproduction *(3–5)*. An inadequate amount of angiogenesis contributes to ulcer formation *(6)*, and excessive angiogenesis contributes to the pathology of a number of conditions including arthritis, psoriasis, and solid tumors. In a series of now classic experiments, Folkman and colleagues demonstrated that solid tumors could not grow any larger than 2 to 3 mm in diameter without being able to induce their own blood supply *(7)*. Whether or not angiogenesis occurs in a particular tissue depends on the balance between the relative amounts of molecules that induce and molecules that inhibit angiogenesis *(8)*. In normal tissues, blood vessels are usually quiescent and cells usually secrete low levels of inducers and high levels of inhibitors.

The expression of the angiogenic phenotype is a complex process that requires several cellular and molecular events to occur in both a spatial and temporal pattern. Some of these activities include the degradation of the surrounding basement membrane, the migration of the endothelial cells through the connective-tissue stroma, cell proliferation, the formation of tubelike structures, and the maturation of these endothelial-lined tubes into new blood vessels *(9,10)*. Because there are so many different identifiable steps to in vivo

From: *Methods in Molecular Medicine, vol. 78: Wound Healing: Methods and Protocols*
Edited by: Luisa A. DiPietro and Aime L. Burns © Humana Press Inc., Totowa, NJ

angiogenesis, a number of different in vitro assays have been developed as predictors of in vivo blood vessel growth.

1.1. In Vitro Angiogenesis Assays (see Note 1)

In vitro assays of angiogenesis have several distinct advantages over in vivo assays. For example, assays have been developed for many of the individual phenotypic responses that are required for endothelial cells to form new vessels. In vitro assays are also attractive because the results can be quickly and accurately quantified. Examples of this type of quantification would include endothelial cell chemotaxis assays, cell proliferation, cell motility, matrix degradation, and tube formation.

1.1.1. Endothelial Cell Proliferation

Many investigators rely on predicting in vivo angiogenesis by simply measuring the ability of a given compound to induce or inhibit the proliferation of endothelial cells in vitro *(11,12)*. While cell proliferation is clearly important in angiogenesis, this type of assay has several shortcomings. First, data have shown that one can stimulate angiogenesis that will result in functional new blood vessels in the absence of cell proliferation. Second, not all inducers or inhibitors of angiogenesis positively or negatively affect cell proliferation. As such, using a proliferation assay to predict in vivo biology may overlook potential substances that may be either an inducer or inhibitor.

1.1.2. In Vitro Wound Model

Under normal in vivo circumstances, endothelial cells do not proliferate as a result of their contact inhibition within the context of a vessel. In fact, endothelial cells are thought to have one of the longest turnover times of all cells in the body. Similarly, when grown in a monolayer in culture, primary endothelial cells become contact inhibited when grown to confluence. However, if a portion of the tissue culture plate is denuded, the endothelial cells at the edge of the wound will migrate to close this space. The rate at which the space is closed can be quantified as a measurement of in vitro *(13–15)* wound healing. While this is a rapid assay, there are a few shortcomings. First, while it can be performed on gridded plates, quantification can be problematic. Second, it does not represent a definitive assay for directed migration (chemotaxis), which is presumed to be an important factor in in vivo angiogenesis.

1.1.3. In Vitro Capillary Formation

A popular in vitro assay for predicting in vivo angiogenesis is the capillary formation, or "tube," assay. Endothelial cells are plated on various substrates including collagen and Matrigel in the presence or absence of various factors that may stimulate or inhibit tube formation (16–18). In the presence of an angiogenic factor, the monolayer of endothelial cells will invade the substrate below and form capillary-like structures, which may demonstrate either cord-like or patent tubelike configurations. The assay is attractive in the sense that one can demonstrate the presence or absence of capillary-like structures and therefore suggest the likelihood of in vivo vessel formation. However, the assay is primarily a qualitative one and is not particularly amenable to quantification.

1.1.4. Chemokinesis

Zetter (19) have showed that one can investigate cell migration using colloidal gold-plated cover slips (19). Since endothelial cells will migrate toward angiogenic factors, one can then measure increased/decreased motility in response to various factors. Similarly, this technique has been modified to provide a more quantitative measure of directed migration by using "tracks" (20). This assay has been further modified for high throughput screening in 96-well culture plates using polystyrene beads (21,22). The quantification of cell migration is known to be important for the development of vessels in vivo and, as such, an assay measuring chemokinesis may be predictive of in vivo biology. However, a disadvantage is that this type of assay measures only cell movement only and not directed migration. Biologically speaking, endothelial cells undergo specific directed migration in vivo when responding to cells that are secreting angiogenic factors. Therefore, an assay that can quantify the directed response of endothelial cell migration (chemotaxis) toward a stimulus would be very desirable.

1.1.5. Chemotaxis

Since its original description, the chemotaxis assay, using a modified Boyden chamber, has been used for many years to measure quantitatively the directed migration of different cells types toward a test substance (23,24). Since the initial description, the "migration assay" has been used extensively to evaluate various substances for their ability to stimulate or inhibit endothelial cell migration. Some of these uses have included, but are certainly not limited to, identification of novel inducers or inhibitors of angiogenesis (25–27), characterization of the antiangiogenic activity of peptides derived from the parent molecule (28,29), identification of the key angiogenic factors present in wounds or produced by tumors (30–33), and demonstration of synergistic activity of various antiangiogenic agents (34). The chamber consists of precision-machined acrylic top and bottom plates, assembly hardware, and a silicone gasket. The bottom plate has 48 wells, each with a 25 -µL vol. Corresponding holes in the top plate form the upper wells when the chamber is assembled. The upper chamber has a volume of 50 µL. A single 25 × 80 mm piece of filter membrane is placed between the top and bottom plates, and a gasket is positioned over the filter to create a seal. Narrow raised rims around mating surfaces of top and bottom wells enhance the seal. The migration chamber has cells attached to one side of a semiporous gelatinized membrane with test substances on the other side. In this type of arrangement, the cells can respond to either positive or negative regulators of chemoattraction. The cells and their test substances are incubated together for a period of time sufficient to allow the cells to be induced or inhibited from migrating from one side of the membrane to the other. There are several distinct advantages to this assay. First, it is a rapid assay in which as many as 12 substances (including controls) can be screened in quadruplicate in a very short period of time. Second, small amounts of test substances are needed to perform the assay, which can be critically important when dealing with novel or limited amounts of a given compound. Third, we have found that it has consistently been the most accurate predictor of in vivo angiogenesis.

2. Materials

1. Human microvascular endothelial cells (HMVECs): There are a number of vendors, including Cell Systems (Kirkland, WA) and Clonetics/Biowhittaker (Walkersville, MD), that sell HMVECs (*see* **Note 2**).
2. Growth media: Cells are grown in Endothelial Growth Medium (EGM) (Clonetics/ Biowhittaker). The EGM product consists of the basal medium (EBM) plus the "bullet," which contains several growth supplements. Premade EGM can be purchased. However, the medium has a longer shelf life if purchased as EBM with the bullet.
3. Trypsin/EDTA and Trypsin Neutralizing Solution (TNS): ReagentPack Subculture Reagents (CC-5034; Biowhittaker).
4. Neuro Probe AP48 Chemotaxis Chamber from Neuro Probe, Gaithersburg, MD.
5. Membranes: Semiporous, 5-µm pore membranes (PFC5) from Neuro Probe.
6. 0.5 *M* Acetic acid: Add 3 mL of acetic acid (no. A0808; Sigma, St. Louis, MO) to 97 mL of MilliQ H_2O.
7. Stock solution of 1% gelatin: Add 1 g of gelatin (no. G9391; Sigma) to a final volume of 100 mL of MilliQ H_2O. Autoclave the solution and store at 4°C.
8. Stock solution of 10% bovine serum albumin (BSA): Mix 1 g of BSA (Sigma) with 10 mL of PBS. Filter sterilize with a 0.4-µ*m* filter and store at 4°C.
9. Staining kit: Diff-Quick Stain Set (Dade-Behring, Duluth, GA).
10. Glass slides (no. 48311-703; VWR, Westchester, PA).
11. Cover slips (no. 12-548-5M; Fisher, Pittsburgh, PA).
12. Mounting medium (no. 8310-4; Stephens, Riverdale, NJ).
13. Cryopreservation medium (Cellvation; Celox, St. Paul, MN).
14. Phosphate-buffered saline (PBS).
15. Hank's balanced salt solution (HBSS).

3. Methods

3.1. Propagation and Freezing of Endothelial Cells

1. Culture human dermal microvascular endothelial cells (HMVECs) in EGM and grow in a 37°C incubator containing 5% CO_2. Split and passage the cells as follows (*see* **Note 2**):
   a. Gently rinse the cells with 5 mL of HBSS.
   b. Detach the cells with 3 mL of trypsin until the cells "round up."
   c. Immediately inactivate trypsin with TNS.
   d. Spin down the cells at 800g and remove all of the medium via suction using glass borate Pasteur pipets.
   e. For propagation of cells, split a T-25 flask by adding 20 mL of EGM and placing 5 mL in four flasks (1:4 split).

3.2. Freezing of HMVECs

To ensure maximum number of passages, it is recommended that the cells be split before they reach confluence (*see* **Note 3**).

1. To freeze, wash, trypsinize, quench, and centrifuge the cells as described in **Subheading 3.1.**
2. Remove the media via suction and add 1 mL of Cellvation/10^6 cells.
3. Transfer to 2-mL cryogenic vials.
4. Store the vials at room temperature for 30 min.
5. Place ampoules in an insulated container at –20°C for 60 min.
6. Remove the vials from insulated container and place at –70°C for 60 min.
7. Transfer the vials to the vapor phase of a liquid nitrogen container for 24 h.
8. Store in liquid nitrogen.

3.3. Preparation of Membranes

1. Place 50 mL of the 0.5 M acetic acid solution in a plastic 150-mm dish with six to eight membranes overnight on an orbital shaker at room temperature.
2. The next day, rinse the membranes with MilliQ H_2O three times for 1 h each.
3. Make 50 mL of a 1:100 dilution of the 1% gelatin stock and incubate with the membranes overnight on an orbital shaker (*see* **Note 4**).
4. Rinse the membranes briefly in MilliQ H_2O, briefly blot between paper towels to dry, and store between pieces of Whatman paper in a dry location.

3.4. Migration Assay

1. Remove the EGM from the HMVECs, rinse with 10 mL of PBS, and refeed the cells with EBM + 0.1% BSA overnight.
2. The next morning, pipet 26 µL of PBS into the bottom of the migration chambers to briefly rinse the cells.
3. Trypsinize the HMVECs and resuspend the cells at 1×10^6 cells/mL in Dulbecco's Modified Eagle Medium (DME) + 0.1% BSA (you need approx 1.4 mL of cells per chamber, and no less than 1.3 mL).

4. Place 26 µL of the HMVEC suspension into each well. A slightly positive meniscus should be present when the well has been properly loaded. This will prevent the introduction of air bubbles when the membrane is placed on top. Be sure to mix constantly the cell suspension to ensure equal loading. In addition, it is advisable to load the wells in a checkerboard pattern to decrease differences in cell concentrations.

5. Cut what will represent the upper left-hand corner of the membrane so that the orientation of the samples can be maintained.

6. Carefully place the membrane on top of the wells making sure that you do not introduce air bubbles (*see* **Note 5**).

7. Place the rubber gasket, with its cut upper left corner, on top of the membrane. Place the top portion of the chamber on top of the gasket and membrane. Holding the top chamber firmly in place, screw on each of the bolts until tightened (*see* **Note 6**).

8. Turn the chamber upside down and loosely cover it completely with aluminum foil and place the chamber upside down in a tissue culture incubator for 90 min (*see* **Note 7**).

9. Retrieve the chamber, turn it right side up, and fill each upper chamber with the test substances. Pipet 50 µL of each test substance into the wells in quadruplicate down the vertical rows. To avoid bubbles, lower the tip of the pipet at a steep angle to the bottom of the chamber and slowly pipet the test substance into the well. Check for trapped air bubbles by holding the chamber up to the light. If air bubbles are present, remove the substance from the chamber and repipet the liquid into the well.

10. Cover the chamber with aluminum foil again and place in a tissue culture incubator for 4 h. We have found that a 4-h incubation is the most appropriate to balance between random migration and induced/inhibited migration.

11. At the end of the incubation, carefully remove the thumb nuts, and remove the upper chamber and gasket from the gelatinized membrane.

12. Using a pair of forceps, place the membrane into a 100-mm dish containing PBS. Rinse thoroughly to remove all the proteinaceous material.

13. Incubate the membrane in each successive solution of the Diff-Quick Stain Set for approx 30 s each (Fixative, Stain I, Stain II).

14. Rinse in PBS again, place between a folded paper towel or between two pieces of Whatman filter paper, and allow to dry.

15. Using scissors, cut the membrane in half, such that there are 24 wells (six columns) on each piece of the membrane. Trim the edges of the membrane so that it can completely fit on a glass slide, mount onto glass slides with mounting media, cover with cover slips, and allow to dry overnight.

3.5. Quantification of Results

There are several options for quantifying the results of this type of migration. However, we have found that the most effective technique is the traditional

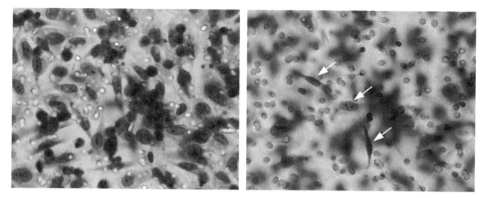

Fig. 1. Images from a stained filter with adherent HMVECs on lower (**left**) and upper (**right**) chamber surfaces. Arrows indicate several cells that have migrated successfully across the membrane on the upper chamber surface.

method of using a microscope to quantify the number of cells that have physically migrated from one side of the membrane to the other (**Fig. 1**).

1. Place the glass slide on the microscope stage and view with the ×100 objective using oil.
2. At 10 *random* locations within each collection of cells that constituted a well in the chamber, count the number of cells per high-power field (hpf) that have migrated from one side of the membrane to the other (*see* **Note 8**).
3. Continue this process for the other three "wells" for each test substance. Therefore, you will count 40 random spots for each test substance.
4. Calculate the mean migration for each test substance and express the data as the mean number of cells migrated/10 hpf.

3.6. Cleaning and Sterilization of Chamber

The chamber is fabricated from an acrylic. As such, protein and other substances will accumulate in the chambers. To minimize this from happening, the entire apparatus should be soaked in MilliQ H_2O immediately after completion of the assay. However, over time, there will likely be a buildup of potential contaminants. To prevent this, the chamber can be cleansed by soaking it in Terg-A-Zyme (VWR) for 3 h. If the chamber is contaminated with pathogens, it can be sterilized by soaking the entire apparatus in a solution consisting of 1 tablespoon of Clorox bleach and 2 L of MilliQ H_2O.

4. Notes

1. As discussed under **Subheading 1.1.5.**, the use of the endothelial cell migration assay is an excellent in vitro tool for testing the angiogenic potential of purified

compounds, conditioned media, or serum samples. However, while we and others have found that the migration assay is the most consistent predictor of in vivo biology, it is becoming increasingly evident that the expression of the angiogenic phenotype is considerably more complicated than previously envisioned. For example, the interplay between tumor cells and the various constituents of the surrounding stroma are thought to be critically important in various aspects of tumor biology including angiogenesis *(35,36)*. In addition, we now know that there is even a great deal of heterogeneity between endothelial cells, depending on their anatomical location. As such, the use of dermal microvascular endothelial cells to study physiological or pathological conditions of the kidney or liver is likely to be inappropriate. Therefore, it should be emphasized that in vitro angiogenesis assays, regardless of the type chosen, should not be used exclusively as a measure of angiogenesis. Rather, they should be part of a two-pronged assay system that includes an in vivo assay as well.

2. Microvascular endothelial cells are the most appropriate cell type to use in assays for angiogenesis. Capillaries, rather than larger vessels (arteries, arterioles, veins, and venules), are the main source of cells for both physiological and pathological angiogenesis. In addition, research has increasingly demonstrated that the phenotypes of large-vessel endothelial cells are considerably different from endothelial cells derived from small vessels. We prefer the Cells Systems cells, because they are not hyperstimulated with vascular endothelial growth factor during the expansion process.

3. We recommend that cultured endothelial cells be used prior to passage six in migration assays. It is our experience that their responsiveness to both inducers and inhibitors is markedly reduced with increased passage of the cells.

4. The gelatinized membranes will last no more than 1 mo. After this period of time, the investigator will notice a decreased amount of endothelial cell attachment.

5. We recommend gently bending the membrane in half and initially placing the center of the membrane onto the lower chamber. Once the center portion is in contact with the chamber, slowly lower the remaining portion of the filter onto the chamber working from the center of the membrane to the edges. In this manner, you will decrease the likelihood of introducing bubbles.

6. Do not vigorously screw the bolts down; this will damage the chamber.

7. The investigator can place the HMVECs in either the top or bottom chamber. We routinely place the cells in the bottom chamber and then invert the chamber to allow the endothelial cells to attach to the membrane. We prefer this method because it measures the migration of endothelial cells that are actually in contact with the membrane and are, therefore, presumably in more direct contact with the stimulators/inhibitors that are in the chamber on the other side of the membrane.

8. This aspect of the migration assay is perhaps the most challenging to investigators unaccustomed to observing subtle microscopic changes, such as the migration of individual cells from one side of a membrane to the other. However, with careful consideration and practice, one can begin to easily observe the cells. In all cases, the side of the membrane containing the migrated cells will have far fewer than

the side on which the cells were plated. The best way to observe the migrated cells is to slowly focus up and down until you see the side of the membrane that contains the majority of the cells. Subsequent to finding that side of the membrane, a very slight adjustment in focus will bring the opposite side of the membrane (the side with the migrated cells) into focus.

Acknowledgment

This work was supported in part by National Institutes of Health grants DE12322 (MWL), DE00470 (MWL), and CA79403 (Cardinal Bernardin Cancer Center).

References

1. Flamme, I., Frolich, T., and Risau, W. (1997) Molecular mechanisms of vasculogenesis and embryonic-angiogenesis. *J. Cell Physiol.* **173,** 206–210.
2. Arnold, F. and West, D. C. (1991) Angiogenesis in wound healing. *Pharmacol. Ther.* **52,** 407–422.
3. Welsh, A. O. and Enders, A. C. (1991) Chorioallantoic placenta formation in the rat: Angiogenesis and maternal blood circulation in the mesometrial region of the implantation chamber prior to placenta formation. *Am. J. Anat.* **192,** 347–365.
4. Torry, R. J. and Rongish, B. J. (1992) Angiogenesis in the uterus: potential regulation and relation to tumor angiogenesis. *Am. J. Reprod. Immun.* **27,** 171–179.
5. Rogers, P. A., Abberton, K. M., and Susil, B. (1991) Endothelial cell migratory signal produced by human endometrium during the menstrual cycle. *Hum. Reprod.* **7,** 1061–1066.
6. Folkman, J., Szabo, S., Stovroff, M., McNeil, P., Li, W., and Shing, Y. (1991) Duodenal ulcer: discovery of a new mechanism and development of angiogenic therapy that accelerate healing. *Ann. Surg.* **214,** 414–425.
7. Folkman J. (1995) Tumor angiogenesis, in *The Molecular Basis of Cancer* (Mendelsohn, J., Howley, P. M., Israel, M. A., and Liotta, L. A., eds.), W.B. Saunders, Philadelphia, pp. 206–232.
8. Bouck, N., Stellmach, V., and Hsu, H. (1995) How tumors become angiogenic. *Adv. Cancer Res.* **69,** 35–174.
9. Risau, W. (1990) Angiogenic growth factors. *Prog. Growth Factor Res.* **2,** 71–79.
10. Risau, W. (1997) Mechanisms of angiogenesis. *Nature* **386,** 671–674.
11. Folkman, J. and Ingber, D. E. (1987) Angiostatic steroids: Method of discovery and mechanism of action. *Ann. Surg.* **206,** 374–383.
12. Folkman, J. and Klagsburn, M. (1987) Angiogenic factors. *Science* **235,** 442–447.
13. Pepper, M. S., Vassalli, J. D., Montesano, R., and Orci, L. (1987) Urokinase-type plasminogen activator is induced in migrating capillary endothelial cells. *J. Cell. Biol.* **105,** 2535–2541.
14. Pepper, M. S., Spray, D. C., Chanson, M., Montesano, R., Orci, L., and Meda, P. (1989) Junctional communication is induced in migrating capillary endothelial cells. *J. Cell. Biol.* **109,** 3027–3038.

15. Pepper, M. S., Belin, D., Montesano, R., Orci, L., and Vassalli, J. D. (1990) Transforming growth factor beta 1 modulates basic fibroblast growth factor-induced proteolytic and angiogenic properties of endothelial cells in vitro. *J. Cell. Biol.* **111,** 743–755.

16. Maciag, T., Kadish, J., Wilkins, L., Stemerman, M. B., and Weinstein, R. (1982) Organizational behavior of human umbilical vein endothelial cells. *J. Cell Biol.* **94,** 511–520.

17. Madri, J. A. and Pratt, B. M. (1986) Endothelial cell-matrix interactions: in vitro models of angiogenesis. *J. Histochem. Cytochem.* **34,** 85–91.

18. Nicosia, R. F. and Ottinetti, A. (1990) Growth of microvessels in serum-free matrix culture of rat aorta: a quantitative assay of angiogenesis in vitro. *Lab. Invest.* **63,** 115–122.

19. Zetter, B. R. (1987) Assay of capillary endothelial cell migration. *Meth. Enzym.* **147,** 135–144.

20. Rupnick, M. A., Stokes, C. L., Williams, S. K., and Lauffenburger, D. A. (1988) Quantitative analysis of random motility of human microvessel endothelial cells using a liner under agarose assay. *Lab. Invest.* **59,** 363–372.

21. Obeso, J. L. and Auerbach, R. (1984) A new microtechnique for quantitating cell movement in vitro using polystyrene bead monolayers. *J. Immunol. Meth.* **70,** 141–152.

22. Furcht, L. T. (1996) Critical factors controlling angiogenesis: cell products, cell matrix, and growth factors. *Lab. Invest.* **55,** 505–509.

23. Falk, W., Goodwin, R. H. Jr., and Leonard, E. J. (1980) A 48-well micro-chemotaxis assay for rapid and accurate measurement of leukocyte migration. *J. Immunol. Meth.* **33,** 239–247.

24. Harvath, L., Falk, W., and Leonard, E. J. (1980) Rapid quantification of neutrophil chemotaxis: use of polyvinylpyrrolidone-free polycarbonate membrane in a multiwell assembly. *J. Immunol. Meth.* **37,** 39–45.

25. Rastinejad, F., Polverini, P. J., and Bouck, N. P. (1989) Regulation of the activity of a new inhibitor of angiogenesis by a cancer suppressor gene. *Cell* **56,** 345–355.

26. Dawson, D. W., Volpert, O. V., Gillis, P., Crawford, S. E., Xu, H., Benedict, W., and Bouck, N. P. (1999) Pigment epithelium-derived factor: a potent inhibitor of angiogenesis. *Science* **285,** 245–248.

27. Koch, A. E., Polverini, P. J., Kunkel, S. L., Harlow, L. A., DiPietro, L. A., Elner, V. M., Elner, S. G., and Strieter R. M. (1992) Interleukin-8 as a macrophage-derived mediator of angiogenesis. *Science* **258,** 1798–1801.

28. Tolsma, S. S., Volpert, O. V., Good, D. J., Frazier, W. A., Polverini, P. J., and Bouck, N. (1993) Peptides derived from two separate domains of the matrix protein thrombospondin-1 have anti-angiogenic activity. *J. Cell Biol.* **122,** 497–511.

29. Dawson, D. W., Volpert, O. V., Pearce, S. F., Schneider, A. J., Silverstein, R. L., Henkin, J., and Bouck, N. P. (1999) Three distinct D-amino acid substitutions confer potent antiangiogenic activity on an inactive peptide derived from a thrombospondin-1 type 1 repeat. *Mol. Pharmacol.* **55,** 332–338.

30. Nissen, N. N., Polverini, P. J., Koch, A. E., Volin, M. V., Gamelli, R. L., and DiPietro, L. A. (1998) Vascular endothelial growth factor mediates angiogenic activity during the proliferative phase of wound healing. *Am. J. Pathol.* **152,** 1445–1452.

31. Nissen, N. N., Polverini, P. J., Gamelli, R. L., and DiPietro, L. A. (1996) Basic fibroblast growth factor mediates angiogenic activity in early surgical wounds. *Surgery* **119,** 457–465.

32. Lingen, M. W., Polverini, P. J., and Bouck, N. P. (1996) Retinoic acid induces cells cultured from oral squamous cell carcinomas to become anti-angiogenic. *Am. J. Pathol.* **149,** 247–258.

33. Lingen, M. W., DiPietro, L. P., Solt, D. B., Bouck, N. P., and Polverini, P. J. (1997) The angiogenic switch in hamster buccal pouch keratinocytes is dependent on TFGβ-1 and is unaffected by ras activation. *Carcinogenesis* **18,** 329–338.

34. Lingen, M. W., Polverini, P. J., and Bouck, N. P. (1998) Retinoic acid and interferon alpha act synergistically as antiangiogenic and antitumor agents against human head and neck squamous cell carcinoma. *Cancer Res.* **58,** 5551–5558.

35. Dvorak, H. F., Nagy, J. A., Dvorak, J. T., and Dvorak, A. M. (1994) Identification and characterization of the blood vessels of solid tumors that are leaky to circulating macromolecules. *Am. J. Pathol.* **145,** 510–514.

36. Liss, C., Fekete, M. J., Hasina, R., Lam, C. D., and Lingen, M. W. (2001) Characterization of a paracrine loop for the expression of the angiogenic phenotype in head and neck cancer. *Int. J. Cancer* **93,** 781–785.

27

Analysis of Collagen Synthesis

Robert F. Diegelmann

1. Introduction

The process of wound healing consists of an orderly sequence of events characterized by the specific infiltration of specialized cells into the wound site. The platelets and inflammatory cells are the first cells to arrive, providing key functions and "signals" needed for the influx of connective-tissue cells and a new blood supply. These chemical "signals" are known as growth factors or cytokines. The fibroblast is the connective-tissue cell responsible for the collagen deposition needed to repair tissue injury. Collagen is the most abundant protein in the animal kingdom, accounting for nearly 30% of the total protein in the human body. In normal tissues, collagen provides strength, integrity, and structure. When tissues are disrupted following injury, collagen is needed to repair the defect and to restore structure and thus function. If too much collagen is deposited in the wound site, normal anatomical structure is lost, function is compromised, and the problem of fibrosis results. Conversely, if insufficient amounts of collagen are deposited, the wound is weak and may dehisce or result in a chronic, nonhealing ulcer. Therefore, in many of our studies of the wound-healing process, it is important to analyze collagen synthesis.

In the past there have been a variety of methods used to measure collagen synthesis. The classic assays have been based on quantifying hydroxyproline in protein hydrolysates (1). Hydroxyproline is a unique amino acid found almost exclusively in collagen. The activity of the enzyme prolyl hydroxylase has also been used as an indirect method to measure collagen synthesis during wound healing (2). In addition, histological analysis using trichrome (3) and Sirius red staining (4) and immunohistochemistry (5) have been used to detect collagen

From: *Methods in Molecular Medicine, vol. 78: Wound Healing: Methods and Protocols*
Edited by: Luisa A. DiPietro and Aime L. Burns © Humana Press Inc., Totowa, NJ

as well. Furthermore, there is a commercially available Sirius red colorimetric assay to measure collagen (Sircol™ Collagen Assay; www.biocolor.co.uk/sircol.htm). Tensile strength *(6)* measurements have also been used as an indirect method to measure the function of collagen in healing tissues *(see* Chapter 3). Expression of collagen mRNA has been observed using *in situ* hybridization *(7)* and measured using Northern blot analysis *(8)* and RNase protection assays *(9)*.

The procedure described in this chapter is designed for the specific quantification of newly synthesized collagen. The assay is based on the selective digestion of the newly produced radioactive collagen using highly purified bacterial collagenase *(10)*. Tissue samples obtained by direct biopsy or recovered from polyvinyl alcohol sponges *(see* Chapter 6) or ePTFE implants *(see* Chapter 19) are incubated in vitro with radioactive proline, and then the newly synthesized collagen is solubilized using bacterial collagenase digestion. The amount of radioactive collagen can be compared to the total amount of protein synthesized to obtain a percentage of collagen synthesis (relative collagen synthesis). Alternatively, the amount of collagen and total protein synthesized can be based on sample weight or DNA to obtain an absolute collagen synthesis value.

The technique involves two separate methods. The first method (method A) describes the procedure for obtaining biopsy tissue for study and the incubation of the specimen with radioisotopes to label newly synthesized proteins. The second method (method B) outlines the technique for quantifying collagen and total protein synthesis in the labeled material by using purified bacterial collagenase digestion. **Figure 1** provides an overview of the complete procedure.

2. Materials

2.1. Method A: Radiolabeling Tissue Biopsies

1. Isotopes: Proline L-[2,3-³H]- (cat. no. NET 323) or proline L-[2,3,4,5-³H]- (cat. no. NET 483) (Perkin-Elmer, Boston, MA, www.perkinelmer.com). **Caution:** If the multilabeled ³H-proline is used, some of the ³H label on the fourth carbon will be lost when the proline hydroxylation step occurs.
2. Incubation medium: It is best to use a minimal salt solution such as Krebs-Ringer medium *(11)* or Earle's basic salt solution (cat. no. 24010-068; Life Technologies, Carlsbad, CA) because there will be enhanced isotope incorporation. Minimal essential medium (cat. no. 11095-080; Life Technologies) can also be used, but total isotope incorporation may be less. See the Life Technologies Web site for additional information regarding incubation media (www.lifetech.com). The amount of total proline in the incubation medium can be adjusted to maximize ³H-proline uptake and incorporation *(12)*. These incubation media can be modified by adding fresh ascorbate (0.01 mM) to ensure complete prolyl hydroxylation and maximal collagen expression, if that is a concern *(13)*. However, ascorbate

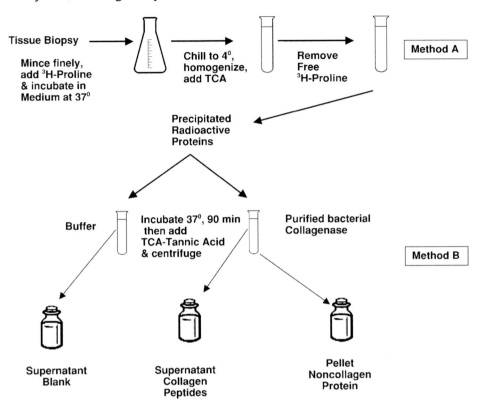

Fig. 1. Schematic representation of techniques for labeling tissue biopsies and analyzing collagen synthesis.

is unstable in culture medium and needs to be added fresh on a daily basis *(14)*. In addition, buffers such as tricine (25 mM, pH 7.4) can be incorporated into the incubation medium, if control of pH is a concern.

3. Biopsy instruments: Dermal skin punch device (trephine) and a small pair of surgical scissors. These instruments can be purchased from Roboz Surgical (Gaithersburg, MD). Disposable biopsy punches (Tru-Punch) can be purchased from Sklar (West Chester, PA). The biopsy punches come in a variety of sizes ranging from 2 up to 8 mm.

2.2. Method B: Assay of Newly Synthesized Collagen (15)

1. Chromatographically purified bacterial (*Clostridium histolyticum*) collagenase (Code: CLSPA; Worthington, Lakewood, NJ), (www.worthington-biochem.com/manual/C/CLS.html). Purified bacterial collagenase is also available from Advanced Biofactures (Lynbrook, NY). This method is absolutely dependent on highly purified collagenase to ensure that only collagen is digested during the

assay (*see* **Note 1** for a description of assays to check on collagenase specificity and purity).

2. Enzyme buffer: A solution of 0.05 M Tris-HCl, pH 7.6, containing 5 mM CaCl$_2$.
3. HEPES buffer: 1 M, pH 7.2. Dissolve 23.83 g of HEPES (cat. no. 391340; Calbiochem, San Diego, CA) in 80 mL of water. Gradually add 10 N NaOH to bring the pH to 7.2. Then adjust the volume to 100 mL with deionized water and store at –20°C.
4. 10% Tricholoracetic acid (TCA)/0.5% tannic acid; stable at 4°C for up to 1 wk. If it develops an intense yellow, indicating oxidation, do not use.
5. 0.2 N NaOH: Store in small aliquots at –20°C.
6. 0.15 N HCl: Store in small aliquots at –20°C.
7. 62.5 mM N-ethylmaleimide (NEM) (cat. no. 34115; Calbiochem): Adjust the pH to approx 6.0 by adding small amounts of solid NaHCO$_3$ and mixing well. Store in small aliquots at –20°C.
8. 50% TCA. Store at 4°C.
9. 5% TCA containing 1 mM proline. Make fresh once a week and store at 4°C.
10. Protease-free ribonuclease (RNase) (Type 1-A, cat. no. R 4875; Sigma, St. Louis, MO); 2.0 mg/mL in enzyme buffer (*see* **item 2**) to give a 100X stock solution.
11. Polypropylene conical bottomed centrifuge tubes (cat. no. 60818-099; VWR, West Chester, PA). Similar tubes that can withstand at least 1000g can be substituted.
12. 6 N HCl.
13. CaCl$_2$.

3. Methods

3.1. Method A: Radiolabeling Tissue Biopsies

1. Obtain samples of tissues to be analyzed by standard surgical biopsy technique *(11,16,17)*. Basically, clean the area to be biopsied of any foreign material, or if hair is present, shave the area. Then use appropriate anesthetics if needed, clean the area with a skin cleanser, dry and use a skin biopsy device (trephine) to obtain a sample of tissue ranging from 3 to 6 mm in diameter.
2. Place the biopsy in incubation medium on ice (minus the isotope) and rinse to remove excessive blood.
3. Obtain a wet weight of the sample, and place the biopsy in a vessel or tube large enough to allow mincing with a small pair of surgical scissors.
4. Add incubation medium to give approx 50 mg/mL and then mince tissue finely and uniformly.
5. Add ^{3}H-proline to give a final concentration of 50 µCi/mL and incubate with gentle shaking at 37°C for 3 h.
6. Terminate the incubation by rapid freezing in a dry ice–acetone bath. The radiolabeled tissues can be stored frozen until analyzed for collagen and total protein synthesis at a later time.

3.2. Method B: Assay of Newly Synthesized Collagen (15)

1. When ready to analyze the specimens, remove them from the freezer and place in a 100°C water bath to rapidly thaw and also to destroy proteolytic enzymes. *Note:* Pyrex® or heat-safe tubes or vessels must be used.

2. Repeat freezing and thawing the samples a total of three times to facilitate the disruption of cells. From this point forward all preparations should be maintained at 4°C.

3. Homogenize the sample. If it has a fine consistency, a glass tissue grinder or a Dounce homogenizer can be used. If the incubation material is of a firmer consistency, a motor-driven device such as a HandiShear® handheld homogenizer (VirTis®) needs to be used. Care should be taken to recover all tissue fragments from the instrument by rinsing with small amounts of chilled enzyme buffer.

4. Add stock RNase to give a final concentration of 20 µg/mL, and incubate at 37°C for 5 min to cleave the ^{3}H-prolyl transfer RNA *(10)*.

5. Again chill The incubation homogenate to 4°C, and add 50% cold TCA to give a final concentration of 10%.

6. After 10 min at 4°C, precipitate the insoluble radioactive protein by centrifuging at 1000g for 5 min at 4°C and remove the supernate.

7. Resuspend the radioactive protein pellet in 1 to 2 mL of cold 5% TCA containing 1 mM proline and recentrifuge. Remove the supernatant and repeat the washing procedure at least three more times to ensure that all of the nonincorporated ^{3}H-proline is removed.

8. Remove excess TCA by either careful aspiration or draining and dissolve the pellet in 0.5–1.0 mL of 0.2 N NaOH. Careful heating in a water bath up to 100°C may be needed to help solubilize the protein precipitate (*see* **Note 2**).

9. Once the protein is solubilized, distribute it in equal amounts to two 4-mL conical centrifuge tubes.

10. Neutralize the NaOH by adding 0.1 mL of the 1 M HEPES buffer (pH 7.2), mix, and add 0.15 N HCl to adjust the pH to 6.8–7.4 (*see* **Note 3**).

11. Place the samples on ice and prepare two incubation "cocktails" as given in **Table 1** *(10,15)*. Then add 40 µL of the minus cocktail to the minus or "blank" tube and 40 µL of the plus cocktail to the plus tube.

12. Mix thoroughly and incubate for 90 min at 37°C with occasional mixing.

13. At the end of the incubation, place the tubes on ice for 5 min, then add an equal volume (usually about 0.5 mL) of cold 10% TCA/0.5% tannic acid, and mix thoroughly.

14. Separate the supernates by centrifuging at 1000g at 4°C, and transfer them to scintillation counting vials.

15. Resuspend the pellets in 0.5 mL of 5% TCA/0.25% tannic acid (4°C), mix thoroughly, centrifuge as before, and add the second supernates to the first.

16. Add an appropriate aqueous scintillation fluid and measure the radioactivity. Appropriate quenching standards containing the same amount of TCA–tannic

Table 1
Incubation Cocktails for Method B

	(−) minus enzyme	(+) plus enzyme	Final concentration in incubation reaction
CaCl$_2$ (25 mM)	1	1	0.5 mM
NEM (62.5 mM)	2	2	2.5 mM
Enzyme buffer	1	0	
Purified collagenase (600–800 µg/mL)	0	1	12–16 µg/mL

NEM, N-ethylmaleimide.

    are needed to convert the cycles-per-minute (cpm) values to disintegrations-per-minute (dpm) units.

17. To quantitate the amount of noncollagen protein synthesized, resuspend the pellet of the plus tube in 1 mL of 6 N HCl, mix, and transfer to a scintillation vial.

18. Rinse the tube with an additional 0.5 mL of 6 N HCl and add to the same vial. Be sure the material is dissolved before adding the scintillation fluid and counting the radioactivity (*see* **Note 4**).

19. Once again set up some appropriate counting standards with 1.5 mL of 6 N HCl so that the counting efficiency can be determined and the cpm values can be converted to dpm units.

20. One of the biggest problems in these types of analyses is deciding on the appropriate denominator so that values can be compared from sample to sample. There are two basic approaches to consider. One determines an *absolute* amount of collagen and total protein synthesized by first measuring the protein or DNA in a small portion of the NaOH-solubilized substrate. A number of suitable assays are available for these measurements (*see* **Note 5**). A more convenient value to obtain is the *relative* amount of collagen synthesized based on the total amount of protein synthesized by the particular tissue. This quantification is not affected by any possible loss of biopsy material during the sample preparation. The relative percentage of collagen synthesis reflects how specialized or dedicated a particular tissue is for collagen synthesis. During wound healing, this value will increase with time to a certain point, then decrease. To calculate the relative percentage of collagen synthesis, determine the difference in the dpm between the minus incubation supernate (enzyme blank) and the plus incubation supernate (tube containing collagenase). Next determine the total dpm in the plus enzyme pellet and multiply that value by 5.4 to correct for the enriched proline and hydroxyproline content of collagen compared to noncollagenous proteins (*18*). With these values, use the following formula to obtain the relative percentage of collagen synthesized:

$$\% \text{ Collagen} = \frac{\text{dpm in plus supernate (minus the blank)}}{\text{dpm in pellet} \times 5.4 + \text{dpm in plus supernate (minus the blank)}} \times 100$$

These basic techniques have been used to analyze collagen synthesis during embryonic development *(18)*, during wound healing in the dermis *(17)*, in isolated portions of wounds *(19)*, in human keloids *(20)*, in wounds where there are foreign bodies *(21)*, in steroid-impaired wounds *(22)*, and around breast tumors *(23)*. In addition, these techniques can be used to analyze collagen in tissue culture *(24)* and cell culture systems *(15,25)* (*see* **Note 6**).

4. Notes

1. It is absolutely critical that the bacterial collagenase used in this assay be pure and free of other, nonspecific proteolytic activity. Assurance assays such as the one that follows should be used. These assays are reprinted with permission from Worthington. See Worthington's Web site for additional information (www.worthington-biochem.com/manual/C/CLS.html):

    Reagents

    - 0.05 M TES [tris(hydroxymethyl)-methyl-2-aminoethane sulfonate] buffer with 0.36 m*M* calcium chloride, pH 7.5.
    - 4% Ninhydrin in methyl cellosolve.
    - 0.2 *M* Sodium citrate with 0.71 m*M* stannous chloride, pH 5.0.
    - Ninhydrin-citric acid mixture: Prepare by mixing 50 ml of the 4% ninhydrin in methyl cellusolve with 50 mL of 0.2 *M* citrate with 0.71 m*M* stannous chloride, pH 5.0. Allow mixture to stir for 5 minutes.
    - 50% n-Propanol.
    - Substrate: Worthington bovine achilles tendon collagen (Code: CL) and vitamin-free casein.
    - 50% (w/v) Trichloroacetic acid.

    Enzyme

    - Dissolve enzyme [the collagenase] at a concentration of 1 mg/ml in 0.05 *M* TES [TES-CaCl$_2$ buffer] with a 0.36 m*M* calcium chloride, pH 7.5. Dilutions run are 1/10 and 1/20 in the above buffer.

    Procedure

    Weigh 25 mg of Worthington bovine collagen into each of four test tubes [use ones with caps]. Include at least two tubes to serve as blanks which will contain no enzyme. Add 5.0 ml of 0.05 *M* TES [TES-CaCl$_2$] buffer to the tubes and incubate at 37°C for 15 minutes. Start the reaction by adding 0.1 ml of enzyme dilution to appropriate tubes.

    After 5 hours, stop the collagenase reaction by transferring 0.2 ml of solution (leaving behind the collagen) to test tubes containing 1.0 ml of ninhydrin-citric acid mixture. Include an enzyme blank (collagen incubated with 0.1 ml TES [TES-CaCl$_2$] buffer in place of enzyme). Heat (the capped test tubes) for 20 minutes in a boiling water bath. After cooling, dilute with 5 ml of 50% n-propanol. Let stand for 15 minutes and read absorbance at 600 nm. From an L-leucine standard curve determine micromoles amino acid equivalent to leucine liberated.

Non-specific protease activity (i.e. caseinase activity) is determined using the above assay and substituting 25 milligrams vitamin-free casein for collagen. The reaction is stopped after 5 hours by the addition of 0.5 ml of 50% trichloroacetic acid. After centrifugation, 0.2 ml of the supernatant is transferred to 1.0 ml of ninhydrin and treated as above. Caseinase activity is calculated as collagenase activity.

Calculation

$$\text{Units/mg} = \frac{\text{micromoles L-leucine equivalents liberated}}{\text{mg enzyme in digestion mixture}}$$

If the bacterial collagenase is found to have nonspecific proteolytic enzyme activity, it may be necessary to purify it through a molecular sieve column to remove the contaminant *(10)*. A Sephacryl G-200 column can be used in place of the Sephadex G-200 column as described originally. The bacterial collagenase available from Advanced Biofactures (ABC collagenase Form III; Lynbrook, NY) has already been purified and therefore costs more and may have a lower specific activity compared to preparations that can be prepared in an individual's laboratory. Nevertheless, it is imperative that the enzyme digests only collagen.

2. If the protein pellet is very large, it may be necessary to extract the TCA using two ethanol/ether (3:1 [v/v]) washes followed by an ether wash. The residue can then be dried to a powder before solubilization in the NaOH as above. One advantage of this drying technique is that the dried powder can be weighed and the absolute collagen and total protein data can be expressed per units of dry weight tissue.

3. Adjusting the pH is one of the most difficult and time-consuming parts of this assay. A small pH probe works well. Do not use pH paper to test the pH because varying amounts of sample will be lost and contribute to inaccurate results. The HEPES buffer (0.2 mL) can be added and the pH can be adjusted prior to dispensing the sample into two equal aliquots.

4. It is important to be sure that all of the precipitate is solubilized before counting the radioactivity in the sample. Hydrolysis *(15)* prior to counting or the use of a specialized tissue solubilizer may be required. This problem will vary from tissue to tissue and should be determined prior to an experiment.

5. Caution must be taken, however, if a comparison is being made between two tissues that may have a different cellular content. For example, DNA would not be a good denominator to compare normal skin (low cellular density) with a wound or dermal ulcer biopsy where there may be a high density of inflammatory cells contributing to the DNA content. An absolute quantitation can also be

obtained using the starting wet weight of the tissue. However, wet weights can be highly variable and difficult to obtain unless standard humidity conditions are used. In addition, there may be loss of some sample along the way during preparation, which would contribute to variable results. If a dry powder is prepared prior to incubation, that value can be used to calculate the absolute amount of collagen and total protein per tissue dry weight.

6. Obviously, these basic procedures will need to be adapted when used with various tissues. Dense tissues containing highly crosslinked collagen are more difficult to work with, whereas tissues that are easily dissociated will be easier to homogenize and analyze. Like every other method that we use, this technique has certain limitations and drawbacks. Once these are recognized and understood by the researcher, the analysis of collagen synthesis can proceed smoothly.

Acknowledgment

This chapter is dedicated to Dr. Beverly Peterkofsky, my dear friend and mentor.

References

1. Udenfriend, S. (1966) Formation of hydroxyproline in collagen. *Science* **152,** 1335–1340.
2. Mussini, E., Hutton, J. J., and Udenfriend, S. (1967) Collagen proline hydroxylase in wound healing, granuloma formation, scurvy, and growth. *Science* **157,** 927–929.
3. Kuo, T., Speyer, M. T., Ries, W. R., and Reinisch, L. (1998) Collagen thermal damage and collagen synthesis after cutaneous laser resurfacing. *Lasers Surg. Med.* **23,** 66–71.
4. Anderson, S. M., McLean, W. H., and Elliott, R. J. (1991) The effects of ascorbic acid on collagen synthesis by cultured human skin fibroblasts. *Biochem. Soc. Trans.* **19,** 48S.
5. Graham, M. F., Diegelmann, R. F., Elson, C. O., Lindblad, W. J., Gotschalk, N., Gay, S., and Gay, R. (1988) Collagen content and types in the intestinal strictures of Crohn's disease. *Gastroenterology* **94,** 257–265.
6. Hambley, R., Hebda, P. A., Abell, E., Cohen, B. A., and Jegasothy, B. V. (1988) Wound healing of skin incisions produced by ultrasonically vibrating knife, scalpel, electrosurgery, and carbon dioxide laser. *J. Dermatol. Surg. Oncol.* **14,** 1213–1217.
7. Barnes, J. L. (1998) In situ hybridization in the study of remodeling in proliferative glomerulonephritis. *Toxicol. Pathol.* **26,** 43–51.
8. Rosenblat, G., Willey, A., Zhu, Y. N., Jonas, A., Diegelmann, R. F., Neeman, I., and Graham, M. F. (1999) Palmitoyl ascorbate: selective augmentation of procollagen mRNA expression compared with L-ascorbate in human intestinal smooth muscle cells. *J. Cell. Biochem.* **73,** 312–320.
9. Ujike, K., Shinji, T., Hirasaki, S., Shiraha, H., Nakamura, M., Tsuji, T., and Koide, N. (2000) Kinetics of expression of connective tissue growth factor gene during liver regeneration after partial hepatectomy and D-galactosamine-induced liver injury in rats. *Biochem. Biophys. Res. Commun.* **277,** 448–454.

10. Peterkofsky, B. and Diegelmann, R. (1971) Use of a mixture of proteinase-free collagenases for the specific assay of radioactive collagen in the presence of other proteins. *Biochemistry* **10,** 988–994.
11. Uitto, J. (1970) A method for studying collagen biosynthesis in human skin biopsies in vitro. *Biochim. Biophys. Acta* **201,** 438–445.
12. Peterkofsky, B. and Prather, W. (1979) Increased proline transport resulting from growth of normal and Kirsten sarcoma virus-transformed BALB 3T3 cells in the presence of N(6), O(2')-dibutyryl cyclic adenosine 3',5'-monophosphate. *Arch. Biochem. Biophys.* **192,** 500–511.
13. Blanck, T. J. and Peterkofsky, B. (1975) The stimulation of collagen secretion by ascorbate as a result of increased proline hydroxylation in chick embryo fibroblasts. *Arch. Biochem. Biophys.* **171,** 259–267.
14. Peterkofsky, B. (1972) The effect of ascorbic acid on collagen polypeptide synthesis and proline hydroxylation during the growth of cultured fibroblasts. *Arch. Biochem. Biophys.* **152,** 318–328.
15. Peterkofsky, B., Chojkier, M., and Bateman, J. (1982) Determination of collagen synthesis in tissue and cell culture systems, in *Immunochemistry of the Extracellular Matrix: Volume II Applications* (Furthmayr, H., ed.), CRC Press, Boca Raton, FL, pp. 19–47.
16. Stein, H. D. and Keiser, H. R. (1971) Collagen metabolism in granulating wounds. *J. Surg. Res.* **11,** 277–283.
17. Diegelmann, R. F., Rothkopf, L. C., and Cohen, I. K. (1975) Measurement of collagen biosynthesis during wound healing. *J. Surg. Res.* **19,** 239–243.
18. Diegelmann, R. F. and Peterkofsky, B. (1972) Collagen biosynthesis during connective tissue development in chick embryo. *Dev. Biol.* **28,** 443–453.
19. Cohen, I. K., Moore, C. D., and Diegelmann, R. F. (1979) Onset and localization of collagen synthesis during wound healing in open rat skin wounds. *Proc. Soc. Exp. Biol. Med.* **160,** 458–462.
20. Cohen, I. K., Diegelmann, R. F., and Keiser, H. R. (1976) Collagen metabolism in keloid and hypertrophic scar, in *The Ultrastructure of Collagen* (Longacre, J. J., ed.), Thomas, Springfield, IL, pp. 199–212.
21. Cohen, I. K., Diegelmann, R. F., and Wise, W. S. (1976) Biomaterials and collagen synthesis. *J. Biomed. Mater. Res.* **10,** 965–970.
22. Cohen, I. K., Diegelmann, R. F., and Johnson, M. L. (1977) Effect of corticosteroids on collagen synthesis. *Surgery* **82,** 15–20.
23. Diegelmann, R. F. and Cohen, I. K. (1978) Elevated collagen synthesis in dimethylbenz(a)-anthracene rat breast tumors and the effect of beta-amino propionitrile on tumor growth. *Surg. Forum* **29,** 176–178.
24. Cohen, I. K. and Diegelmann, R. F. (1978) Effect of N-acetyl-cis-4-hydroxyproline on collagen synthesis. *Exp. Mol. Pathol.* **28,** 58–64.
25. Diegelmann, R. F., Cohen, I. K., and McCoy, B. J. (1979) Growth kinetics and collagen synthesis of normal skin, normal scar and keloid fibroblasts in vitro. *J. Cell. Physiol.* **98,** 341–346.

28

Method for Detection and Quantitation of Leukocytes During Wound Healing

Iulia Drugea and Aime L. Burns

1. Introduction

The wound repair process is a highly ordered series of events that encompasses hemostasis, inflammatory cell infiltration, tissue regrowth, and remodeling. An important component of normal wound healing is the generation of an inflammatory reaction, which is characterized by the sequential infiltration of neutrophils, macrophages, and lymphocytes *(1)*. Neutrophils are the first leukocyte in the wound, entering within hours after initial injury. The function of neutrophils within wounds is most generally believed to be protective against wound infection *(2,3)*. However, more recent observations suggest that neutrophils may also produce growth factors that promote tissue repair *(4)*. Following neutrophil influx, macrophages are recruited to sites of injury by various chemoattractants, including chemokines *(5,6)*. Previous studies have demonstrated that macrophages perform two distinct functions vital to the healing process. Initially, macrophages engulf and phagocytose wound debris and senescent cells, clearing the way for the growth of new dermal matrix. Subsequently, macrophages produce angiogenic and fibrogenic growth factors that promote the growth phase of repair *(7–9)*. As neutrophil and macrophage levels decrease, the late inflammatory phase of wound healing is typified by the ingress of T-lymphocytes *(10)*. Specific subpopulations of T-lymphocytes have been demonstrated to either promote or inhibit repair, but the overall importance of lymphocytes to successful tissue repair remains somewhat unclear *(11–13)*.

Because of the interest in elucidating the function of leukocytes during wound healing, various methods have been developed to quantitate and localize

From: *Methods in Molecular Medicine, vol. 78: Wound Healing: Methods and Protocols*
Edited by: Luisa A. DiPietro and Aime L. Burns © Humana Press Inc., Totowa, NJ

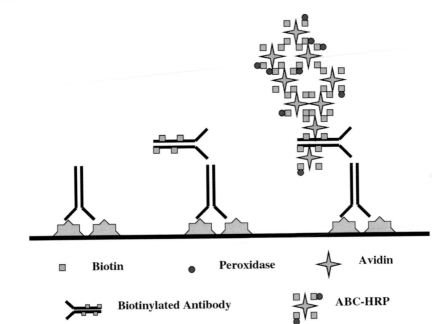

Fig. 1. Schematic of three principal steps in avidin-biotinylated enzyme complex (ABC-HRP) protocol. First, the primary antibody binds to its cellular antigen. Second, a biotinylated secondary antibody binds to the primary reagent. Third, ABC-HRP complexes bind to the secondary antibody and are visualized with a substrate reaction.

these cells. The current protocol describes a method to quantitate cell numbers at sites of injury using an immunoenzymatic staining method. This protocol utilizes a preformed avidin-biotin-enzyme complex (ABC) method on frozen skin sections (14). Briefly, the sequence of reagents is a primary antibody (15–17), biotinylated secondary antibody, ABC-horseradish peroxidase (HRP) followed by incubation with diaminobenzidine (DAB) (**Fig. 1**). One sample method of quantitation is also included with the protocol.

2. Materials
2.1. Sample Collection and Sectioning

1. TBS tissue-freezing media (Triangle Biomedical Science, Durham, NC).
2. Base molds.
3. Liquid nitrogen.
4. Dewar flask.
5. Dry ice.
6. –80°C Freezer.

7. Cryostat (e.g., Jung CM 3000 Cryostat; Leica Instruments GmbH, Nussloch, Germany).

2.2. Immunostaining

1. Coplin or other staining racks and jars.
2. Acetone.
3. Whatman #1 qualitative filter papers.
4. Modified Harris hematoxylin solution (Sigma, St. Louis, MO). Store at room temperature and filter through filter paper prior to counterstaining.
5. 10X Phosphate-buffered saline (PBS): 18.6 mM NaH$_2$PO$_4$, 84.1 mM Na$_2$HPO$_4$, 1.5 M NaCl; pH 7.4 in dH$_2$O. Store at room temperature.
6. 1X PBS: Dilute 10X stock with dH$_2$O. Store at room temperature.
7. PAP Pen (Kiyota International, Elk Grove Village, IL).
8. Kimwipes® (Kimberly-Clark, Roswell, GA).
9. 30% H$_2$O$_2$. Store at 4°C.
10. Methanol: H$_2$O$_2$ bath. Dilute H$_2$O$_2$ 1 : 100 in methanol to produce a 0.3% solution. Make fresh prior to use.
11. Normal mouse serum (Sigma). Aliquot and store at –20°C. Dilute 1 : 10 in 1X PBS immediately prior to use.
12. Normal goat serum (Sigma). Aliquot and store at –20°C. Dilute 1 : 10 in 1X PBS immediately prior to use.
13. Primary antibody to stain neutrophils: Rat anti–mouse Ly-6G/GR-1 monoclonal antibody (RB6-8C5) (PharMingen, San Diego, CA). Dilute 1 : 100 (5 µg/mL) in 1X PBS just prior to use (*see* **Note 1**).
14. Primary antibody to stain macrophages: Rat anti–mouse macrophages/monocytes antibody (MOMA-2) (Serotec, Kidlington, Oxford, UK). Dilute 1 : 600 (1.7 µg/mL) just prior to use.
15. Primary antibody to stain T-lymphocytes: Rabbit anti–human T-cell, CD3ε antibody (Dako, Carpinteria, CA). Store at 4°C. Dilute 1 : 250 (2 µg/mL) in 1X PBS just prior to use.
16. Secondary reagent for staining macrophages and neutrophils: Biotinylated mouse anti–rat IgG (H+L) (Jackson Immunoresearch Lab, West Grove, PA). Dilute 1 : 200 (10 µg/mL) in 1X PBS just prior to use.
17. Secondary reagent for staining T-lymphocytes: Biotinylated goat anti–rabbit IgG (H + L) (Vector, Burlingame, CA). Aliquot and store at –20°C. Dilute 1 : 200 (7.5 µg/mL) with 1X PBS just prior to use.
18. Vectastain ABC kit, peroxidase standard (ABC-HRP; Vector). Store at 4°C. Thirty minutes prior to use mix one drop of solution A with one drop of solution B in 5 mL of 1X PBS and mix well. Prepared ABC solution may be stored at 4°C and used for up to 1 wk.
19. DAB solution (Kirkegaard & Perry, Gaithersburg, MD). Store at 4°C. Make working DAB reagent immediately before use: Thoroughly mix 100 µL of DAB with 5 mL of 0.1 M Tris-HCl, pH 7.6. Combine 1.7 µL of 30% H$_2$O$_2$ with 100 µL of dH$_2$O. Add 100 µL of diluted H$_2$O$_2$ to the DAB/Tris solution and mix well.

Use immediately. Inactivate any leftover working DAB reagent prior to disposal with at least 1 vol of bleach (*see* **Note 2**).
20. 95% Ethanol.
21. 100% Ethanol.
22. Cytoseal 280 (Stephens Scientific, Kalamazoo, MI).
23. Glass cover slips.

2.3. Analysis

1. Light microscope for counting stained cells (e.g., Leitz Laborlux S; Leica Mikroskopie und Systeme GmbH, Wetzlar, Germany).
2. Image analysis system, to assess wound size, comprising the following components:
   a. Microscope with camera mounting (e.g., Zeiss Axioskop 20 with phototube; Carl Zeiss, Thornwood, NY).
   b. Charge-coupled device camera and camera control unit (e.g., DEI-750D; Optronics, Goleta, CA).
   c. A color video monitor (e.g., Sony Trinitron PVM-14N1U; Sony, San Jose, CA).
   d. Computer system.
3. Computer software including image acquisition software (e.g., Optronics Acquisition for Windows 95) and image analysis software (e.g., Scion Image from Scion, Frederick, MD; or NIH Image from National Institutes of Health, Bethesda, MD).

3. Methods

3.1. Sample Collection and Sectioning

1. Collect and embed wound tissues to be analyzed in TBS tissue-freezing media in base molds of the appropriate size.
2. Immediately snap-freeze all samples in liquid nitrogen and store on dry ice or at –80°C (long term) for sectioning.
3. Prepare 10-μm frozen sections for staining (*see* **Notes 3** and **4**). Keep the sections at –80°C until the time of analysis.

3.2. Immunostaining

This protocol is specific for use on 10-μm-thick frozen murine dermal wound sections. All incubations and washes are carried out at room temperature.

1. Thaw the slides at room temperature for 5 min (*see* **Notes 5** and **6**) and label them with a pencil or appropriate pen (*see* **Note 7**).
2. Place the samples in a slide rack (or Coplin jar, depending on the number of slides), and fix in an acetone bath for 15 min.
3. While the slides are being fixed, filter the hematoxylin through the Whatman filter paper (*see* **Note 8**).

4. Wash the slides in a 1X PBS bath for 3 min. Repeat twice using fresh PBS each time.

5. If you are staining for T-cells, skip to **step 9** (*see* **Note 9**).

6. Place the slides in a methanol-H_2O_2 bath for 30 min to quench endogenous peroxidase activity.

7. Prepare the diluted normal mouse serum (macrophage or neutrophil staining only).

8. Wash the slides three times in 1X PBS for 3 min each.

9. Remove the slides from the last wash, and tap each one on a layer of paper towels to remove the excess PBS (*see* **Note 10**). If you are staining for T-cells, at this time prepare the diluted normal goat serum.

10. Circle the tissue samples with a PAP Pen in order to produce a hydrophobic barrier around each section (*see* **Note 11**).

11. Lay each slide flat and add 25–50 µL of diluted serum to each circled sample. The volume will depend on the size of the section (*see* **Note 12**). Incubate for 30 min.

12. Remove the excess liquid from the slides by holding them perpendicular to the bench and tapping them gently on a layer of paper towels. Some serum will remain on the sections. Wipe off any serum that traverses the PAP Pen barrier with a Kimwipe, which may otherwise provide a channel for leakage of the primary antibody.

13. Lay each slide flat and pipet 25–50 µL of primary antibody diluted appropriately for the samples (*see* **Note 13**). Incubate for 30 min.

14. Wash the slides three times in 1X PBS for 3 min each.

15. If you are staining for macrophages or neutrophils, skip to **step 18**. For T-cell staining continue with **step 16**.

16. Place the slides in a methanol-H_2O_2 bath for 30 min to quench endogenous peroxidase activity (*see* **Note 9**).

17. Wash the slides three times in 1X PBS for 3 min each.

18. Lay each slide flat and add 25–50 µL of diluted biotinylated secondary antibody. Incubate for 30 min.

19. While the samples are incubating, prepare the ABC-HRP according to the protocol provided by the manufacturer. Let the complexes form for 30 min before use (*see* **Note 14**).

20. Wash the slides three times in 1X PBS for 3 min each.

21. Apply 25–50 µL of ABC-HRP to each sample. Incubate the slides for 30 min.

22. Wash the slides three times in 1X PBS for 3 min each.

23. Add 25–50 µL of prepared DAB solution to the samples and incubate for 5 min (neutrophils) or 10 min (macrophages and T-cells) in the dark (*see* **Note 15**). Inactivate unused DAB solution with bleach (1 vol : 1 vol) before disposal.

24. Wash the slides for 5 min in dH_2O.

25. Counterstain the slides with one quick dip in filtered hematoxylin (*see* **Note 16**).

26. Immediately immerse the slides in a tap water bath and dip two to four times. Repeat this washing twice in fresh tap water baths working as quickly as possible.

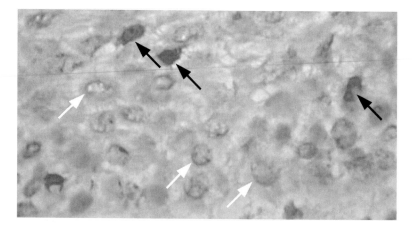

Fig. 2. Cross section of a d 7 postinjury murine dermal wound stained for T-cells (×650). Black arrows indicate several CD3-positive cells; white arrows indicate unstained cells.

Then place the slides in a bath under gently running tap water to remove excess hematoxylin.

27. Dehydrate the slides in 95% ethanol for 1 min. Repeat twice.
28. Place the slides in 100% ethanol for 1 min. Repeat once.
29. Let the slides air-dry.
30. Cover slip the sections with Cytoseal 280.
31. Analyze after at least 1 h to allow mounting medium to dry (**Fig. 2**).

3.3. Analysis

1. Count the total number of stained cells in the wound bed (*see* **Notes 17** and **18**).
2. Determine the wound bed area using the Image Analysis system. First capture the section image using the camera-specific image acquisition software.
3. Save the image in the TIF format.
4. Open the image file using Scion Image (PC) or NIH Image (Mac) software.
5. Demarcate the wound bed using the wand tool.
6. Measure the area in pixels.
7. To transform the data from pixels to area in square millimeters, measure the area of a known object (e.g., a micrometer) in pixels at the same magnification used for the sample measurement.
8. Calculate the number of cells per square millimeter for each wound (**Fig. 3**).

4. Notes

1. Be aware that this antibody also recognizes granulocytes and some monocyte lineages in the bone marrow.
2. DAB is toxic; always wear gloves.

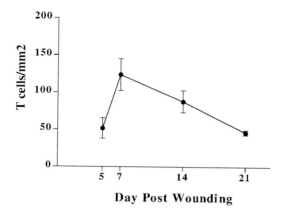

Fig. 3. Time course of T-cell infiltration in a murine 3-mm dermal excisional punch wound model (*see* **ref. 5** for model). Data are expressed as mean (±SEM) number of T-cells per square millimeter. At each time point $n = 8$ except for d 21, $n = 5$.

3. Dermal wound and control skin sections are prepared in a Leica cryostat with an object temperature of –18°C and cabinet temperature of –28°C. Optimal section thickness will depend on the tissue being stained. During sectioning, samples are stored in a slide box placed on dry ice.

4. Samples are collected in duplicate on positively charged Superfrost Plus Microscope slides (Fisher, Pittsburgh, PA) to ensure adherence during processing.

5. It is suggested that various controls be run initially to test for antibody specificity including both positive (e.g., 4-μm frozen mouse spleen sections for T-cells) and negative tissue controls, staining samples both ± primary antibody and ± secondary antibody, as well as reagent substitutions (e.g., irrelevant antibody), and so forth.

6. Although this protocol is specific for frozen sections, cell staining can also be done on paraffin sections. An antigen retrieval step may be needed at the beginning of the protocol after deparaffinization (an example is provided in **ref. 18**).

7. Incubations in acetone and methanol will cause most laboratory-type pens to run. It is best to label the slides with either a pencil or a pen specifically made for histological processing (e.g., Securline Marker II; Precision Dynamics, San Fernando, CA).

8. For filtering, place a glass or plastic funnel on top of a glass beaker. Shape the round filter paper into a triangle by folding it in half once (half circle), and then in half again. Open one side of the fold and place the paper inside the funnel. Pour the hematoxylin over the filter paper.

9. Most staining protocols include a peroxidase activity quenching step prior to incubation with the primary antibody. This works fine for macrophage and neutrophil staining but was found to *prohibit* T-cell staining with this particular

anti-CD3 primary antibody. Make sure that the methanol-H_2O_2 step occurs *after* the incubation with the anti-T-cell primary antibody.

10. Process only a small batch of slides at one time. Since the samples should never be allowed to dry out or sit out uncovered, keep the majority of the slides in the final PBS wash. Remove four or five slides, tap them gently to remove excess PBS, lay them flat on the bench, make circles with the PAP Pen, and immediately cover the sections with diluted serum. Slides may also be carefully dabbed with a Kimwipe to remove excess droplets of PBS, as needed.

11. Placing the slides on a black background (e.g., construction paper) makes it easier to visualize the samples for application of the PAP Pen and other reagents.

12. The volume needed to cover each sample is determined by both the size of the section and the size of the waxy ring made with the PAP Pen. Try to make the ring as small as possible without damaging the sample. Completely cover the section with enough reagent so that the samples will not dry out from evaporation during any of the incubations. To limit evaporation, slides may be kept in a humidified chamber or even on a layer of damp paper towels in a closed plastic container, if available. If serum or antibody leaks outside the PAP Pen ring, first rinse the slides in 1X PBS, then reapply more wax to seal the barrier, and finally add the reagent again. Also note that PAP Pens come in two sizes that vary in thickness.

13. When starting a new staining project, changing tissue types, or even switching between frozen and paraffin samples, it is often best to do a titration with both the primary and secondary antibodies. This will help to determine the best concentrations or dilutions to use for a specific set of conditions. The dilutions to be tested depend on the initial concentration of the antibody. For example, the anti-CD3 primary antibody was tested over a range from 1:50 to 1:1000 (0.5–10 µg/mL) concurrently with the secondary anti–rabbit antibody, which was tested between dilutions from 1:100 to 1:500 (3–15 µg/mL).

14. Several cells and tissues including red cells, monocytes, muscle, liver, and kidney have high levels of endogenous peroxidase activity. If this causes interference with the staining protocol, an alternate enzyme label, such as alkaline phosphatase (AP), should be employed *(19)*. If using ABC-AP, samples can be treated with levamisole (Vector) to quench endogenous phosphatase activity.

15. Incubation times may be varied to improve staining contrast as well as decrease any background. This may be especially important when working with various tissue types. It is suggested that test samples be initially incubated for 5, 10, and 15 min to determine the best level of staining.

16. There are other counterstains that may be used depending on the tissue being stained and the substrate used for staining. These include methyl green, eosin, and nuclear fast red. Vector provides a partial table that outlines counterstain/ substrate compatibility (see the Vector catalog or www.vectorlabs.com/Protocols/ Counterstains/cstaincomp.pdf).

17. Initially, the wound bed margins are visually determined under low power (×100). The total number of DAB-stained cells in the wound bed are counted using a

high power that provides the best resolution for ease of counting (×400–1000). A 10 × 10 square ocular graticule is used to provide both a guide for counting and a guide for moving over the complete wound bed. Within each field, count the stained cells moving across and down the graticule in a specific pattern. This ensures that all the cells within the grid are in fact counted and eliminates the possibility that a cell is counted more than once. Additionally, since the cells must be counted at a high power at which visualization of the complete wound bed is not possible, the grid is used to line up adjacent fields when moving left to right and up and down until all the cells in the complete wound bed have been counted.

18. As an alternate to counting all the cells in the wound bed (or all the cells in an extremely dense sample), an average count per high-power field can be made. The area of each high-power field can be determined via micrometer. Data may be presented as cells per high-power field or, preferentially, cells per square millimeter.

References

1. Ross, R. and Benditt, E. P. (1962) Wound healing and collagen formation: fine structure in experimental scurvy. *J. Cell. Biol.* **12**, 533–551.
2. Detmers, P. A., Powell, D. E., Walz, A., Clark-Lewis, I., Baggiolini, M., and Cohn, Z. A. (1991) Differential effects of neutrophil-activating peptide 1/IL-8 and its homologues on leukocyte adhesion and phagocytosis. *J. Immunol.* **147**, 4211–4217.
3. Simpson, D. M. and Ross, R. (1972) The neutrophilic leukocyte in wound repair a study with antineutrophil serum. *J. Clin. Invest.* **51**, 2009–2023.
4. Taichman, N. S., Young, S., Cruchley, A. T., Taylor, P., and Paleolog, E. (1997) Human neutrophils secrete vascular endothelial growth factor. *J. Leukoc. Biol.* **62**, 397–400.
5. DiPietro, L. A., Polverini, P. J., Rahbe, S. M., and Kovacs, E. J. (1995) Modulation of JE/MCP-1 expression in dermal wound repair. *Am. J. Pathol.* **146**, 868–875.
6. DiPietro, L. A., Burdick, M., Low, Q. E., Kunkel, S. L., and Strieter, R. M. (1998) MIP-1alpha as a critical macrophage chemoattractant in murine wound repair. *J. Clin. Invest.* **101**, 1693–1698.
7. Hunt, T. K., Knighton, D. R., Thakral, K. K., Goodson, W. H. D., and Andrews, W. S. (1984) Studies on inflammation and wound healing: angiogenesis and collagen synthesis stimulated in vivo by resident and activated wound macrophages. *Surgery* **96**, 48–54.
8. Leibovich, S. J. and Ross, R. (1975) The role of the macrophage in wound repair. A study with hydrocortisone and antimacrophage serum. *Am. J. Pathol.* **78**, 71–100.
9. Polverini, P. J., Cotran, P. S., Gimbrone, M. A. Jr., and Unanue, E. R. (1977) Activated macrophages induce vascular proliferation. *Nature* **269**, 804–806.
10. Ross, R. and Odland, G. (1968) Human wound repair. II. Inflammatory cells, epithelial-mesenchymal interrelations, and fibrogenesis. *J. Cell. Biol.* **39**, 152–168.

11. Barbul, A., Shawe, T., Rotter, S. M., Efron, J. E., Wasserkrug, H. L., and Badawy, S. B. (1989) Wound healing in nude mice: a study on the regulatory role of lymphocytes in fibroplasia. *Surgery* **105,** 764–769.
12. Boyce, D. E., Jones, W. D., Ruge, F., Harding, K. G., and Moore, K. (2000) The role of lymphocytes in human dermal wound healing. *Br. J. Dermatol.* **143,** 59–65.
13. Schaffer, M. and Barbul, A. (1998) Lymphocyte function in wound healing and following injury. *Br. J. Surg.* **85,** 444–460.
14. Hsu, S. M., Raine, L., and Fanger, H. (1981) Use of avidin-biotin-peroxidase complex (ABC) in immunoperoxidase techniques: a comparison between ABC and unlabeled antibody (PAP) procedures. *J. Histochem. Cytochem.* **29,** 577–580.
15. Fleming, T. J., Fleming, M. L., and Malek, T. R. (1993) Selective expression of Ly-6G on myeloid lineage cells in mouse bone marrow. RB6-8C5 mAb to granulocyte-differentiation antigen (Gr-1) detects members of the Ly-6 family. *J. Immunol.* **151,** 2399–2408.
16. Kraal, G., Rep, M., and Janse, M. (1987) Macrophages in T and B cell compartments and other tissue macrophages recognized by monoclonal antibody MOMA-2. An immunohistochemical study. *Scand. J. Immunol.* **26,** 653–661.
17. Mason, D. Y., Cordell, J., Brown, M., Pallesen, G., Ralfkiaer, E., Rothbard, J., Crumpton, M., and Gatter, K. C. (1989) Detection of T cells in paraffin wax embedded tissue using antibodies against a peptide sequence from the CD3 antigen. *J. Clin. Pathol.* **42,** 1194–1200.
18. Mason, D. Y., Krissansen, G. W., Davey, F. R., Crumpton, M. J., and Gatter, K. C. (1988) Antisera against epitopes resistant to denaturation on T3 (CD3) antigen can detect reactive and neoplastic T cells in paraffin embedded tissue biopsy specimens. *J. Clin. Pathol.* **41,** 121–127.
19. Ormanns, W. and Schaffer, R. (1985) An alkaline-phosphatase staining method in avidin-biotin immunohistochemistry. *Histochemistry* **82,** 421–424.

29

Detection of Reactive Oxygen Intermediate Production by Macrophages

Jorge E. Albina and Jonathan S. Reichner

1. Introduction

The reparative phenomena that follow sterile tissue injury are an ordered sequence of partially overlapping events and include the macrophage as a key cell type in orchestrating the process of repair. Several studies suggest that the wound-derived macrophage acquires a functional phenotype that is congruent with its specialized role in repair, and that this phenotype is determined by factors within the wound milieu. This phenotype distinguishes the wound macrophages from macrophages obtained at other anatomical sites. Evidence in support of this hypothesis includes the findings that wound-derived macrophages are more phagocytic and fungicidal than resident or immune-elicited peritoneal macrophages *(1)*. Wound macrophages demonstrate a substantially greater capacity to suppress splenocyte proliferation in a nitric oxide (NO)–dependent mechanism but fail to kill NO-sensitive tumor cells that readily succumb to immune activated cells *(2,3)*. Wound macrophages also demonstrate differential responsiveness to activation signals. Exposure of wound macrophages to anoxia results in an increase in arginase activity not seen by similar exposure of immune-elicited or resident peritoneal cells *(4)*. Wound macrophages are deficit in their capacity to generate reactive oxygen intermediates (ROIs) even when challenged with classic activators of the respiratory burst oxidase system (**Figs. 1–4**) *(5)*. Several assays for measuring ROI production in inflammatory cells are provided in this chapter.

From: *Methods in Molecular Medicine, vol. 78: Wound Healing: Methods and Protocols*
Edited by: Luisa A. DiPietro and Aime L. Burns © Humana Press Inc., Totowa, NJ

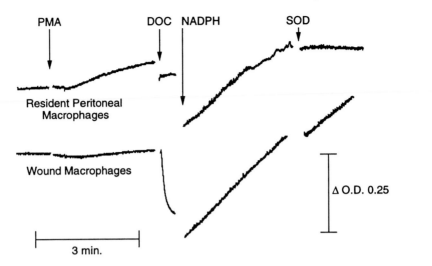

Fig. 1. Evidence that wound-derived macrophage lysates do not demonstrate NADPH oxidase activity as determined by reduction of ferricytochrome-*c* recorded at 550 nm. Arrows indicate the times of addition for PMA (200 n*M*), deoxycholate/Tween (DOC), NADPH (0.6 m*M*), and SOD (300 U/mL). (Reproduced with permission from **ref. 5**).

2. Materials
2.1. Superoxide Release

1. Flat-bottomed 96-well plate.
2. Phenol red–free Hank's balanced salt solution (HBSS).
3. Superoxide dismutase (CuZn-SOD; from bovine erythrocytes) (S-2515; Sigma, St. Louis, MO).
4. Cytochrome-*c* solution containing phorbol 12-myristate 13-acetate (PMA): Make stock solutions of 320 μ*M* ferricytochrome-*c* (horse heart, Type VI, C-7752; Sigma) in phenol red–free HBSS and 20 μ*M* PMA (P-1680; LC Laboratories, Woburn, MA) in phenol red–free HBSS. Add PMA to cytochrome-*c* for a final working concentration of 400 n*M*.
5. Spectrophotometric plate reader (e.g., model EL340; Biotek, Winooski, VT).

2.2. Superoxide Formation in Cell-Free Lysates

1. Reaction buffer: 17 m*M* potassium phosphate buffer with 1.2 m*M* magnesium chloride, 5 m*M* potassium chloride, 123 m*M* NaCl, 160 m*M* ferricytochrome-*c*, 6 m*M* sodium azide, and 5 m*M* glucose.
2. PMA (200 n*M*) (P-1680; LC Laboratories).
3. Sodium deoxycholate (0.06% [w/v]) and Tween-20 (0.06% [v/v]) solution.
4. NADPH (0.6 m*M*, N-1630; Sigma).
5. SOD (300 U/mL final concentration, CuZn-SOD) (S-2515; Sigma).

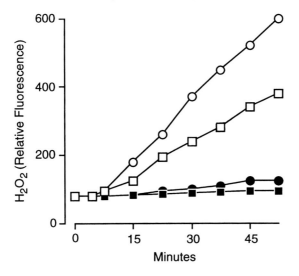

Fig. 2. H$_2$O$_2$ release by peritoneal lavage or wound-derived macrophages. H$_2$O$_2$ release after PMA stimulation (200 n*M*) was measured over time using 4-OH phenyl-acetic acid and HRP. When indicated, SOD (300 U/mL) was present in the cuvets prior to the addition of PMA. Wound-derived macrophages: (–) SOD (■); (+) SOD (●). Peritoneal lavage cells: (–) SOD (□), (+) SOD (○). (Reproduced with permission from **ref. 5**.)

2.3. H$_2$O$_2$ Release

1. Reaction buffer: 50 m*M* potassium phosphate (pH 8.0), 1 m*M* EDTA, 1 m*M* sodium azide, 1 m*M* 4-OH phenylacetic acid (H-4377; Sigma), and 8 U/mL of horseradish peroxidase (HRP) (P-6782; Sigma).
2. SOD (300 U/mL final concentration, CuZn-SOD) (S-2515; Sigma).
3. Luminescence spectrometer (e.g., model LS-50B; Perkin-Elmer, Newton Center, MA).

2.4. Lucigenin-Dependent Chemiluminescence Assay

1. Phenol red–free HBSS containing 1% heat-inactivated (56°C, 30 min) fetal bovine serum (FBS).
2. 400 µ*M* Lucigenin (bis-*N*-methylacridinium nitrate) (M-8010; Sigma).
3. Luminometer (Chem-Glo II photometer).
4. PMA (20 µ*M*) (P-1680; LC Laboratories).
5. SOD (300 U/mL final concentration, CuZn-SOD) (S-2515; Sigma).

2.5. Oxygen Consumption

1. Instrumentation: Instech Model 203 Dual Channel Oxygen Uptake System (Instech, Plymouth Meeting, PA), which consists of an oxygen electrode, an

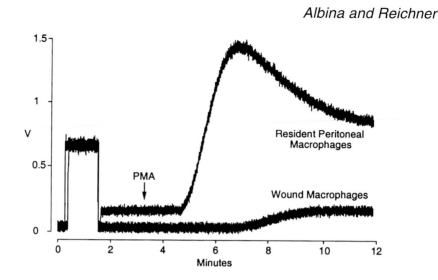

Fig. 3. O_2^--dependent lucigenin chemiluminescence. Peritoneal lavage or wound macrophages were dispensed at 10^7 cells/mL into 0.5 mL of HBSS containing 200 μM lucigenin and placed in the chamber of a Chem-Glo II photometer. Cells were stimulated with PMA (200 nM), and the chemiluminescent signal was recorded and expressed in volts. The square wave was generated using a radioactive standard and indicates similar instrument calibration for both runs. Chemiluminescence was completely abrogated by SOD (300 U/mL) (not shown). (Reproduced with permission from **ref. 5**.)

oxygen amplifier, and a stirred 600-μL oxygen chamber system. In addition, the system permits circulation of temperature-controlled H_2O, which must be maintained at 37°C. The amplifier is connected to a High Performance Data Acquisition System (MacPacq MP100; BIOPAC, Goleta, CA) to convert the digital signal to an analog waveform using Acq*Knowledge* software (**Fig. 4**; *see* **Note 1**).

2. 1 mM Sodium dithionite (S-1256; Sigma).
3. HBSS containing 1% heat-inactivated FBS.
4. PMA: 200 nM in HBSS + 1% fetal calf serum [FCS], prewarmed to 37°C.

3. Methods

3.1. Superoxide Release

This is a well-accepted and straightforward protocol for quantification of superoxide release from viable neutrophils or macrophages as determined by reduction of ferricytochrome-*c* (*6*). Inclusion of SOD lends specificity to this assay regarding demonstrating that reduction of ferricytochrome-*c* is owing to superoxide production and not spurious reductants. SOD catalyzes the conversion of superoxide to H_2O_2 and water.

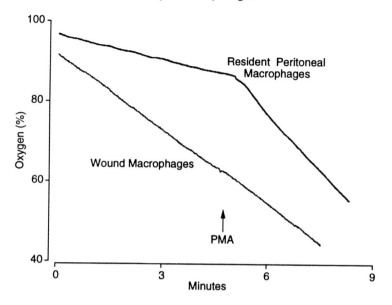

Fig. 4. O_2 consumption by peritoneal lavage or wound-derived macrophages. Cells were placed in the chamber of an Instech 203 O_2 uptake system. Oxygen content in culture media was monitored continuously prior to and after the addition of PMA (200 n*M*). (Reproduced with permission from **ref. 5**.)

1. In a 96-well flat-bottomed plate, add neutrophils or macrophages (*see* **Note 2**) at 3×10^5/well in 100 µL using phenol red–free HBSS (*see* **Note 3**).
2. Into control wells add 10 µL of SOD from a stock of 30,000 U/mL for a final concentration of 300 U/mL (*see* **Note 4**). Add 10 µL of HBSS to the test wells.
3. Add 100 µL of 320 µ*M* cytochrome-*c* solution containing PMA at 400 n*M* (*see* **Notes 5** and **6**).
4. Immediately take a zero-time optical density reading at 550/630 nm (dual wavelength) or 550 nm (single wavelength) in a spectrophotometric plate reader.
5. Place the plate in an incubator at 37°C for 60 min and then read the absorbance.
6. Calculate superoxide production from the difference in absorbance at 550 nm (corrected for absorbance at 630 nm) and the extinction coefficient for the absorbance of reduced ferricytochrome-*c* using the following equations: $\Delta E_{550nm-630nm} = 2.1 \times 10^4\ M^{-1} \bullet cm^{-1}$ (*see* **Note 7**).

3.2. Superoxide Formation in Cell-Free Lysates

This assay can be used to isolate and study specific protein components of the cyanide-insensitive inducible respiratory burst generated by the NADPH oxidase system (**Fig. 1**). Expected temporal results from cells with functional NADPH oxidase activity include demonstration of superoxide production on addition of PMA, suppression of that activity on dissolution of cells, and recovery with addition of NADPH into the lysate. Cytochrome-c reduction by the cell lysate is inhibitable with SOD.

1. Suspend 1×10^6 cells in 1 mL of reaction buffer.
2. Transfer the cells to a standard quartz cuvet and place in a spectrophotometer. Take continuous readings at 550 nm at 37°C with constant stirring within the cuvet. Permit the reaction to occur for several minutes until stabilization is reached.
3. Stimulate with PMA and record the change in absorbance for 5 min. At that time, lyse the cells with a mixture of sodium deoxycholate and Tween-20. Monitor changes in absorption for an additional 45 s.
4. Add NADPH to the cuvet. Record for 3 min.
5. Add SOD. Record.

3.3. H_2O_2 Release

This is a fluorometric assay in which H_2O_2 release is quantitated using a coupled reaction between cell-derived H_2O_2 and 4-OH-phenylacetic acid, which forms a fluorescent product (6,6'-diOH-[1,1'-biphenyl]-3,3'-diacetic acid) when the reaction is catalyzed by HRP (7). Cellular H_2O_2 is formed from the partial reduction of molecular oxygen following the action of SOD on superoxide. In the absence of exogenous SOD, this enzyme may be limiting for the reaction, and the assay can be used as a measure of cellular SOD production. Therefore, in the protocol described next, addition of excess SOD accelerates dismutation of superoxide and enhances detection of H_2O_2 (**Fig. 2**).

1. Place 1.5×10^6 neutrophils or macrophages in 3 mL of reaction buffer. Depending on the experimental conditions, add SOD to the appropriate samples at 300 U/mL final concentration.
2. Measure fluorescence in a luminescence spectrometer with excitation at 318 nm and emission at 405 nm. Results are presented as relative fluorescence intensity.

3.4. Lucigenin-Dependent Chemiluminescence Assay

This assay has the advantage of being unaffected by secreted molecules with the ability to oxidize cytochrome-c such as H_2O_2, NO, and $ONOO^-$ (8). Lucigenin-dependent chemiluminescence is not produced by the myeloperoxidase reaction. Data generated can be expressed either as instantaneous light intensity (mV), total light within a given time period (mVs), or as a rate of light intensity (mVs^{-1}) (**Fig. 3**).

1. Suspend 5×10^6 cells in 0.25 mL of HBSS containing FBS, add 0.25 mL of lucigenin, and place in the chamber of a luminometer.
2. Inject 5 µL of PMA ± 30 µL of SOD or HBSS.

3.5. Oxygen Consumption

A dedicated system including a detector and a device capable of continuous recording and measuring dissolved oxygen content in the medium containing leukocytes is required. An increased rate of oxygen consumption following PMA stimulation indicates NADPH oxidase activity.

3.5.1. Chamber Preparation and Instrument Calibration

1. Rinse the oxygen chamber with at least 10 vol of dH_2O.
2. Inject dH_2O into the chamber and set gain to 140–150.
3. Inject sodium dithionite. If the chamber is properly sealed, the reading of the meter should drop to 0–5. Adjust the zero offset to produce a reading of zero on the amplifier, and lock the control.
4. Reinject fresh water. The meter should return to 140–150. Adjust the computer input to 100%.
5. Flush the chamber with phosphate-buffered saline prior to introduction of cells.

3.5.2. Assay

1. Resuspend 1.7×10^6 cells in 1 mL of HBSS + FCS, prewarmed to 37°C. Place 600 µL in the chamber of an oxygen uptake system and incubate for 3 min before recording. Begin continuous recording to establish baseline consumption (approx 5 min).
2. Initiate stimulation by injecting 5 µL of PMA, and record oxygen concentration for an additional 4 to 5 min (*see* **Notes 8** and **9**).

4. Notes

1. As an alternative to the more costly use of a digital-to-analog converter, the oxygen amplifier may be connected directly to a strip recorder.
2. Inflammatory cells can be derived from wounds by several methods, including isolation from polyvinyl alcohol sponges (*see* Chapter 6).
3. For measurement of ferricytochrome-*c* reduction, all reagents must be free of color capable of absorption at 550 nm such as phenol red or hemoglobin.
4. Diphenyleneiodonium (10 µ*M*) may be used to inhibit NADPH oxidase activity.
5. Stimulants other than PMA can be used such as formyl-met-leu-phe or serum-opsonized zymosan.
6. Loss of assay sensitivity is likely owing to aging of cytochrome-*c*; it is best to use fresh reagent and keep dessicated at –20°C.
7. Results are frequently normalized by cell number.
8. Basal rates of oxygen consumption are largely owing to mitochondrial respiration, which can be revealed by abrogation on injection of KCN (5 m*M* final concentration).
9. The oxygen electrode is sensitive to changes in temperature, which may occur if PMA is injected directly from a stock prepared in dimethylsulfoxide. It is

best to prepare a stock solution in HBSS and make sure it is prewarmed to 37°C prior to injection.

Acknowledgments

This work was supported by National Institute of General Medical Sciences grant GM-42859, the Anita Allard Memorial Fund, and allocations to the Department of Surgery by Rhode Island Hospital.

References

1. Albina, J. E., Caldwell, M. D., Henry, W. L. Jr., and Mills, C. D. (1989) Regulation of macrophage functions by L-arginine. *J. Exp. Med.* **169,** 1021–1029.
2. Albina, J. E. and Henry W. L. Jr. (1991) Suppression of lymphocyte proliferation through the nitric oxide synthesizing pathway. *J. Surg. Res.* **50,** 403–409.
3. Mateo, R. B., Reichner, J. S., and Albina, J. E. (1996) NO is not sufficient to explain maximal cytotoxicity of tumoricidal macrophages against an NO-sensitive cell line. *J. Leukoc. Biol.* **60,** 245–252.
4. Albina, J. E., Henry, W. L. Jr., Mastrofrancesco, B., Martin, B. A., and Reichner, J. S. (1995) Macrophage activation by culture in an anoxic environment. *J. Immunol.* **155,** 4391–4396.
5. Nessel, C. C., Henry, W. L. Jr., Mastrofrancesco, B., Reichner, J. S., and Albina, J. E. (1999) Vestigial respiratory burst activity in wound macrophages. *Am. J. Physiol.* **276,** R1587–R1594.
6. Pick, E. and Mizel, D. (1981) Rapid microassays for the measurement of super-oxide and hydrogen peroxide production by macrophages in culture using an automatic enzyme immunoassay reader. *J. Immunol. Methods* **46,** 211–226.
7. Segura-Aguilar, J. (1993) A new direct method for determining superoxide dismutase activity by measuring hydrogen peroxide formation. *Chem. Biol. Interact.* **86,** 69–78.
8. Aasen, T. B., Bolann, B., Glette, J., Ulvik, R. J., and Schreiner, A. (1987) Lucigenin-dependent chemiluminescence in mononuclear phagocytes: role of superoxide anion. *Scand. J. Clin. Lab. Invest.* **47,** 673–679.

30

Measurement of Chemokines at the Protein Level in Tissue

Robert M. Strieter, Marie D. Burdick, John A. Belperio, and Michael P. Keane

1. Introduction

The recruitment of specific leukocyte subpopulations in response to injury is a fundamental mechanism of acute and chronic inflammation. The elicitation of leukocytes is dependent on a complex series of events, including reduced leukocyte deformability, endothelial cell activation, and expression of endothelial cell–derived leukocyte adhesion molecules; leukocyte-endothelial cell adhesion and leukocyte activation; and expression of leukocyte-derived adhesion molecules, leukocyte transendothelial migration, and leukocyte migration beyond the endothelial barrier along established chemotactic and haptotactic gradients. While the events of leukocyte extravasation may appear intuitive, it has taken more than 150 yr of research to elucidate the molecular and cellular steps involved in the process of leukocyte migration.

Leukocyte chemotaxins are important in leukocyte extravasation; they often lack specificity for particular subsets of leukocytes. The nonspecificity of these chemotactic factors for subsets of leukocytes is interesting. However, it is apparent that the nature of the stimulus and the subsequent spectrum of chemotactic factors produced determine the subpopulation of leukocytes elicited during an inflammatory response. For example, during neutrophil extravasation associated with acute lung injury, neutrophil chemotaxins predominate over other leukocyte chemotactic factors. By contrast, a different set of leukocyte chemotaxins predominate when a specific antigenic stimulus in the lung leads to cell-mediated immunity, resulting in the production of chemotactic factors that recruit exclusively mononuclear cells, leading to

From: *Methods in Molecular Medicine, vol. 78: Wound Healing: Methods and Protocols*
Edited by: Luisa A. DiPietro and Aime L. Burns © Humana Press Inc., Totowa, NJ

chronic inflammation. Thus, a diversity of chemotactic factors must exist with specific activity to target subsets of leukocytes and maintain leukocyte migration.

The salient feature of inflammation and the development of tissue injury is the extravasation of predominately neutrophils followed by mononuclear cells. These extravasating leukocytes contribute to the pathogenesis of inflammation and promote the eradication of the offending agent. In addition, the shear magnitude of increase in infiltrating cells; the activation of these cells; and the release of a variety of mediators, including additional cytokines that interact with resident nonleukocyte cellular populations lead to further amplification of tissue injury. The maintenance of leukocyte recruitment during inflammation requires intercellular communication between infiltrating leukocytes and the endothelium and resident stromal and parenchyma cells. The elicitation of leukocytes during inflammation from the vascular to the extravascular compartment in tissue is determined, in general, by the expression of tissue/cellular-derived chemokines. Although a variety of factors may be involved in mediating inflammation, chemokines are the focus of this chapter. Furthermore, understanding methods to extract and quantifiably measure chemokine protein levels, as compared to mRNA, in tissue provides direct evidence for their potential biological function in the local tissue microenvironment.

1.1. Chemokines

A new classification for chemokines has recently been reported (1) and is used throughout this chapter in conjunction with the older terminology. The human CXC, CC, C, and CX_3C chemokine families of chemotactic cytokines are four closely related polypeptide families that behave, in general, as potent chemotactic factors for neutrophils, eosinophils, basophils, monocytes, mast cells, dendritic cells, natural killer (NK) cells, and T- and B-lymphocytes (**Tables 1** and **2**). The CXC chemokines can be further divided into two groups on the basis of a structure/function domain consisting of the presence or absence of three amino acid residues (Glu-Leu-Arg, the "ELR" motif) that precedes the first cysteine amino acid residue in the primary structure of these cytokines (1–9). The ELR^+ CXC chemokines are chemoattractants for neutrophils and act as potent angiogenic factors (1–12). By contrast, the ELR^- CXC chemokines are chemoattractants for mononuclear leukocytes and are potent inhibitors of angiogenesis (1–9). There is approx 20–40% homology among the members of the four chemokine families (1–9). Chemokines have been found to be produced by an array of cells including monocytes, alveolar macrophages, neutrophils, platelets, eosinophils, mast cells, T- and

Table 1
CXC Chemokine/Receptor Family *(1)*

Systematic name	Human chromosome	Human ligand	Mouse ligand	Chemokine receptor(s)
CXCL1	4q12-q13	GROα/MGSA-α	GRO/KC?	CXCR2 > CXCR1
CXCL2	4q12-q13	GROβ/MGSA-β	GRO/KC?	CXCR2
CXCL3	4q12-q13	GROγ/MGSA-γ	GRO/KC?	CXCR2
CXCL4	4q12-q13	PF4	PF4	Unknown
CXCL5	4q12-q13	ENA-78	LIX?	CXCR2
CXCL6	4q12-q13	GCP-2	Ckα-3	CXCR1, CXCR2
CXCL7	4q12-q13	NAP-2	Unknown	CXCR2
CXCL8	4q12-q13	IL-8	Unknown	CXCR1, CXCR2
CXCL9	4q21.21	Mig	Mig	CXCR3
CXCL10	4q21.21	IP-10	IP-10	CXCR3
CXCL11	4q21.21	I-TAC	Unknown	CXCR3
CXCL12	10q11.1	SDF-1α/β	SDF-1	CXCR4
CXCL13	4q21	BLC/BCA-1	BLC/BCA-1	CXCR5
CXCL14	Unknown	BRAK/bolekine	BRAK	Unknown
(CXCL15)	Unknown	Unknown	Lungkine	Unknown

B-lymphocytes, NK cells, keratinocytes, mesangial cells, epithelial cells, hepatocytes, fibroblasts, smooth muscle cells, mesothelial cells, and endothelial cells. These cells can produce chemokines in response to a variety of factors that trigger the innate immune response, including microorganism molecular patterns, interleukin-1 (IL-1), tumor necrosis factor (TNF), C5a, LTB4, and interferons. The production of chemokines by both immune and nonimmune cells supports the contention that these cytokines may play a pivotal role in further orchestrating the inflammatory response of innate immunity and promote acute lung injury.

An ideal leukocyte chemotactic factor is one that demonstrates longevity at the site of inflammation within tissue. For example, whereas C5a is rapidly inactivated to its des-arg form in the presence of serum/plasma peptidases and loses a significant portion of its neutrophil chemotactic activity, IL-8 (CXCL8) *(1)* in the presence of serum maintains 100% of its activity *(13)*. Thrombin and plasmin have been found to convert IL-8 (CXCL8) from the 77 to the 72 amino acid form, whereas urokinase and tissue-type plasminogen activator are unable to induce NH_2-terminus truncation *(11)*. Moreover, IL-8 (CXCL8) incubated

Table 2
CC Chemokine/Receptor Family *(1)*

Systematic name	Human chromosome	Human ligand	Mouse ligand	Chemokine receptor(s)
CCL1	17q11.2	I-309	TCA-3, P500	CCR8
CCL2	17q11.2	MCP-1/MCAF	JE?	CCR2
CCL3	17q11.2	MIP-1α/LD78α	MIP-1α	CCR1, CCR5
CCL4	17q11.2	MIP-1β	MIP-1β	CCR5
CCL5	17q11.2	RANTES	RANTES	CCR1, CCR3, CCR5
(CCL6)		Unknown	C10, MRP-1	Unknown
CCL7	17q11.2	MCP-3	MARC?	CCR1, CCR2, CCR3
CCL8	17q11.2	MCP-2	MCP-2?	CCR3
(CCL9/10)		Unknown	MRP-2, CCF18 MIP-1γ	Unknown
CCL11	17q11.2	Eotaxin	Eotaxin	CCR3
(CCL12)		Unknown	MCP-5	CCR2
CCL13	17q11.2	MCP-4	Unknown	CCR2, CCR3
CCL14	17q11.2	HCC-1	Unknown	CCR1
CCL15	17q11.2	HCC-2/Lkn-1/MIP-δ	Unknown	CCR1, CCR3
CCL16	17q11.2	HCC-4/LEC	LCC-1	CCR1
CCL17	16q13	TARC	TARC	CCR4
CCL18	17q11.2	DC-CK1/PARC AMAC-1	Unknown	Unknown
CCL19	9p13	MIP-3β/ELC/exodus-3	MIP-3β/ELC/exodus-3	CCR7
CCL20	2q33-q37	MIP-3α/LARC/exodus-1	MIP-3α/LARC/exodus-1	CCR6
CCL21	9p13	6Ckine/SLC/exodus-2	6Ckine/SLC/exodus-2/TCA-4	CCR7
CCL22	16q13	MDC/STCP-1	ABCD-1	CCR4
CCL23	17q11.2	MPIF-1	Unknown	CCR1
CCL24	7q11.23	MPIF-2/eotaxin-2	Unknown	CCR3
CCL25	19p13.2	TECK	TECK	CCR9
CCL26	7q11.23	Eotaxin-3	Unknown	CCR3
CCL27	9p13	CTACK/ILC	ALP/CTACK/ILC ESkine	CCR10[*]

in the presence of neutrophil granule lysates and purified proteinase-3 can undergo significant conversion from the 77 to 72 amino acid forms of the molecule and enhance its biological activity *(13)*. The 72 amino acid form of IL-8 (CXCL8) binds to neutrophils twofold more than the 77 amino acid form and is two- to threefold more potent in inducing cytochalasin B–treated neutrophil degranulation *(11)*. Other studies have demonstrated similar findings for NH_2-terminal truncations of ENA-78 (CXCL5) *(1,14)*.

Although these findings support the contention that the NH_2-terminus of CXC chemokines is critical for receptor binding and activation, the role of the heparin-binding domain in the COOH-terminus of these molecules may also play an important role in enhancing the response to IL-8 (CXCL8) *(15)*. The combination of IL-8 (CXCL8) and heparin sulfate results in both a significant rise in cytosolic-free Ca^{+2} and a fourfold increase in neutrophil chemotaxis, as compared to IL-8 (CXCL8) alone *(15)*. Interestingly, heparin in combination with IL-8 (CXCL8) enhances its ability to induce a rise in cytosolic-free Ca^{+2}, but not in neutrophil chemotaxis. The effects of these glycosaminoglycans on IL-8 (CXCL8) activity are specific; neither heparin sulfate nor heparin alters the affect of N-Formyl-Met-Leu-Phe (fMLP)-induced neutrophil activation. These findings, together with the importance of the ELR motif in neutrophil binding and activation, support the notion that both the NH_2- and COOH-terminal domains of ELR^+ CXC chemokines interplay in a cooperative fashion to optimize their ability to mediate neutrophil activation and chemotaxis. These findings also suggest that these CXC chemokines can undergo further refinement at the local level of inflammation, enhancing their ability to further amplify recruitment of additional neutrophils.

NH_2-terminal processing of CC chemokines may also play a significant role in modifying their biological function for recruitment of mononuclear cells. The lymphocyte surface glycoprotein CD26/dipeptidyl peptidase IV is a membrane-associated peptidase that has a high degree of specificity for peptides with proline or alanine at the second position and cleaves off dipeptides at the NH_2-terminus *(16)*. Whereas NH_2-terminal truncation of the CXC chemokine granulocyte chemotactic protein-2 (CXCL6) *(1)* by CD26 results in no change in chemotactic activity for neutrophils *(16,17)*, NH_2-terminal truncation of regulated-on-activation normal T-cell-expressed and secreted chemokine ([RANTES]; CCL5) *(1)*, eotaxin (CCL11) *(1)*, and macrophage-derived chemokine (CCL22) by CD26 has been shown to markedly impair their ability to bind to their receptors and elicit chemotactic activity *(16,17)*. Interestingly, while CD26 NH2-terminal truncation of RANTES (CCL5) results in reduced binding and activation of two of its CC chemokine receptors, CCR1 and CCR3, RANTES (CCL5) binding to its other receptor, CCR5, is actually preserved *(17)*. This suggests that CD26 modification of RANTES (CCL5) increases its receptor selectivity and may significantly modify its biological behavior during both innate and adaptive immune responses. By contrast, NH_2-terminal processing of LD78β (CCL3) *(1)*, an isoform of macrophage inflammatory peptide-1α (MIP-1α) *(1)*, by CD26 increases its chemotactic activity *(18)*. This effect is mediated through both of its major CC chemokine receptors, CCR1 and CCR5 *(18)*.

These studies are important to local chemokine biology, since further extracellular processing of these potent leukocyte chemoattractants can play a major role in positively or negatively modifying their behavior in recruitment of leukocytes during inflammation of the innate host defense. Furthermore, measurement of protein, rather than mRNA, provides further evidence of their biological function in the context of the local tissue microenvironment.

1.2. Chemokine Receptors

Chemokine receptors belong to the largest known family of cell-surface receptors, the G-protein-coupled receptors, which mediate transmission of stimuli as diverse as hormones, peptides, glycopeptides, and chemokines *(19)*. The functional unit consists of a seven-transmembrane receptor coupled to the heterotrimeric G-protein. Currently, at least 11 cellular CC chemokine receptors, 6 CXC chemokine receptors, 1 C chemokine receptor, and 1 CX_3C receptor have been cloned, expressed, and identified to have specific ligand-binding profiles (**Tables 1** and **2**) *(1,7,8,20–25)*. The expression of these receptors on specific cells in the context of the temporal expression of their respective chemokine ligands will play an important role in mediating the initial and subsequent leukocyte infiltration during the evolution of the inflammatory response of innate immunity.

1.3. Measurement of Chemokine Protein Levels in Tissue

While reverse transcriptase polymerase chain reaction, Northern blot analysis, and *in situ* hybridization for mRNA have been universally used to detect the expression of mRNA in tissue, the ability to quantitatively detect protein has been more difficult. We and others have devised a strategy to homogenize and sonicate tissue using an antiproteinase buffer system to extract protein and analyze the quantitative levels of chemokines using conventional enzyme-linked immunosorbent assays (ELISAs) that are specific for these proteins. We have effectively utilized this technique for the analysis of lung tissue in several studies. The lung is an ideal organ/tissue environment to measure chemokines and their receptors during inflammatory and immunological responses. Moreover, the methods to measure chemokine ligands in the lung are analogous to measuring chemokines in any organ/tissue (e.g., skin and liver). The ability to detect chemokines in a quantifiable manner at a protein level provides immediate feedback on their temporal importance in promoting inflammatory/immunologically mediated processes. Furthermore, the ability to measure chemokine protein, as compared to mRNA levels, provides the additional fidelity of placing this expression in the context of its biological function. The future of proteomics will further enhance our ability to detect quantifiable levels of proteins in tissue specimens.

2. Materials

1. 1X Phosphate-buffered saline (PBS).
2. Antiproteinase buffer (*see* **Note 1**).
3. Tissue tearor (BioSpec, Bartlesville, OK).
4. Sonicater (microtip).
5. Centrifuge.
6. Syringe filters (1.2 µm) (Gelman, Ann Arbor, MI).
7. ELISA kits.

3. Methods

1. Homogenize tissue specimens used for analysis in sterile 1X PBS in the presence of antiprotease buffer (*see* **Note 1**) at 4°C using a tissue tearor until the tissue is fully homogenized. Approximately 0.2 g of tissue can be homogenized in 1 mL of antiprotease buffer. This may require some adjustment depending on the tissue being analyzed. We routinely homogenize mouse or rat lungs in 1 and 3 mL, respectively.
2. Sonicate (microtip) the homogenized tissue for 30 s at 50% duty cycle, output set at four, and at 4°C under sterile conditions.
3. Following sonication, centrifuge the tissue specimens at 1000*g* for 10 min, and filter through 1.2-µm syringe filters.
4. Aliquot the prepared homogenate, and store at –70°C until measured in a conventional ELISA for a specific chemokine (*see* **Notes 2** and **3**). Chemokine levels are standardized to total protein.

4. Notes

1. While a number of buffer systems can be used to extract tissue chemokines for analysis in a conventional ELISA, we have determined that the optimal antiproteinase buffer system is the following: One tablet of Complete® (Boehringer Mannheim) is dissolved in in 50 mL of 1X PBS. The amount of 1X PBS and Complete used in homogenization of a tissue specimen depends on the size of the tissue specimen. For example, mouse or rat lungs are placed in 1 and 3 mL of 1X PBS and Complete, respectively, and then homogenized with the tissue tearor. **Table 3** illustrates the differences in proteinase buffers used in homogenization and the importance of sonication using lung tissue from a rat. In this experiment, donor lung allografts (Brown Norway) were harvested at d 4 from Lewis recipient animals as previously described *(26)* and then subjected to homogenization

Table 3
Comparison of Antiprotease Buffers and Importance of Sonication

Buffer[a]	KC/CXCL1 (ng/mL)	IP-10/CXCL10 (ng/mL)	MIG/CXCL9 (ng/mL)
1X PBS alone	0.000	0.071	0.899
1X PBS + sonication	0.084	0.171	1.600
Antiprotease cocktail	0.099	0.120	1.500
Antiprotease cocktail + sonication	0.121	0.181	1.900
Complete and 1X PBS	0.159	0.421	2.600
Complete and 1X PBS + sonication	0.165	1.400	4.800

[a]Antiprotease cocktail consists of 1X PBS + 2 mM phenylmethylsufonyl fluoride (Sigma) + 1 µg/mL of each of the following: antipain (Sigma), aprotinin (Sigma), leupeptin (Sigma), and pepstatin A (Sigma). Complete (Boehringer Mannheim) is a proprietary antiprotease cocktail in tablet form.

as just described in the presence or absence of an antiprotease buffer with or without associated sonication. The results of these studies demonstrate that the use of combined antiprotease buffer (Complete) together with the addition of sonication leads to the greatest extraction of all three chemokines from the lung tissue as analyzed by conventional ELISA.

2. This same sample can also be used to detect the expression of chemokines by semiquantitative means, such as by Western blot analysis using conventional strategies.

3. Two examples of how this technique for the measurement of chemokines can be used to understand lung inflammation are as follows:

a. Measurement of chemokines in pneumonia: Inflammatory sequestration in the lung is the hallmark of the host response to infection related to a number of microbial organisms. In a model of *Aspergillus fumigatus* pneumonia in mice, TNF-α protein levels were highly associated with the production of murine MIP-2 (CXCL2/3), MIP-1α (CCL3), and MCP-1 (CCL2). Furthermore, neutralization of TNF-α resulted in marked attenuation of the expression of murine MIP-2 (CXCL2/3), MIP-1α (CCL3), and MCP-1 (CCL2) that was paralleled by a reduction in the infiltration of inflammatory cells and associated with increased mortality *(27)*. In these experiments, mice were infected with *A. fumigatus* conidia. Both lungs of a mouse were processed as described above in 1 mL of Complete and 1X PBS to generate tissues specimens for quantitative measurement of TNF-α and chemokine protein levels. There was a rapid increase in lung TNF-α protein levels, which reached a plateau by 24 h (~2 ng/mL) as measured by specific ELISA, whereas levels of TNF-α were essentially undetectable from control vehicle-treated animal lungs *(27)*. The levels of TNF-α were paralleled by the production of MIP-2 (CXCL2/3; 2.75 ng/mL), MIP-1α (CCL3; 0.67 ng/mL), and MCP-1 (CCL2; 0.6 ng/mL) protein as measured by specific ELISAs. Similar to TNF-α, MIP-2 (CXCL2/3), MIP-1α (CCL3), and MCP-1 (CCL2) protein levels were essentially undetectable in control treated animals. Passive immunization with neutralizing TNF-α antibodies resulted in marked attenuation of the inflammatory response with an associated decline in measurable protein levels of MIP-2 (CXCL2/3), MIP-1α (CCL3), and MCP-1 (CCL2), and increased mortality of the animals. The study represents a model system to not only measure quantitative chemokine protein levels in a kinetic manner under conditions of tissue inflammation, but to understand further the dynamic relation of other cytokines (i.e., TNF-α) that mediate the expression of chemokines in vivo and on a protein level.

b. Measurement of chemokines in lung allograft rejection: Acute lung allograft rejection is a major complication of lung transplantation and is characterized by the infiltration of activated mononuclear cells. The CC chemokines, RANTES (CCL5), MIP-1α (CCL3), and MIP-1β (CCL4), are potent mononuclear cell chemoattractants. To assess their role in mediating lung allograft rejection, rat lung allografts were processed as described in **Subheading 3** for protein measurement of these chemokines *(26)*. Lung allografts demonstrated a marked time-dependent increase in protein levels of RANTES (CCL5) and MIP-1α (CCL3), as compared to syngeneic control lungs (**Fig. 1**). By contrast, MIP-1β (CCL4) protein levels were found to decline during lung allograft rejection (**Fig. 1**). RANTES protein levels, however, were 160-fold higher than MIP-1α in this model system. RANTES protein levels correlated with the temporal recruitment of mononuclear cells and the expression of RANTES-related receptors CCR1 and CCR5. To determine whether RANTES was involved in promoting lung allograft rejection, lung allograft recipients were passively immunized with either anti-RANTES or control antibodies. In vivo neutralization of RANTES markedly attenuated allograft rejection, mononuclear cell infiltration, and expression of CCR1 and CCR5. These experiments not only support the notion that RANTES protein and the expression of its receptors have an important role in the pathogenesis of acute lung allograft rejection, but using strategies of protein isolation and measurement with conventional and specific ELISAs can provide evidence for quantifiable levels of chemokines in tissue during an immunologically mediated process.

Acknowledgment

This work was supported, in part, by grants from the National Institutes of Health (CA87879, HL66027, P50HL67665, P50CA90388, HL04493, and HL03906).

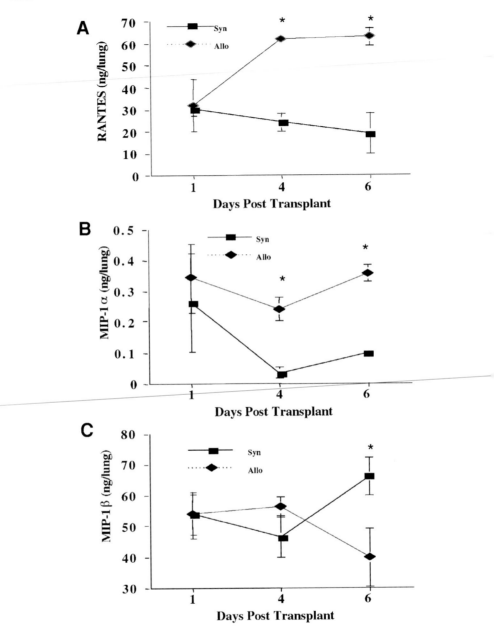

Fig. 1. (**A**) RANTES (CCL5), (**B**) MIP-1α (CCL3), and (**C**) MIP-1β (CCL4) protein levels in rat lung transplants. Syn = syngeneic control; allo = allograft; * = p < 0.05.

References

1. Zlotnik, A. and Yoshie, O. (2000) Chemokines: a new classification system and their role in immunity. *Immunity* **12**, 121–127.
2. Strieter, R. M., Lukacs, N. W., Standiford, T. J., and Kunkel, S. L. (1993) Cytokines. 2. Cytokines and lung inflammation: mechanisms of neutrophil recruitment to the lung. *Thorax* **48**, 765–769.
3. Strieter, R. M., Koch, A. E., Antony, V. B., Fick, R. B. Jr., Standiford, T. J., and Kunkel, S. L. (1994) The immunopathology of chemotactic cytokines: the role of interleukin-8 and monocyte chemoattractant protein-1. *J. Lab. Clin. Med.* **123**, 183–197.
4. Strieter, R. M. and Kunkel, S. L. (1994) Acute lung injury: the role of cytokines in the elicitation of neutrophils. *J. Investig. Med.* **42**, 640–651.
5. Strieter, R. M. and Kunkel, S. L. (1997) Chemokines in the lung, in *Lung: Scientific Foundations* (Crystal, R., West, J., Weibel, E., and Barnes, P., eds.), Raven, New York, pp. 155–186.
6. Strieter, R. M., Kunkel, S. L., Keane, M. P., and Standiford, T. J. (1999) Chemokines in lung injury: Thomas A. Neff Lecture. *Chest* **116**, 103S–110S.
7. Luster, A. D. (1998) Chemokines—chemotactic cytokines that mediate inflammation. *N. Engl. J. Med.* **338**, 436–445.
8. Rollins, B. J. (1997) Chemokines. *Blood* **90**, 909–928.
9. Locati, M. and Murphy, P. M. (1999) Chemokines and chemokine receptors: biology and clinical relevance in inflammation and AIDS. *Annu. Rev. Med.* **50**, 425–440.
10. Hebert, C. A., Vitangcol, R. V., and Baker, J. B. (1991) Scanning mutagenesis of interleukin-8 identifies a cluster of residues required for receptor binding. *J. Biol. Chem.* **266**, 18,989–18,994.
11. Hebert, C. A. and Baker, J. B. (1993) Interleukin-8: a review. *Cancer Invest.* **11**, 743–750.
12. Clark-Lewis, I., Dewald, B., Geiser, T., Moser, B., and Baggiolini, M. (1993) Platelet factor 4 binds to interleukin 8 receptors and activates neutrophils when its N terminus is modified with Glu-Leu-Arg. *Proc. Natl. Acad. Sci. USA* **90**, 3574–3577.
13. Padrines, M., Wolf, M., Walz, A., and Baggiolini, M. (1994) Interleukin-8 processing by neutrophil elastase, cathepsin G and proteinase-3. *FEBS Lett.* **352**, 231–235.
14. Walz, A., Strieter, R. M., and Schnyder, S. (1993) Neutrophil-activating peptide ENA-78. *Adv. Exp. Med. Biol.* **351**, 129–137.
15. Webb, L. M., Ehrengruber, M. U., Clark-Lewis, I., Baggiolini, M., and Rot, A. (1993) Binding to heparan sulfate or heparin enhances neutrophil responses to interleukin 8. *Proc. Natl. Acad. Sci. USA* **90**, 7158–7162.
16. De Meester, I., Korom, S., Van Damme, J., and Scharpe, S. (1999) CD26, let it cut or cut it down. *Immunol. Today* **20**, 367–375.

17. Proost, P., Struyf, S., Schols, D., Durinx, C., Wuyts, A., Lenaerts, J. P., De Clercq, E., De Meester, I., and Van Damme, J. (1998) Processing by CD26/dipeptidyl-peptidase IV reduces the chemotactic and anti-HIV-1 activity of stromal-cell-derived factor-1alpha. *FEBS Lett.* **432,** 73–76.

18. Proost, P., Menten, P., Struyf, S., Schutyser, E., De Meester, I., and Van Damme, J. (2000) Cleavage by CD26/dipeptidyl peptidase IV converts the chemokine LD78beta into a most efficient monocyte attractant and CCR1 agonist. *Blood* **96,** 1674–1680.

19. Iacovelli, L., Sallese, M., Mariggio, S., and de Blasi, A. (1999) Regulation of G-protein-coupled receptor kinase subtypes by calcium sensor proteins. *FASEB J.* **13,** 1–8.

20. Broxmeyer, H. E. and Kim, C. H. (1999) Regulation of hematopoiesis in a sea of chemokine family members with a plethora of redundant activities. *Exp. Hematol.* **27,** 1113–1123.

21. Nibbs, R. J., Wylie, S. M., Pragnell, I. B., and Graham, G. J. (1997) Cloning and characterization of a novel murine beta chemokine receptor, D6. Comparison to three other related macrophage inflammatory protein-1alpha receptors, CCR-1, CCR-3, and CCR-5. *J. Biol. Chem.* **272,** 12,495–12,504.

22. Premack, B. A. and Schall, T. J. (1996) Chemokine receptors: gateways to inflammation and infection. *Nat. Med.* **2,** 1174–1178.

23. Imai, T., Chantry, D., Raport, C. J., Wood, C. L., Nishimura, M., Godiska, R., Yoshie, O., and Gray, P. W. (1998) Macrophage-derived chemokine is a functional ligand for the CC chemokine receptor 4. *J. Biol. Chem.* **273,** 1764–1768.

24. Liao, F., Alderson, R., Su, J., Ullrich, S. J., Kreider, B. L., and Farber, J. M. (1997) STRL22 is a receptor for the CC chemokine MIP-3alpha. *Biochem. Biophys. Res. Commun.* **236,** 212–217.

25. Liao, F., Alkhatib, G., Peden, K. W., Sharma, G., Berger, E. A., and Farber, J. M. (1997) STRL33, a novel chemokine receptor-like protein, functions as a fusion cofactor for both macrophage-tropic and T cell line-tropic HIV-1. *J. Exp. Med.* **185,** 2015–2023.

26. Belperio, J. A., Burdick, M. D., Keane, M. P., Xue, Y. Y., Lynch, J. P. 3rd, Daugherty, B. L., Kunkel, S. L., and Strieter, R. M. (2000) The role of the CC chemokine, RANTES, in acute lung allograft rejection. *J. Immunol.* **165,** 461–472.

27. Mehrad, B., Strieter, R. M., and Standiford, T. J. (1999) Role of TNF-alpha in pulmonary host defense in murine invasive aspergillosis. *J. Immunol.* **162,** 1633–1640.

31

Methods of Measuring Oxygen in Wounds

Harriet W. Hopf, Thomas K. Hunt, Heinz Scheuenstuhl,
Judith M. West, Lisa M. Humphrey, and Mark D. Rollins

1. Introduction

Accurate measurement of tissue oxygen tension has led to an understanding of the crucial role of oxygen in wound healing and the degree to which oxygen supply in wounded tissue is often the limiting factor in healing. This, in turn, has led to studies demonstrating that activation of the sympathetic nervous system by such common perioperative stressors as hypothermia, pain, and hypovolemia decreases wound oxygen tension and impairs wound healing. In the past 6 to 7 yr, these observations have led to several large, randomized, controlled trials to increase wound oxygen tension management of surgical patients (e.g., maintenance of normothermia and administration of high oxygen concentrations to the patient) that yielded dramatic improvements in wound healing and resistance to infection. Tissue oxygen measurements are relatively simple to make, particularly with current highly stable probes, and their use will undoubtedly lead to further advances in wound care.

The first measurements of tissue oxygen levels were made with microelectrodes. Because tissue perfusion tends to be heterogeneous, multiple measurements over small incremental distances were required to create a map of tissue oxygen gradients. The resulting histogram indicated mean or median tissue oxygen levels. Microelectrodes are not practical for measurements in humans under most circumstances, since they require multiple needle punctures. Therefore, in the 1970s Thomas K. Hunt and others began to develop techniques to measure average tissue oxygen levels from a single site. In this chapter, we detail six of the most important and commonly used methods for oxygen measurement, ranging from quantifying oxygen levels in cell culture, to

From: *Methods in Molecular Medicine, vol. 78: Wound Healing: Methods and Protocols*
Edited by: Luisa A. DiPietro and Aime L. Burns © Humana Press Inc., Totowa, NJ

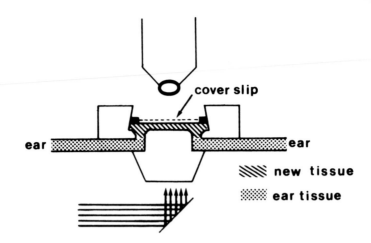

Fig. 1. Schematic of ear chamber. Note that the healing tissue grows up into the chamber through several round holes. (Reprinted with permission from **ref. 28**).

microelectrode measurements of wound oxygen gradients, to clinically useful measurements in humans.

2. Materials

2.1. Rabbit Ear Chamber Model

1. Ear chamber: Refer to **Figs. 1** and **2** showing cross-sections of a chamber as fashioned and used by Ian Silver. The chamber body is transparent Lucite (Perspex). Many designs can be used. They can be simple or sophisticated. There is no commercial source. The upper membrane, held in place by a circlip, may be glass, Teflon, or both. The easiest to use for oxygen measurement is two membranes that have interlocking holes: a permeable Teflon membrane on the inside, topped by an impermeable glass one (*see* **Note 1**). The healing tissue grows from the ear cartilage up through the holes into and across the chamber.

2. Oxygen probes: These must have fine tips, a few microns for best resolution. They can be handmade by drawing out a fine glass capillary tube over a platinum wire, usually about 25 μ in diameter. It is then electro-polished to as small a tip as possible. Experts can make them <2 μ. Assembled, membrane-covered, oxygen probes that contain both electrodes and are as small as 0.5 mm can be purchased. Licox (GMS, Germany; and Integra Neurosciences, NJ) makes the best of that size (*see* **Notes 2** and **3**).

3. Cathode: a silver/silver chloride wire of any description.

4. A potentiometer that can be set to 0.6 V.

5. Nanoammeter.

6. Lop-eared rabbit (*see* **Note 4**).

7. Sedating drugs: These may be useful to keep the animal still, but any interference with ventilation will lower the measured oxygen tensions.

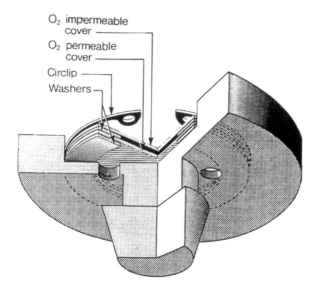

O₂ impermeable cover
O₂ permeable cover
Circlip
Washers

Fig. 2. Partial cross-section of ear chamber as used by Silver. The material can be any material that is transparent to light. (Reprinted with permission from **ref. *1***).

8. Punch.
9. Bandaging material.
10. Mineral oil (liquid petrolatum).
11. Holding device to keep the animal still—must be handmade.
12. Dissecting microscope with a stage assembly that holds the lower pole of the Lucite plug firmly.
13. Micromanipulator.
14. Faraday cage: This is useful if microelectrodes are used (*see* **Note 5**). If handled with care, the same animal and chamber can be used many times.

2.2. Wire Mesh Cylinder Model

1. Stainless steel mesh: This can be purchased from Cambridge Wire Cloth (Cambridge, MA). The material is 316SS with 0.010-in. diameter spacing. The type of metal alloy is important. Perforated plastic tubing is not satisfactory, though thin-meshed plastic of approximately the same properties as just described might be useful. We have used silicone mesh for studies requiring magnetic resonance imaging:
   a. For rabbit: 55×61 mm mesh rolled around a 3-cm cork borer (steel rod).
   b. For rat or guinea pig: 28×33 mm mesh rolled around a 7 to 8-mm rod.
   c. For mouse: 14×17 mm mesh rolled around a 2-mm rod.
2. Polyethylene or polypropylene test tubes with caps the same size as the cylinders. Alternately, the caps of Nunc® internal threaded cryovials are useful.

3. Silicone elastomer: This is manufactured by Dow Corning (Midland, MI) (MDX4-4210) and purchased from Factor II (Lakeside, AZ).
4. Silastic, as an alternate to MDX polymer.
5. Oven.
6. Glass rod.
7. Cork borer large enough to contain the cylinders but no larger.
8. Surgical instruments.
9. Suture.
10. Syringes.
11. Spinal needle (12–19 g), for introducing oxygen electrode.

2.3. Subcutaneous Wound Tissue Oximetry

2.3.1. Preparation of Tonometer

1. Silicone tubing (1.2 mm od, 0.76 mm id) (no. 508-004; Dow Corning). Available from Fisher, cat. no. 11-189015C (*see* **Note 6**).
2. Intravenous catheter (20 gauge, 1-in) with introducer needle (*see* **Note 7**).
3. Spinal needle (19 gauge), obturator in place with hub cut off, or 12 to 14-g spinal needle.

2.3.2. Placement of Tonometer

1. Powder-free, sterile gloves.
2. Sterile tonometer.
3. Indelible ink marker.
4. Ruler.
5. 1% Lidocaine (without epinephrine).
6. Bottle of Betadine®.
7. Bottle of alcohol.
8. Four sterile towels.
9. No. 11 Blade scalpel.
10. Sterile 4 × 4 gauze, 3 packages.
11. Two small squares of Tegaderm (3M, Minneapolis, MN).

2.3.3. Measurement of Psqo$_2$

1. Licox Po$_2$ computer (Integra Neuroscience/GMS).
2. C1 Licox oxygen probe (length: 15–20 cm; measuring tip: 5–8 mm; OD: 0.5–0.8 mm) (*see* **Notes 8** and **9**).
3. C8 Licox temperature probe.
4. Small bottle of normal saline, sterile.
5. Syringe (10 mL).
6. Needle (16 g) or filter straw.
7. Intravenous tubing with Y connector, including stopcock on one limb (**Fig. 3**; *see* **Note 10**).
8. 1-in. Dermapore, silk, or paper tape.

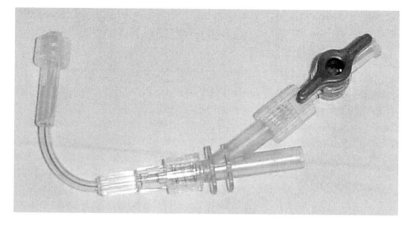

Fig. 3. Y adapter. This consists of iv tubing with a Luer connector at the distal end, and a Y connector at the proximal end. One limb has a stopcock, used for flushing. The oxygen probe is inserted through the other limb.

9. Nonsterile gauze 4×4s and 2×2s.
10. Chux or towel.
11. Oxygen supply.
12. Simple face mask.
13. Pulse oximeter.

2.4. Measurement of Transcutaneous Oxygen in Patients with Ulcers of Lower Extremity

1. Electrolyte solution.
2. Transcutaneous oximeter, including oxygen sensors (*see* **Notes 11** and **12**).
3. Attachment device (double stick ring for Novametrix, ring with attachment well for Radiometer).
4. Alcohol wipes.
5. 1-in. Dermapore, paper, or silk tape.
6. Chux or towel.
7. Foam wedge for elevating leg.
8. Oxygen supply.
9. Simple face mask or nonrebreather face mask.
10. Pulse oximeter.

3. Methods

3.1. Rabbit Ear Chamber Model

Healing has six main components: inflammation, epithelialization, angiogenesis, contraction, collagen deposition, and resistance to infection. All are influenced by oxygen supply. None of them occur at very low oxygen tension. Collagen synthesis rises to a peak at about a Po_2 of 250 mmHg. Resistance to infection peaks at about 600 mmHg. Each of the cells involved in wound healing, including epithelial, inflammatory, endothelial, and fibroblast, has a range of oxygen tensions at which it functions best.

The gradients of oxygen from a point in the vasculature to the center space of a wound are closely packed and steep. The Po_2 falls from near arterial levels at the capillary to near zero at the farthest distance from the capillaries and zero at the avascular center of the wound. These gradients can best be quantified using the rabbit ear chamber. This method is by far the most difficult to perform, but no other technique so clearly defines the heterogeneity of wound oxygen concentrations. It creates a living, healing wound in thin cross-section in an apparatus that allows point-by-point Po_2 measurement. Many other substances, particularly those that change on manipulation of oxygen, may be measured in this system. Measurements using the rabbit ear chamber form the basis for the understanding of oxygen delivery in wounds that has led to improved wound outcomes in surgical patients and those with chronic wounds. **Figure 4** shows a profile of oxygen tensions and lactate concentrations in a rabbit ear chamber (*see* **Notes 13–15**).

Ear chamber wounds are made by punching a hole in a lop-eared rabbit's ear into which a transparent "plug" or module is inserted. This plug becomes fixed in place and guides healing of the tissues at the edge of the hole through a space about 2 cm in diameter and 60–200 μ thick. Since it is transparent, the module can be mounted on a microscope stage and the growth of vessels through the engineered space can be observed. The top of the "wound space" that the new tissue traverses is a removable transparent membrane made of a material appropriate to the experiment to provide access to the tissue, if desired. Magnification can be more than sufficient to see red blood cells flowing through vessels.

The method was most frequently used by Ian Silver PhD, DVM, of Bristol University, UK. Most of his articles on this subject were published before 1965 and are difficult to find. A few that describe the method best are listed in **refs. *1–4***. Most of the equipment must be handmade. Recently, Suzuki and colleagues in Japan and London have used ear chambers, though not for measuring oxygen *(5–6)* (*see* **Note 16**).

1. Gas sterilize the entire ear chamber apparatus and implant it using a semisterile technique.
2. Punch a hole in the rabbit's ear in a place that has the least apparent large vessels (*see* **Fig. 5**).

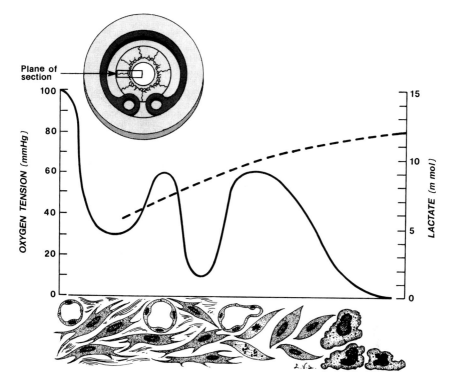

Fig. 4. Cross-section of wound module in rabbit ear chamber (upper left). Note that Po₂, depicted graphically above the cross-section by the solid line, is highest next to the vessels, with a gradient dropping to zero at the wound edge. Note also that the lactate gradient denoted by the dotted line is highest in the dead space and lower (but still above plasma) closer to the vasculature. (Reprinted with permission from **ref. 28**.)

3. Elevate the inner skin from the cartilage. Implant the device by placing the Dacron "skirt" under the inner skin to provide mechanical stability. Rearrange the skin to fit comfortably. No sutures are placed.
4. Bandage the ear securely.
5. At any time after the vessels first appear, the chamber can be used (*see* **Note 17**). First, remove the circlip. Next, carefully lift out the glass cover (usually leaving the Teflon membrane in place) or align the holes in the two glass membranes.
6. Fill the well of the assembly with mineral oil to prevent access of air.
7. Sedate the rabbit and confine in a holder. Place the ear chamber in the fixation plate on a dissecting microscope.
8. Select the sites for measurement and set the electrodes, mounted on a micromanipulator, in place. The electrodes either can be placed on the surface of the oxygen-permeable Teflon or can pierce through it (*see* **Note 18**).

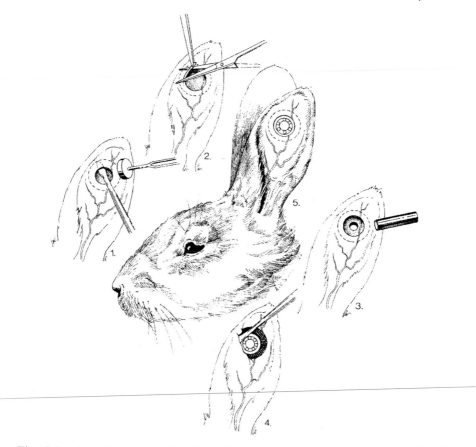

Fig. 5. Implantation of ear chamber. (1) make a small hole in the inner skin of ear in a place with relatively few visible vessels. (2) undermine the skin to give a space for the Dacron skirt that is fixed to the Lucite plug. (3) mark a spot, and punch a hole through the cartilage and dorsal skin. (4) insert the chamber with the inner skin of ear over the Dacron skirt, cutting away some skin if necessary. (5) Final appearance. (Reprinted with permission from **ref. *1*.**)

9. When studies are finished for the day, replace the glass cover or seal with a large plug that precisely fills the well to prevent any exposure to air, even with the Teflon in place, which will stop the angiogenesis.

3.2. Wire Mesh Cylinder Model

One of the criticisms of the ear chamber model is the large amount of data generated that are difficult to interpret statistically. One way to avoid the problems of complexity, too much data, and too much diversity is to measure the P_{O_2} in the dead space, at one definable point, and then calculate the gradients as from arterial or midcapillary level to wound-space level. This is done in what is called a "dead-space" wound. This model is perhaps the simplest and least expensive of wound models and can be used in any animal, including humans. Gases, electrolytes, lactate, glucose, cytokines, growth factors, protein, and ingrown collagen (after 14–21 d) have been measured, making this probably the most frequently used model in wound healing *(7–13)*. Arterial or venous levels drawn at about the same time with serial draws from the wound can be done if wound fluid samples are small in comparison with the volume of the cylinder. This allows studies of the total gradients. Flow of substances both into and out of the wound can be studied. Regarding P_{O_2} measurements, the P_{O_2} in the wound is sensitive to the arterial P_{O_2}, but the response time for full equilibrium is long, perhaps as long as 45–60 min. An unlimited number of substances can be measured using this model. The cylinders and the implantation method are shown in **Fig. 6**.

3.2.1. Preparation of Cylinder (see **Note 19**)

3.2.1.1. STANDARD RAT CYLINDERS

1. Cut the steel mesh into 28 × 33 mm rectangles.
2. Roll on the long axis around a 7- or 8-mm-diameter steel rod, and maintain the cylindrical shape by placing in the cap of a polyethylene or polypropylene test tube of appropriate diameter.
3. Mix MDX polymer with curing agent according to the manufacturer's specifications, and inject into the cap with the cylinder removed. Replace the cylinder and centrifuge the assembly at about 900*g* for 10 min. This removes nascent air bubbles in the Silastic as well as forces the material into the pores of the steel mesh.
4. Incubate the assembly at 75°C for 30 min, cool, and repeat the process for the opposite end of the cylinder. Cylinders are autoclaved to sterilize.

3.2.1.2. SPECIALTY RAT CYLINDERS

1. Specialty cylinders are made from the same dimension mesh rectangles. Tease three wires out of one end along the 28-mm axis, roll the cylinder, and polymerize. Place Silastic at the opposite end from the free wires as outlined in **Subheading 3.2.1.1.** After autoclaving, solid materials may be placed in the cylinder through the open end.
2. Close the open end by pressing a disk of Silastic cut from a 3-mm-thick sheet of polymerized material over the protruding wires. The free wires grasp the disk strongly enough to use the cylinder like those produced with two polymerized plastic ends (*see* **Subheading 3.2.1.1.**). Sizes and shapes are not critical for most purposes. The major issue is that they not erode through the skin of the animal.

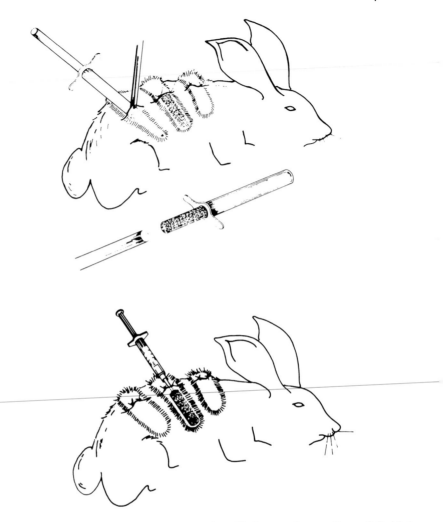

Fig. 6. Method for insertion of wire mesh cylinders and sampling of fluid (*see* **Subheading 3.2.2.** for full details of placement). Incisions are made in the dorsal skin. A rod is used to insert the cylinder and the incision is closed. After a few days, a syringe is used to sample wound fluid percutaneously. (Reprinted with permission from **ref. 2**.)

3.2.1.3. RABBIT CYLINDERS

Rabbit cylinders are manufactured in the same fashion as the rat cylinders from 55 × 61 mm mesh rolled along the short axis. This size of cylinder has also been used in sheep and dogs.

3.2.2. Implantation

Four cylinders are implanted in rabbits, guinea pigs, and large rats; two in small rats or mice. The implantation procedure is done under semi-sterile conditions with the animals under general anesthesia. On awakening, the animals seem unaware of the cylinders provided they are not so large that they erode the skin. Dressings are not necessary.

1. Make a dorsal, longitudinal incision large enough to insert the cylinder end on.
2. Open the plane between the sc muscle and the deep fascia for 1 or 2 cm by gently spreading a pair of surgical scissors.
3. Insert a glass rod or pointed pipet of about the same diameter as the cylinder to enlarge the hole between the fascia and the sc muscle.
4. Insert a cork borer just large enough to easily hold the cylinder over the glass rod, and use reciprocating motion of the borer and the tube to make a space large enough to hold the cylinder.
5. Remove the glass tube and use it to push the cylinder into position through the cork borer. Enough space from the medial cylinder to the midline should be left so that the skin wound can be closed easily.
6. Repeat the process on the other side through the same incision.
7. Pull the skin down to the spinal ligament using one or two closure sutures during closure of the midline wound so as to separate the cylinders on the two sides. It is important to be sure that the cylinders on each side do not touch. If the cylinders do touch, their spaces will communicate and they will lose their identity for statistical purposes.
8. Insert a small needle and syringe through the skin and the Silastic plug to withdraw fluid for analysis (*see* **Notes 20** and **21**). Placement of a second, venting needle minimizes bleeding into the cylinder.
9. Measure oxygen tension within the cylinder by introducing an oxygen electrode of the type described in **Subheading 3.3.** through a 19-g spinal needle (*see* **Notes 22–24**).

3.3. Subcutaneous Wound Tissue Oximetry

In the 1970s Thomas K. Hunt and others began to develop techniques to measure average tissue oxygen from a single site in humans. Hunt developed the silicone tonometer for this purpose (**Fig. 7**). Silicone is freely permeable to oxygen. When a length of silicone tubing (1 mm OD) is placed subcutaneously, the Po_2 within the tonometer equilibrates with that of a cylinder of surrounding tissue, thus providing a mean wound tissue oxygen tension equivalent to the mean of the microelectrode-generated histograms. Initially, Hunt infused saline slowly through the tonometer and measured the Po_2 of the effluent (microdialysis). A much more convenient method, however, is to place an

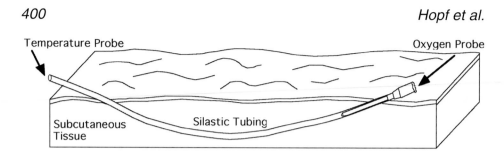

Fig. 7. Schematic drawing of silicone sc oxygen tonometer. The oxygen probe is inserted through the catheter hub. The temperature probe is inserted into the protruding end of the tonometer. Adapted from: Musculoskeletal Infection *(14)*.

oxygen probe within the tonometer to get a continuous measure of tissue oxygen. The tonometer is filled with saline to speed equilibration with surrounding tissue. Temperature is measured at the same site concurrently, because Po_2 is temperature dependent.

Two main types of oxygen probes are currently available: polarographic (Clark) electrodes and optical electrodes (optodes) *(15)*. The polarographic electrodes are based on the observation that when a negatively charged metal and a reference electrode are placed in an electrolyte solution, current flows in proportion to oxygen concentration, with no current flow in the absence of oxygen. Current technology corrects many of the problems that plagued early polarographic probes, including drift, excessive oxygen consumption at the cathode, and poisoning by substances such as halothane. The electrodes are highly accurate even to oxygen tensions in excess of 800 mmHg, although their accuracy diminishes somewhat as current decreases toward zero (no oxygen). Optical electrodes use a fluorescent dye (usually ruthenium) in which the fluorescence is quenched by oxygen. Thus, the fluorescent output is inversely proportional to oxygen tension. Optodes are highly accurate at low oxygen tensions, but lose accuracy at higher oxygen concentrations (around 100–300 mmHg, depending on the design).

Our laboratory currently uses a polarographic electrode, and the methods described pertain specifically to the Licox probe that we use. However, these methods can easily be adapted to any probe that can be placed securely in the tonometer. Most currently manufactured tissue oxygen electrodes are intended for direct implantation and thus are embedded in a sheath of silicone to increase the averaging area around the electrode. These probes work in a tonometer as well. We continue to use the tonometer because: (1) if there is a question of probe drift or malfunction, the probe can be removed to check the calibration and then can be replaced without causing pain to the subject, whereas with a direct implant, a new stick with a sterile probe is required; (2) the probe does not directly contact the subject, so the probe need not be sterile, only clean; and (3) multiple measurements can be made over the course of several days without having to leave the probe in place the entire time (the tonometer is easy to secure).

Although the methods described here are for measurement in sc tissue *(16–20)*, the same probes can be used with essentially the same technique in a number of tissues, including gut, heart, liver, brain, muscle, and bone.

3.3.1. Preparation of Tonometer

1. Cut silicone tubing into 15-cm lengths.
2. Gently wedge one end of the tubing onto the iv catheter. Wedge the other end onto the 19-g spinal needle (if using a 12 to 14-g spinal needle, omit this step) (*see* **Notes 25–27**).
3. Gas sterilize (do not autoclave).

3.3.2. Placement of Tonometer

3.3.2.1. METHOD 1

The tonometer should be in place for at least 30 min before actual measurements begin (this can include equilibration time). For about 30 min after the tonometer is placed, readings may reflect arterial Po_2 because of minor bleeding around the tube. The tonometer may be implanted under general or local anesthesia. Placement is identical, except that local anesthetic is not required for placement during general anesthesia.

1. Inspect the lateral upper arm for a site without obvious veins, bruises, or broken skin. Mark an entry and exit site measured 7 cm apart (this is to ensure that the probe tip is at least 2 cm from the exit site and there is no possibility of diffusion of room air to the probe tip).
2. Raise a skin wheal with 1% lidocaine (*without* epinephrine) at the planned entry and exit sites; the wheal should be at least 1.5 cm in diameter. It is not necessary to inject local anesthetic into the sc tissue between the skin wheals.
3. Prep the arm with Betadine paint solution in a circular fashion.
4. After 1 to 2 min, use alcohol to wash off the betadine. Drape the site with sterile towels.
5. Make a small stab wound with a no. 11 blade at the planned entry and exit sites. The stab wound should be large enough to allow easy passage of the catheter, but as small and superficial as possible, in order to minimize bleeding. Make the stab wound in line, with skin lines to minimize or eliminate scarring.
6. Immediately hold point pressure over the sites until the bleeding stops, usually 1 to 2 min.
7. Using the spinal needle, pull the tonometer through just under the skin, so that the catheter is in up to the hub. You want the tonometer to be superficial, but if you see skin puckers, you are too shallow and should pull back and go

deeper. The subject should not feel pain; if the subject does, you are probably too shallow (in the dermis).

8. Cut the silicone tubing close to the spinal needle, leaving a fairly long distal segment of silicone tubing. Wipe off any blood with either alcohol or saline. Dry the catheter hub.

9. Cover the tonometer with two small Tegaderm dressings. One should cover the exit site, with about 2 cm covering the silicon tubing. Cut the silicon tubing about 1 cm beyond the Tegaderm edge. The second Tegaderm should cover the entrance site, with about 0.5 cm of the iv catheter hub uncovered. Usually the two Tegaderm dressings will overlap somewhat. If a significant amount of blood accumulates, the dressing should be removed, the site dried, and a fresh dressing applied in the same fashion. Write on the Tegaderm: "Do not remove."

3.3.2.2. METHOD 2

1. The tonometer in this case consists just of silicone tubing wedged onto the iv catheter. Prepare the entrance and exit sites as outlined in **Subheading 3.3.2.1.**
2. Insert a 12 to 14-g spinal needle (*see* **Note 28**).
3. Thread the tonometer through the sharp end of the needle (hubless). Remove the spinal needle, leaving the tonometer in place.

3.3.3. Measurement of Psqo$_2$

Each probe has been calibrated at the factory in both nitrogen and room air. Calibration values are listed on the probe package, including the IcO$_2$ (current during room air calibration), IcN$_2$ (current during nitrogen calibration), and TS (temperature coefficient for the probe). These should be input into the proper places on the monitor. Barometric pressure at your site should be entered (760 mmHg at sea level), along with 209 for oxygen concentration in room air (*see* **Note 29**). The calibration temperature and tissue temperature settings should be 00, since you will be measuring actual temperature during both calibration and oxygen measurement. Calibration is performed with both the temperature and oxygen probes in room air by pushing the blue calibration button (*see* **Notes 30** and **31**). For quality assurance, record room air Po$_2$ and temperature immediately after calibration, and again after removing the probe from the tonometer (*see* **Notes 32** and **33**).

1. Draw up 10 mL of saline into the 10-mL syringe using the 16-g needle or the filter straw.
2. Carefully place the calibrated probe through the Y adapter (*see* **Note 10**) and flush with saline to remove all bubbles. Then place the assembly into the hub of the tonometer (*see* **Note 34**).
3. Tape the tubing to the patient's arm so that the probe lies flat.
4. Tape the monitor cable or probe/cable connection to the side rail.
5. Flush the assembly with at least 8 mL of normal saline.

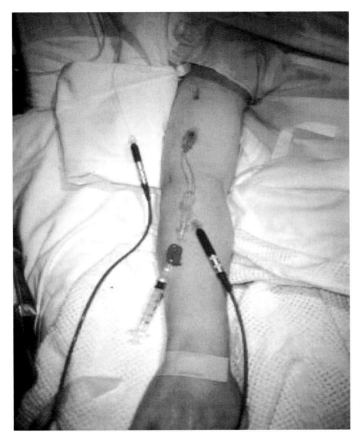

Fig. 8. Tonometer in a patient's arm. The oxygen probe has been placed through the Y connector, and the temperature probe has been inserted through the distal end of the tonometer until the measurement tip is under the skin.

6. Place the thermocouple probe through the distal end of the silicon tubing. Advance it as far as it will go.
7. Flush the system gently with about 0.5 mL of saline. **Figure 8** shows a patient with the entire assembly in place in the arm.
8. Cover the entire arm with a Chux or towel to decrease heat loss.
9. Record the baseline value for Po_2 (sc oxygen) and Tsq (sc temperature) only after the value has changed ≤1 mmHg in 5 min, and it has been at least 25 min since probe insertion (*see* **Notes 36–37**). Data may be recorded continuously or at specified intervals.
10. For the oxygen challenge, administer 7–10 L/min of oxygen via simple face mask (40–60% oxygen). Record the final value after oxygen has been on for at least 25 min and $Psqo_2$ has changed ≤1 mmHg in 5 min (*see* **Note 38**).

11. After the measurements and any interventions are complete, gently remove the probes from the tonometer and replace in their covers.
12. Record the room air Po$_2$ after about 5–10 min, when the value is stable (*see* **Note 39**).
13. Place a 2 × 2 gauze under the catheter hub and tape a 4 × 4 gauze over the catheter hub and the distal tip of the tonometer if reuse is planned.

3.3.4. Removal of Tonometer

1. Remove the Tegaderm.
2. Pull the catheter hub out slightly until you can grasp *both* the catheter hub and the attached silicone tubing. Normally, you will be able to see the silicone at the catheter hub.
3. While holding the silicone as it attaches to the catheter hub, cut the other, free end of the silicone tubing at the exit site, and pull the tonometer out by the hub.
4. If you do not see any silicone on the catheter, grasp the tonometer by both ends and pull; if the tubing and catheter are disconnected, the entire tonometer will come out in two pieces. If this protocol is followed, you will never leave silicone under the skin.
5. If necessary, wash the skin with alcohol before dressing with a fresh Tegaderm.

3.4. Measurement of Transcutaneous Oxygen in Patients with Ulcers of Lower Extremity

Subcutaneous oxygen measurement is accurate and simple, and application of the technique in surgical patients has improved outcomes in acute wounds. Oxygen supply is similarly critical and often impaired in chronic wounds. However, use of an invasive technique is often contraindicated or difficult in patients with chronic wounds. Transcutaneous oximetry is a noninvasive measurement that, although less reliable than sc oximetry, has been used in a parallel fashion in chronic wounds *(21–26)*. Transcutaneous oximeters use a polarographic electrode embedded on a flat sensing surface to measure Po$_2$. Some also contain a carbon dioxide electrode. Normally, diffusion of oxygen through the skin is so slow that noninvasive measurement is impractical. The transcutaneous probe heats the skin (generally a temperature of 42–44°C is selected), which liquefies the stratum corneum and allows increased oxygen diffusion. The probes were originally developed to allow noninvasive measurement of arterial oxygen tension on the trunk. The device is useful in newborns, in whom the skin is quite thin, but not in adults, in whom tissue oxygen consumption becomes a larger factor and variability of skin thickness makes correction impossible. However, it was discovered that in tissue with impaired perfusion (e.g., on the leg of a patient with peripheral vascular disease), transcutaneous oximetry is a fairly good measure of skin/sc/wound oxygen tension.

A number of studies *(21–25)* have demonstrated that healing is impaired at transcutaneous oxygen levels <40 mmHg, and that healing almost certainly will not occur at levels <20 mmHg. A few studies have demonstrated improved healing when tissue oxygen is raised above 20 or 40 mmHg *(26)*, but the research in this area lags behind that in acute wounds. However, it seems clear that the results of large, randomized, controlled trials will be similar to those seen in acute wounds.

1. Have the subject lie supine on a comfortable surface (*see* **Notes 40–42**). Choose six or seven sites: two to three around the ulcer, one on each calf, and one on each foot.
2. Cover the sensors with an electrolyte solution and a gas-permeable membrane. The membrane must be replaced periodically but can otherwise be cleaned with alcohol between uses. The manufacturer provides clear directions for membrane application. Warm the sensors for about 10 min prior to application (*see* **Note 43** and **44**). Calibration of the sensors may be done in room air for some probes, whereas others require placement in a calibration chamber with controlled gas concentrations.
3. Wipe the sites clean with alcohol to improve adherence (*see* **Note 45**).
4. Place the attachment device on the site or on the probe, depending on your preference, and then apply to the site. Place a drop of solution on the sensor (or on the skin) prior to application of the sensor. The sensor cable can be secured with tape (*see* **Note 46**). Cover the leg with a Chux, towel, or single bath blanket to minimize heat loss (*see* **Note 47**).
5. Equilibration requires 10–20 min. Do not record values until changes are <1 mmHg in 5 min. Choosing a standard equilibration time (such as 10 min) instead of waiting for true equilibration will increase inaccuracy.
6. After the baseline is reached, have the subject undergo an oxygen challenge. The concentration used should be standardized within your laboratory, although various concentrations have been used in published studies. One option is to administer 40–60% oxygen using a simple face mask, with oxygen flow set at 7–10 L/min. To achieve a higher FiO_2, a nonrebreather mask with 15 L/min oxygen flow may be used.
7. Make measurements with the subject supine, with legs elevated, and with legs dependent, breathing room air and supplemental oxygen at each position.

3.5. Additional Methods

3.5.1. Microdialysis

Microdialysis is much the same technique as sc oximetry *(27)*. In this case, however, the "tonometer" measures small water-soluble substances as well as gases. It is less convenient, but it has been used extensively in brain research. Strangely, few investigators have recognized its potential for wound research, and although we know of investigators who have used it, we can find no publication detailing its use in wounds. One publication refers to its use for oxygen and lactate measurement in ischemic tissue *(28)*. We mention it here because it should be used more to take advantage of the potential for kinetic, dynamic assays.

The method relies on the principle of fluid and solute exchange across a semipermeable membrane. It is possible to use tubing made of a wide range of molecular weight cutoffs. Dialysis tubes about 0.5 mm in diameter are often used, but for wound healing, size is not critical. Perfusion fluid is pumped slowly though the implanted semipermeable membrane and collected in an impermeable collecting device for assay. Additionally, substances can be added to the *dialysis fluid*, and the metabolic consequences of their presence can be measured in the effluent. For instance, epinephrine in the pumped fluid would be expected to lower the Po_2 in the effluent.

Oximetric devices of various sorts have been attached to these devices. The advantage is that changes in a wide variety of other, related substances such as glucose, lactate, oxidant derivatives, pH, Pco_2, and other low molecular weight substances can be measured and correlated with changes in oxygen tension.

A wide variety of materials have been used. The most pertinent published work in an sc "wound" was done with a 0.5-mm catheter and a 30-mm membrane (CMA 60; CMA, Solna, Sweden). An isotonic perfusion fluid (147 mEq/L Na$^+$, 4 mEq/L K$^+$, 2.3 mEq/L Ca^{2+} 156 mEq/L Cl$^-$; osmolality 290 mosm/kg) was used, and glucose, pyruvate, and lactate were measured by the CMA 600 Microdialysis Analyzer (CMA). However, a variety of microanalytic techniques can be used. A precision, low-volume pump with capacity to pump accurately at rates as low as 0.1 μL/min is necessary. However, one advantage of the technique is its adaptability. Virtually any part of it can be changed. Even the probe itself can be varied, and various modifications can be hand fabricated. The manner of insertion can also be varied. An electronic temperature sensor as well as a surface heater, perhaps an infrared lamp, will be useful for skin and sc tissue work. For oxygen measurements, a transcutaneous sensor may be useful for superficial wounds. The dialysis fluid can be captured in a glass capillary tube and measured in a Radiometer blood gas analyzer that is equipped with a holding device for it. Alternatively, a platinum electrode can be placed in the exit tube under the skin surface with the cathode; an Ag/AgCl electrode can be placed at any convenient point in the fluid stream. Gold and carbon electrodes "painted" on the outside of the catheter have also been constructed, but we are unaware of any such commercially available devices. If oxygen is to be measured in the effluent alone, a relatively large unit and fairly rapid pump rate will be helpful, although oxygen-consuming cells are not expected to enter the device.

The dialysis tube is implanted either at surgery or under local anesthesia. It can be placed inside a steel slit cannula and inserted percutaneously. The steel cannula is then withdrawn. Any number of devices can be implanted. The device mentioned here has an impermeable exit fluid collector. For oxygen, a glass capillary tube is connected to the exit line, and, when full enough, it is transferred to the blood gas analyzer.

Most microdialysis devices have been made for brain measurements. They are designed to minimize tissue injury. However, this is not what is desired in wound work. The easiest method is to use a loop-shaped device or to lay the device in a full-thickness wound that is then closed. For measuring wounds of greater maturity, a Teflon or Silastic "form" can be surgically implanted and later removed and replaced by a dialysis catheter, or the like. One must take care to minimize air or fluid interfaces; air contaminates and slows the assay, and the more fluid, the slower the response time.

Fluid is passed through the dialysis tube at about 0.1–5 µL/min, collected at the exit end, and stored as appropriate for analysis. The time needed to collect samples depends on the rate of perfusion. The device will equilibrate to the tissue values after varying periods of time depending mainly on the perfusion rate. The easiest way to deal with this is to start with very slow perfusion rates and increase slowly. The slowest is closest to the equilibrium value. Correction factors can be calculated so that more rapid perfusion rates can be used, if necessary.

The principle has a wide range of applications. Glucose, lactate, pH, and Po_2 present no problems. Theoretically, fair-sized peptides can be detected immunologically. One of the attractive possibilities is to perfuse with radical acceptors, such as hydroxyl ion and nitric oxide, so that the reduction product is made in the dialysis tube and assayed outside. On the other hand, oxidant production during infusion of diphenyl iodonium in the dialysis tube could estimate the contribution of the NADPH-linked oxidase to total amount of oxygen consumed for oxidant production. To measure long-term trends in wounds, the dialysis tube can be left in place until it no longer perfuses, or it can be inserted into a larger "dead space wound" that has been healing around an inert implant, such as Silastic or Teflon, at appropriate intervals.

3.5.2. Measurement of Oxygen in Cell Culture

Much wound-healing work is done in culture. Since oxygen is so critical to the phenotypes of wound cells, it is mandatory either to control the Po_2 in the cells carefully or, at least, to measure it.

Traditional cell culture on impermeable plastic dishes limits the ability to control and maintain dissolved gases. Indeed, the fact that cell culture systems work at all is dependent on their limited permeability to oxygen and the development of a reduced oxygen concentration at the surface of the monolayer. Animal cells do poorly at oxygen tensions >100 mmHg for any length of time over 24 h or so.

In a standard polystyrene dish or flask, the oxygen concentration in the atmospheric phase of a CO_2 incubator is approx 20%. With a medium depth of 3 mm or greater, a gradient develops wherein the concentration at the cell (i.e., monolayer) level drops to about 5%, or about 35 mmHg. In general, cells grow best in the atmosphere most similar to their natural habitat. Fibroblasts, endothelial cells, keratinocytes, and so on thrive in cell cultures as monolayers on polystyrene substrate held in standard incubators.

Another factor in the dissolving of gases in the medium is agitation. Most incubators experience a mild vibration effect, which can be seen as standing circular waves in culture dishes. This effect helps mobilize dissolved gases, but it can be deleterious to cell cultures because it creates uneven plating on the plastic substrate. This creates areas of confluence surrounded by areas devoid of cells, giving a mixed cellular response to stimuli. Fortunately, most modern incubators do not vibrate sufficiently to create a real problem, but then neither do gases mix adequately in the dishes or flasks.

To increase the oxygen concentration in a standard vessel, the ambient concentration must be raised above that of air. This requires an oxygen source and an incubator capable of maintaining high O_2. By this method, oxygen concentrations at the monolayer level of up to 15% (Po_2 of about 100 mmHg) can be accomplished by raising the atmosphere in the incubator to 80–90% O_2. Likewise, reduced oxygen atmospheres require the replacement of atmospheric O_2 with something inert, such as nitrogen. Since these methods require the oxygen to be dissolved in the medium for its effect, and because most plastic substrates can contain high levels of dissolved oxygen naturally, anoxic conditions are difficult to achieve and maintain.

It is possible to use a plastic tissue culture material with high oxygen permeability. Permanox dishes can be purchased from Nalge Nunc (cat. no. 17888) in a 60-mm dish format. In a standard CO_2 incubator, the oxygen concentration at the monolayer approximates that of the ambient atmosphere in the incubator chamber. Fibroblasts will not thrive in Permanox dishes that are incubated in ambient air, since the oxygen concentration of about 20% is toxic to their metabolism. Conversely, vascular endothelium and monocytes (macrophages) grow well at this concentration, and this phenomenon can be used to differentially culture cells from a mixed population of endothelium and fibroblasts (vascular cells), or monocytes and fibroblasts (bone marrow). At the other end of the spectrum, Permanox plates are necessary to control cultures at low oxygen tensions as well.

In addition to the oxygen-permeable culture dishes, a small chamber capable of maintaining a fixed atmosphere for several days comes in handy in such protocols. Such a chamber is manufactured by Billups Rothenberg and is available from Markson or other distributors. These chambers can be flushed with gas mixtures of any appropriate concentrations, provided that CO_2 is maintained at 5% for media requiring it, and 10% for Dulbecco's modified Eagle's medium. Oxygen concentration is controlled by a flow meter, with nitrogen as the other gas. Using three flow meters leading into a mixing chamber, it is possible to mix O_2, CO_2, and N_2 in any desired combination. Alternatively, equipment that automatically delivers any gas at the desired level is commercially available. Incubators with such equipment built in are also available, even ones with hyperbaric capacity.

Last, but most important, is the verification of the oxygen concentration in the experimental conditions in the laboratory. Various researchers in our laboratory have measured the oxygen at the monolayer level in cell cultures on Permanox dishes using a modified culture chamber. Licox probes (*see* **Subheading 3.3.**) are threaded into the culture and the concentration is monitored constantly while the flushing gas mixture is modified at will. In this way, it has been determined that the monolayer Po_2 closely approximates the atmospheric Po_2 within the chamber utilizing Permanox dishes. Once these measurements have been completed and validated for a particular chamber setup, it becomes possible to measure only the atmospheric Po_2 using a sensor in the outflow, and to extrapolate the culture concentration. Before performing definitive experiments, each laboratory should verify the culture conditions present in its situation. *One cannot rely on assumptions when it comes to oxygen concentrations in cultures.* This principle can be extended further. Oxygen is invisible and odorless, easily penetrates most syringes and many plastics, and leaks in glass vessels are common. Thus, it *must* be measured at every critical step. We often see articles in which air-equilibrated dishes and flasks are termed *normoxic*. Biologically, this usually means *hyperoxic*. Worse, experimentally it means *uncertain*.

4. Notes

1. Wound healing will not progress if a Teflon membrane is used alone.
2. The same technology can be used to measure other substances. To measure lactate, e.g., a larger glass capillary tube is drawn down over a platinum wire and cut so as to leave a small opening at the tip. In this space a small piece of filter paper saturated with a solution of lactate oxidase is placed. The oxidase produces a current proportional to the oxygen derived.
3. Other ion-sensitive electrodes can be made for measurement of glucose, CO_2, and so on. Any microprobe that can sense through or under a Teflon membrane is acceptable. It is also possible to remove the entire membrane and replace it without disturbing the anatomy, if necessary.
4. During studies, the rabbit and its ear should be kept warm. If the animal or the ears become cool, tissue oxygen will rapidly decrease. The effect of temperature is a recurring theme in tissue oxygen measurements.

5. The tiny oxygen probes produce so little current that even a person walking into the room during a measurement may produce an error. A Faraday cage is useful to minimize stray currents.

6. Availability of silicone tubing of the recommended size varies. Inner diameter should be no less than 0.7 mm; outer diameter should be no more than 1.4 mm. Thickness of silicone should be <0.4 mm, or equilibration will be delayed.

7. Any brand of iv catheter is fine. Depending on silicone tubing size, an 18-g catheter may be a better fit. The iv catheter can be cut shorter by up to 1 cm, using a no. 20 scalpel. This may be required to accommodate probe length (*see* **Note 8**).

8. Note that any oxygen electrode system may be substituted for the Licox device, as long as it is stable and fits the tonometer. The manufacturer of the Licox probes, GMS, recently licensed its technology to Integra Neurosciences in the US. We have found the GMS probes to be more reliable and still purchase from Germany. There may be other distributors of GMS probes in the US. Thus, these directions will have to be adapted to the actual probe dimensions.

9. Make sure you purchase a probe system that allows you to calibrate the probes in room air (rather than requiring that you use a factory-determined calibration value). Otherwise, you will not be able to adjust for drift, which may occur with storage of the probes. The probes must be stored in a saline-filled sheath to prolong shelf life. However, they must be calibrated in air (ideally 100% humidity) or they will drift. We shake most of the saline out of the sheath, and then place the oxygen and temperature probes side by side within the sheath, about 2 cm above the saline.

10. The company that custom built the Y connector/iv extension shown in **Fig. 3** (Burron, Bethlehem, PA) is either no longer in business or no longer willing to custom build the connector for us. However, it should be possible to build these connectors from commercially available products. The iv extension tubing for the Y connector should be of appropriate length so that when the probe is placed through the Y connector, tubing, and iv catheter into the silicone tubing, the probe tip is fully within the silicone tubing (not the iv catheter) but <1.5 cm past the tip of the iv catheter (**Fig. 8**).

11. Radiometer and Novametrix both make excellent transcutaneous oximeters (including oxygen probes) specifically intended for evaluation of the adequacy of lower-extremity perfusion and oxygenation.

12. Transcutaneous probes can contain a single oxygen electrode or both oxygen and carbon dioxide electrodes. Most studies have been published using only oxygen values, but carbon dioxide may be worth evaluating.

13. The ear chamber model is remarkably versatile. Gradients across the edges can be demonstrated. The effects of hypovolemia, oxygen breathing, and various drugs or gases can be measured. Bone slices or other materials have been implanted to record the architecture and rate of progress of the invading or surrounding vasculature. Additionally, wounds have been allowed to mature, and the new tissue, at the chamber's largest diameter, has been reincised. By replacing the

cover slip the evolving vasculature can be studied. Perfusion patterns change; initially the flow is parallel to the new wound and then later runs across the site of the new wound as the vessels mature. Blood flow often reverses itself from day to day in the new vessels.

14. These data show the problems inherent in blindly placing electrodes into wound tissue, no matter how well the electrodes are engineered. Histograms are needed to analyze such results, and statistical analysis becomes difficult. One weakness of the method is that it is very difficult to apply conventions to the exact site of measurement.

15. It is important to note that in one respect **Fig. 4** is misleading. There are areas of zero Po_2 to be found on or in healing tissue, but the mean Po_2 in the space is higher. In other models, the Po_2 in the wound space may be quite low. For example, levels are about 5–20 mmHg in wounds with a significant dead space (e.g., the wire mesh cylinder model; *see* **Subheading 3.2.**); however, Po_2 in incised wounds is generally higher than that in the cylinder model.

16. This method is almost an art form. If it is to be undertaken, considerable study and practice are required. Silver and Niinikoski (Turku, Finland) have the greatest experience. The team of Nakata, Takada, Komori, Taguchi, Fujita, and Suzuki of the Department of Anesthesiology, Tokyo Women's Medical College, Japan, are the most recent users of the ear chamber technique although they did not use it for oxygen measurements. Their device is similar but not identical to the Silver device.

17. Fluid displaces the air in the chamber after a few days. About a week later, semicircular areas of angiogenesis will appear in the dorsal window as the healing tissue enters the chamber through the holes between the ear cartilage and the chamber. These will grow inward and coalesce into a ring of new vessels that is analogous to a growth ring, and these eventually will fill the entire chamber. Some vessels will enlarge, and others will drop out until a mature circulation is developed with only a few vessels of about 0.3 mm running across it.

18. Using the electrode on the membrane avoids poisoning the probe with protein. Penetrating it usually means that measurements have to be made quickly and results are likely to be the victim of electrode drift.

19. Instructions are given for preparation of cylinders for use in rats or guinea pigs. Preparation of cylinders for use in rabbits and mice is identical, except for the size of the mesh rectangle and the diameter of the rod. These dimensions are specified in **Subheading 2.2., items 1a** and **1c**.

20. Fluid enters the cylinders slowly, and the skin adheres to them in a few days. In rabbits, adequate fluid for most purposes can be obtained after 3 d. Rats take a little longer. In these respects, guinea pigs are not as good to work with since it may take up to 10 d to fill the chambers. Chambers in guinea pigs are also more often infected.

21. Wound fluids are usually clear tan or brown. Any gross blood or turbidity invalidates most results. In rats and rabbits infections are rare. Guinea pigs are less immune. It takes an injection of almost a million organisms to infect a rabbit

chamber, but almost any bacteria will infect a guinea pig. If the fluid is turbid, it is well to measure the Po_2 in a sample several times over a period of about 10 min. Rapid decline of the Po_2 indicates potential infection. Cells float in the wound-space fluid and use a significant amount of oxygen. Oxygen levels should be measured within a few minutes of fluid withdrawal. If consumption appears to be an issue, one can describe or account for it merely by recording the decay rate of oxygen in the cuvet of the blood gas instrument as opposed to the decay owing to the electrode itself (measured in a sterile aqueous sample). If rapid decay occurs in the saline control sample, bacteria or white cells are caught in the cuvet, and it should be cleaned.

22. The Po_2 within the wound fluid is usually 7–20 mmHg during room air breathing under general anesthesia, lower on the first days of measurement (mean about 10 mmHg) than later (15 to 18 mmHg). The standard deviation is usually about 30% of the mean.

23. For oxygen, it is necessary to use a blood gas syringe that is impermeable to oxygen. Since no hemoglobin, or very little, is present, any contamination with air represents a significant error. For statistical purposes, it is best to sample each chamber only once during the entire experiment since penetration may alter the wound fluid oxygen as well as many other factors, such as vascular endothelial growth factor. For exploratory purposes, this can be overlooked since the drift with serial penetrations is relatively small. If insufficient fluid is present, fluid can be taken from the dependent end of the cylinder using a needle in the other end as a vent for air to replace the fluid.

24. Alternatively, wound fluid samples can be analyzed for blood oxygen, pH, and carbon dioxide. Such studies must be done with care, however, because the introduction of any air bubbles will falsely raise the Po_2 to about 150 mmHg. Moreover, blood gas analysis is inaccurate in the absence of red cells owing to the loss of buffering capacity. Samples must be analyzed immediately and may still yield inaccurate results.

25. The cut edges of the spinal needle must be smooth or they may tear the silicone tubing.

26. Leave the introducer needle partly in the catheter for stiffening. Make sure you do not cut the tubing with the needle, or kink the catheter. A rolling, pulling motion is most successful. The tubing should reach all the way to the catheter hub or it may come off during placement.

27. The silicone tubing should be at least 3 cm onto the spinal needle or it will slide off during placement. Spinal needle size may need to be adjusted, depending on tubing size.

28. If you use the large bore (12–14 g) spinal needle technique, make sure the silicon tubing is sized to fit easily through the needle tip.

29. Barometric pressure is 760 mmHg at sea level and decreases with increasing altitude. Most hospital blood gas laboratories measure barometric pressure daily. Barometric pressure does not vary much, so once average barometric pressure is determined for your site, there is no need to measure it each day.

30. Make sure you warm up the machine with the probe *connected* for at least 15 min before you calibrate. The oxygen and current values should be stable prior to calibration. Make sure you calibrate with the temperature probe and oxygen probe in close proximity. Check that the room air reading you get makes sense. You can calculate the room air oxygen tension for your barometric pressure using the equation (barometric pressure –47)(0.209), in which 47 is water vapor pressure (saturated at 37°C) and 0.209 is the concentration of oxygen in room air. The value should be in the range of 150–160 mmHg. The calculated value is displayed by the monitor during calibration.

31. The IcO_2 (current) value at the time of calibration should be recorded. The IcO_2 display on the monitor should be updated to reflect the true current rather than the factory calibration value. If there is a need to unplug the machine or disconnect the patient, this can then be done with no loss of calibration. The probes should be left in place in the tonometer and disconnected at the hub from the cable.

32. The oxygen probe should never be left in air for more than a brief period or it will dry out and fail.

33. The probe-cable connection is a straight pull style. Twisting or unscrewing will damage the probe.

34. It is generally easiest to dispel all air bubbles from the Y connector and extension tubing with the assembly in a vertical position, and before connecting it to the tonometer. Make sure the arm with the oxygen probe is also filled with saline. This requires loosening the probe–Y connector connection slightly, injecting a small volume from the syringe, and then retightening. After you insert the probe assembly into the tonometer, flush the tonometer at a fairly rapid rate (to dislodge air bubbles), but without excessive force. If you need to refill the saline syringe (sometimes several flushes are required), before you remove the syringe, turn off the stopcock. Fill the hub with saline before reattaching the syringe and opening the stopcock to prevent the introduction of air bubbles. Place gauze over the open end of the tonometer during flushing to keep the patient's arm dry.

35. When you place the temperature probe in the distal end of the tonometer, make sure you watch the wire disappear under the skin. After the probe is inserted, the measured tissue temperature will slowly rise and then stabilize as the room temperature saline warms to body temperature. If the temperature decreases, check to make sure that the temperature probe has not slipped back; try to advance it again and see if the temperature goes up. The temperature will be displayed only about every minute, so you have to watch for it.

36. It is a good idea to record values every 5 min during equilibration to be sure that a stable baseline has actually been reached.

37. $Psqo_2$ should be 50–70 mmHg if the subject is well perfused, lower if not. It should not be much higher unless the subject is on oxygen at baseline. $Psqo_2$ >100 mmHg (subject breathing room air) suggests an air bubble. If this occurs, the tonometer should be flushed with saline. Routine monitoring of arterial oxygen saturation by pulse oximeter is helpful for data interpretation. Subcutaneous

temperature in well-perfused subjects should be >34.5°C. It may be as low as 30°C in poorly perfused subjects.

38. In well-perfused subjects with normal pulmonary function, administration of 50% oxygen should increase $Psqo_2$ to 90–130 mmHg. The increase will be smaller, or absent, when perfusion is impaired.

39. At the end of the measurement, if the probe is >10% off from the original room air Po_2 reading when it is removed from the patient, the measurement should be rejected or repeated.

40. It is best to have the subject void just before the test, because they will not be allowed to get up once you start.

41. In the past, a reference sensor was advocated on the chest wall to account for variability in arterial oxygen, but the introduction of pulse oximetry renders this site unnecessary. It is not feasible to measure multiple sites with only one probe. If only one probe is used, measure the most distal wound edge.

42. The measurement sites should be flat, without obvious vessels or bruising. Thick skin or callus will give falsely low values. The plantar surface of the foot is rarely an acceptable site. The probe should not be over a bony prominence or a site that will be under pressure. The periwound sites should be as close to the open area as possible, but not on macerated or uneven skin. One site should be at the distal edge of the wound, since this is often the lowest value. Sites should be described in detail on the data sheet so that the same sites may be used for follow-up studies. If the wound is hypoxic, the values at the other sites help to identify etiology. To assist in identifying the etiology of wound hypoxia, measurements should be made with the subject supine, with legs elevated and dependent, with breathing room air and supplemental oxygen at each position. However, if venous or arterial insufficiency is already known to be present, or time is a limiting factor, the supine values are most critical.

43. The sensors are generally preset to heat to 44°C. If the patient has arterial disease or particularly sensitive skin, the heat can be decreased to 42°C as a safety precaution to prevent burns, although this is rarely necessary. The sensors can be left in place for up to 3 h. We have never had a burn and routinely use 44°C. When the sensor is removed, the site will be redder than the surrounding skin because of heat-induced vasodilation, but this resolves rapidly.

44. Some monitors allow measurement of the energy required to maintain the sensor surface temperature at 44°C. Although no study has systematically evaluated this, it may be a useful measure of skin blood flow, since more energy will be required to maintain the temperature at higher blood flow.

45. In some cases, the alcohol may not be sufficient to remove products that have been applied to the skin and it will be impossible to affix the sensor securely. If the seal with the skin is not airtight, air will leak in and throw off the values. Isoflurane, a common vapor anesthetic, is an extremely effective solvent, and we use it when alcohol fails. Isoflurane can be obtained from the anesthesia work room in your operating room. It is an extremely potent vapor, so you should use very little and be sure to replace the cap immediately.

46. Tape should not be applied directly over the probe, because pressure can cause inaccuracy.
47. Covering the skin will raise skin surface temperature an average of 2°C, even in patients with arterial insufficiency.

References

1. Knighton, D. R., Silver, I. A., and Hunt, T. K. (1981) Regulation of wound-healing angiogenesis—effect of oxygen gradients and inspired oxygen concentration. *Surgery* **90**, 262–270.
2. Hunt, T. K., Andrews, W. S., Halliday, B., Greenburg, G., Knighton, D., Clark, R. A., and Thakral, K. K. (1981) Coagulation and macrophage stimulation of angiogenesis and wound healing, in *The Surgical Wound* (Dineen, P. and Hildick-Smith, G., eds.), Lea & Febiger, Philadelphia, pp. 1–18.
3. Knighton, D. R., Hunt, T. K., Thakral, K. K., and Goodson, W. H. III (1982) Role of platelets and fibrin in the healing sequence. *Ann. Surg.* **196**, 379–388.
4. Hunt, T. K., Banda, M. J., and Silver, I. A. (1985) Cell interactions in post-traumatic fibrosis, in *Fibrosis*, CIBA Foundation Symposium 114 (Evered, D. and Whelan, J., eds.), Pitman, London, pp. 127–129.
5. Suzuki, Y., Suzuki, K., and Ishikawa, K. (1994) Direct monitoring of the micro-circulation in experimental venous flaps with afferent arteriovenous fistulas. *Br. J. Plast. Surg.* **47**, 554–559.
6. Nakata, T., Takada, K., Komori, M., Taguchi, A., Fujita, M., and Suzuki, H. (1998) Effect of inhalation of nitrous oxide on rabbit ear chamber microvessels. *In Vivo* **11**, 375–378.
7. Hunt, T. K., Twomey, P., Zederfeldt, B. H., and Dunphy, J. E. (1967) Respiratory gas tensions and pH in healing wounds. *Am. J. Surg.* **114**, 302–307.
8. Zederfeldt, B. H. and Hunt, T. K. (1968) Availability of oxygen in tissue remote from major injury. *Bull. Soc. Int. Chir.* **1**, 15–21.
9. Hunt, T. K. and Dunphy, J. E. (1969) Effects of increasing oxygen supply to healing wounds. *Br. J. Surg.* **56**, 705.
10. Niinikoski, J., Heughan, C., and Hunt, T. K. (1971) Oxygen and carbon dioxide tensions in experimental wounds. *Surg. Gynecol. Obstet.* **133**, 1003–1007.
11. Hunt, T. K. and Pai, M. P. (1972) Effect of varying ambient oxygen tensions on wound metabolism and collagen synthesis. *Surg. Gynecol. Obstet.* **135**, 561–567.
12. Ehrlich, H. P., Grislis, G., and Hunt, T. K. (1972) Metabolic and circulatory contributions to oxygen gradients in wounds. *Surgery* **72**, 578–583.
13. Heughan, C., Grislis, G., and Hunt, T. K. (1974) The effect of anemia on wound healing. *Ann. Surg.* **179**, 163–167.
14. Hopf, H. W. and Hunt, T. K. (1992) The Role of Oxygen in Wound Repair and Wound Infection. In: *Musculoskeletal Infection* (Poss, R., ed.) American Academy of Orthopedic Surgeons, Park Ridge, IL, p. 333.
15. Hopf, H. and Hunt, T. K. (1994) Comparison of Clark electrode and optode for measurement of tissue oxygen tension, in *Adv Exp Med Biol: Oxygen Transport to Tissue XV* vol. 345 (Vaupel, P., ed.), Plenum, NY, pp. 841–847.

16. Chang, N., Goodson, W., Gottrup, F., and Hunt, T. K. (1983) Direct measurement of wound and tissue oxygen tension in postoperative patients. *Ann. Surg.* **197,** 470–478.
17. Gottrup, F., Firmin, R., Rabkin, J., Halliday, B. J., and Hunt, T. K. (1987) Directly measured tissue oxygen tension and arterial oxygen tension assess tissue perfusion. *Crit. Care Med.* **15,** 1030–1036.
18. Hopf, H. W., Hunt, T. K., West, J. M., et al. (1997) Wound tissue oxygen tension predicts the risk of wound infection in surgical patients. *Arch. Surg.* **132,** 997–1004; discussion, 1005.
19. Kurz, A., Sessler, D., and Lenhardt, R. (1996) Perioperative normothermia to reduce the incidence of surgical-wound infection and shorten hospitalization. *N. Engl. J. Med.* **334,** 1209–1215.
20. Greif, R., AkÁa, O., Horn, E. P., Kurz, A., and Sessler, D. I. (2000) Supplemental perioperative oxygen to reduce the incidence of surgical-wound infection. Outcomes Research Group [see comments]. *N. Engl. J. Med.* **342,** 161–167.
21. Wütschert, R. and Bounameaux, H. (1997) Determination of amputation level in ischemic limbs: reappraisal of the measurement of TcPo2. *Diabetes Care* **20,** 1315–1318.
22. Burgess, E. M., Matsen, F., Wyss, C. R., and Simmons, C. W. (1982) Segmental transcutaneous measurements of PO2 in patients requiring below-the-knee amputation for peripheral vascular insufficiency. *J. Bone Joint Surg. [Am.]* **64,** 378–382.
23. Butler, C. M., Ham, R. O., Lafferty, K., Cotton, L. T., and Roberts, V. C. (1987) The effect of adjuvant oxygen therapy on transcutaneous pO2 and healing in the below-knee amputee. *Prosthet. Orthot. Int.* **11,** 10–16.
24. Dowd, G. S. (1987) Predicting stump healing following amputation for peripheral vascular disease using the transcutaneous oxygen monitor. *Ann. R. Coll. Surg. Engl.* **69,** 31–35.
25. Ito, K., Ohgi, S., Mori, T., Urbanyi, B., and Schlosser, V. (1984) Determination of amputation level in ischemic legs by means of transcutaneous oxygen pressure measurement. *Int. Surg.* **69,** 59–61.
26. Smith, B., Desvigne, L., Slade, J., Dooley, J., and Warren, D. (1996) Transcutaneous oxygen measurements predict healing of leg wounds with hyperbaric therapy. *Wound Rep. Reg.* **4,** 224–229.
27. Ungerstedt, U. (1991) Microdialysis—principles and applications for studies in animals and man. *J. Int. Med.* **230,** 365–373.
28. Lundberg, G., Walberg, E., Swedenborg, J., Sundberg, C. J., Ungerstedt, U., and Olofsson, P. (2000) Continuous assessment of local metabolism by microdialysis in critical limb ischemia. *Eur. J. Endovasc. Surg.* **19,** 605–613.
29. Silver, I. A. (1980) The physiology of wound healing, in *Wound Healing and Wound Infection* (Hunt, T. K., ed.), Appleton-Century-Crofts, New York, pp. 11–28.

32

Isolation, Culture, and Characterization of Human Intestinal Smooth Muscle Cells

Martin Graham and Amy Willey

1. Introduction

In vitro models utilizing human mesenchymal cells isolated from normal and pathological tissue have proven very useful for studies of wound repair and fibrosis. We have been studying the pathogenesis of intestinal fibrosis and, over the course of 20 yr, have refined techniques for the isolation, culture, and characterization of smooth muscle cells of the human intestinal muscularis propria *(1)*. These methodologies have been adapted for isolation of similar cell types from liver, gallbladder, and blood vessels *(2)*. In this chapter, we describe techniques for the isolation and culture of these cells (procedure A), for the quantitation of procollagen secretion (procedure B), and for the screening of isolates for the expression of smooth muscle–specific cytoskeletal proteins (procedure C).

2. Materials

2.1. Procedure A: Isolation and Culture of Human Intestinal Smooth Muscle Cells

1. Tissue culture plates.
2. Dulbecco's modified Eagle's medium (DMEM).
3. Nystatin solution: 10,000 U/mL of stock.
4. Penicillin/streptomycin solution (Pen/Strep): 10,000 U/mL of stock.
5. Supplemented DMEM-0: Each 50 mL of DMEM contains 2.5 mL Pen/Strep stock and 0.25 mL of Nystatin stock.
6. Sterile scissors and forceps.
7. Sterile filter paper: Whatman #1 cut in a circle to fit on the stage of a tissue slicer.
8. Tissue slicer (cat. no. 6727C10; Thomas Scientific, Swedesborough, NJ).

From: *Methods in Molecular Medicine, vol. 78: Wound Healing: Methods and Protocols*
Edited by: Luisa A. DiPietro and Aime L. Burns © Humana Press Inc., Totowa, NJ

9. Collagenase solution: 0.5 mg/mL culture medium, sterile filtered (*see* **item 10** and **Note 1**) (cat. no. 4197; Worthington, Freehold, NJ).
10. Syringe filter (0.2 µm) (Acrodisc; Fisher, Pittsburgh, PA).
11. Conical tubes (50 mL).
12. Fetal bovine serum (FBS) (*see* **Note 2**).
13. DMEM supplemented with 10% FBS (DMEM-10).

2.2. Procedure B: Analysis of Procollagen Secretion by Slab Gel Electrophoresis of Radiolabeled Proteins in Culture Medium

1. Tissue culture plates.
2. DMEM-0.
3. FBS (*see* **Note 2**).
4. DMEM-10.
5. L-Ascorbate (Sigma, St. Louis, MO): Make fresh in DMEM at 100 µ*M*.
6. [3,4-^{3}H]-Proline (Amersham, Piscataway, NJ).
7. Glacial acetic acid.
8. Isopropanol.
9. 2X Laemmli's buffer *(3)*.
10. Bio-Rad minigel apparatus.
11. Molecular weight marker (cat. no. RPN756; Amersham).
12. 1 *M* Sodium salicylate enhancing solution.
13. X-ray film (Hyperfilm MP, cat. no. RPN1677L; Amersham).

2.3. Procedure C: Screening of Human Intestinal Smooth Muscle Cells for Smooth Muscle–Specific Cytoskeletal Proteins

1. Tissue culture plates.
2. DMEM-0.
3. FBS (*see* **Note 2**).
4. DMEM-10.
5. RIPA buffer: 1X phosphate-buffered saline, 1% Igepal CA-630 (Sigma), 0.5% sodium deoxycholate, and 0.1% sodium dodecyl sulfate.
6. 21-Gauge needle.
7. Antibodies:
   a. α–Smooth muscle isoactin: 42 kDa (Sigma A2547).
   b. h-Caldesmon: 150 kDa (Sigma C4562).
   c. Vinculin/metavinculin: 116 kDa (Sigma V9131).
   d. Tropomyosin: 36–39 kDa (Sigma T2780).

3. Methods

3.1. Procedure A: Isolation and Culture of Human Intestinal Smooth Muscle Cells

Intestinal tissue harvested in the operating room should be kept on ice in a sterile container and processed on the same day.

1. Filet open the specimen and place the tissue, mucosa side up, in a 100-mm tissue culture plate containing 20 mL if supplemented DMEM. If the specimen is contaminated with fecal material, wash three times in this medium solution.
2. Remove the mucosa from the muscularis using sharp, pointed scissors in the cleavage plane of the submucosa.
3. Cut the muscularis into 2×2 cm squares and place, adventitia side down, on wet, sterile filter paper covering the tissue slicer stage.
4. Slice through the specimen with the blade in the plane of the muscularis, moving from submucosa through to serosa.
5. Discard the initial submucosal and last serosal slices.
6. If desired, culture the innermost circular layer separately from the outer longitudinal layer. The two layers can be differentiated by the difference in grain as viewed from above.
7. Place the sliced tissue in 20 mL of collagenase solution in a clean 100-mm tissue culture plate. Mince with sterile scissors and incubate overnight at 37°C in 8% CO_2.
8. Place the contents of the culture dish in a 50-mL conical tube, add an equal volume of DMEM-10, and centrifuge at $100g$ for 3 min.
9. Remove the supernatant, and resuspend the pellet in 15 mL of DMEM-10. Place 5-mL aliquots of the suspension in three to four 100-mm culture plates and incubate at 37°C in 8% CO_2.
10. Allow the cultures to sit for a minimum of 48 h without disturbance.
11. Carefully aspirate the culture medium, allowing the tissue and cells to remain undisturbed in the plate. Add 5 mL of DMEM-10 to the plate. Again, take care not to disturb the tissue and cells. Repeat medium replacement every 3 d. Individual cells that have been released from the tissue will adhere to the plate, begin to spread, and then begin to proliferate. Small pieces of tissue that have adhered to the dish will begin to sprout cells.
12. The culture plate should be confluent with cells after 4 wk of culture. When cells begin to "ridge" on the bottom of the plate, passage and expand the cells (*see* **Note 1**).

3.2. Procedure B: Analysis of Procollagen Secretion by Slab Gel Electrophoresis of Radiolabeled Proteins in Culture Medium

1. Grow cells to confluence in 100-mm culture dishes in culture medium containing 10% FBS (*see* **Notes 3–5**).
2. Rinse plates two times with 5 mL of DMEM-0 and then add 5 mL of DMEM-0 with fresh L-ascorbate. Incubate overnight.
3. Remove the medium and replace with 5 mL of DMEM-0 containing fresh L-ascorbate and 100 μCi of [3,4-^{3}H]-proline. Incubate for 24 h.
4. Transfer the medium to a tube on ice. Rinse the plate with 5 mL of DMEM-0. Add rinse to the tube. Add glacial acetic acid to achieve a concentration of 0.5 N.
5. Scrape the cells off of the plate in 5 mL of 0.5 N acetic acid into a separate tube at 4°C.

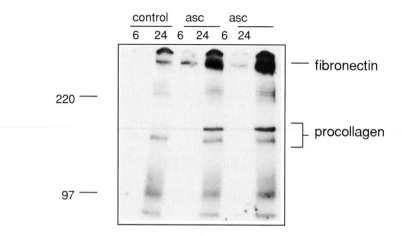

Fig. 1. Example of autoradiogram of procollagen secreted by HISM cells in vitro. HISM cells were incubated with [3,4-³H]-proline for either 6 or 24 h in the absence (control) or presence (asc) of ascorbate. Media were harvested and processed as described in **Subheading 3.2.** The specific upregulation of procollagen secretion induced by ascorbate is seen. Molecular weight markers are shown on the left. (Reprinted with permission from **ref. 7.**)

6. Mix the medium and cell tubes well and incubate at 4°C overnight. Process separately as below in 7–14.
7. Add an equal volume of isopropanol to each tube, vortex, and place at –20°C for 20 min.
8. Centrifuge at 7500g at 4°C for 30 min.
9. Remove the supernatant and dry the pellet in an evaporator or under a stream of nitrogen.
10. Add 100 µL of 2X Laemmli's buffer.
11. Vortex and heat to 100°C for 1 min until the protein is solubilized.
12. Run 20 µL of each sample on 1.5-mm-thick 5% acrylamide gel in the minigel apparatus until the 66 kDa molecular weight marker is at the bottom of the gel. Each well should have approx 20,000 dpm for an adequate signal of procollagen bands. The radioactivity of the samples should be determined prior to running the gel in order to facilitate sample loading.
13. Fix the gel and enhance in sodium salicylate solution.
14. Dry the gel and expose to X-ray film overnight at –80°C. Then quantitate procollagen bands by densitometry (**Fig. 1**) (*4–7*).

3.3. Procedure C: Screening of Human Intestinal Smooth Muscle Cells for Smooth Muscle–Specific Cytoskeletal Proteins

To ensure that the clone of cells isolated from the muscularis is phenotypically "true," it is important that screening for the expression of smooth muscle-specific proteins be performed with each isolate. Using the aforementioned isolation and culture techniques, we find that less than 1 in 20 isolates will not express smooth muscle–specific proteins. Those isolates are then discarded.

The technique involves Western blotting of human intestinal smooth muscle (HISM) cell lysates for α–smooth muscle isoactin, h-caldesmon, metavinculin, and tropomyosin. Since publication of work with α–smooth muscle isoactin *(8)*, we have extended those observations to demonstrate that both h-caldesmon and metavinculin are expressed in vitro by HISM cells. Cells not expressing these proteins are, therefore, considered to have "de-differentiated" in culture.

1. Plate 10^4 HISM cells in a 60-mm culture plate in DMEM-10 (*see* **Note 3**).
2. Allow to grow to confluence. Do not change the medium for 5 d prior to harvest.
3. Rinse the plates two times with 5 mL of DMEM-0. Incubate for 5 h and remove the medium.
4. Scrape the cells into RIPA buffer and force through a 21-gage needle.
5. Quantitate the protein in the lysate.
6. Perform immunoblotting on a Bio-Rad minigel apparatus loading 20 μg of protein/well and utilizing the primary antibodies detailed in **Subheading 2.3., item 7**.

Figure 2 demonstrates a typical screen performed on six lines of HISM cells with a line of human dermal fibroblasts as control. **Figure 2** demonstrates that the fibroblast line does not express any of the markers but does express vinculin. One HISM cell line (lane 4) did not express either metavinculin or h-caldesmon and was considered to have de-differentiated.

4. Notes

1. For the isolation technique, different batches of collagenase should be screened for optimal yield and cell viability. Once a batch is identified as providing a high yield of viable cells, it should be purchased in bulk and stored.
2. For cell culture, different batches of high-quality, low-endotoxin serum should be screened for optimal growth rates. Again, once a batch has been identified as providing good cell growth, it should be purchased in quantity and stored. The importance of high-quality serum cannot be overemphasized.
3. The plating density of cells is critical for efficient growth to confluence; 10–20 $\times 10^3$ cells/cm^2 is usually sufficient. Cells plated at too low a density will not proliferate.
4. HISM cells have the fortuitous property, when confluent, of remaining in robust condition for up to 10 d in culture medium without serum *(9)*. Therefore, for individual experiments of agonist activity, cells should be grown to confluence in medium containing 10% FBS and then placed in serum-free DMEM for 24 h prior to running the experiment. Under these conditions, HISM cells are

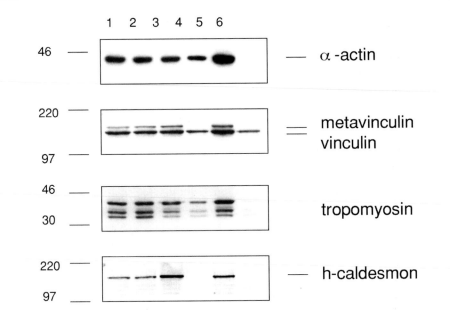

Fig. 2. Screening for expression of smooth muscle–specific cytoskeletal proteins by immunoblotting of cell lysates. Each panel is a separate immunoblot performed with the antibody denoted on the right. Molecular weight markers are shown on the left. Lanes 1–5, five different HISM cell lines; lane 6, control line of human dermal fibroblasts. Note that the fibroblast line does not express any of the markers but does express vinculin. In lane 4 the HISM cell line did not express metavinculin or h-caldesmon and was considered to have de-differentiated.

quiescent, but responsive *(9)*. This technique is important because it allows the investigation of agonists without the contaminating influence of serum, which has relatively high levels of mitogens (platelet-derived growth factor), cytokines (transforming growth factor-β), and other inflammatory mediators.

5. Each isolate should be screened for the expression of smooth muscle cell cytoskeletal markers prior to use (*see* procedure C, **Subheading 3.3.**).

Acknowledgment

This work was supported by National Institutes of Health grant DK34151.

References

1. Graham, M. F., Diegelmann, R. F., Elson, C. O., Bitar, K. N., and Ehrlich, H. P. (1984) Isolation and culture of human intestinal smooth muscle cells. *Proc. Soc. Exp. Biol. Med.* **176,** 503–507.
2. Sanyal, A. J., Contos, M. J., Yager, D., Zhu, Y., Willey, A., and Graham, M. F. (1998) Development of pseudointima and stenosis after transjugular intrahepatic

portosystemic shunts: characterization of cell phenotype and function. *Hepatology* **28,** 22–31.

3. Laemmli, U. K. (1970) Cleavage of structural proteins during the assembly of the head of bacteriophage T4. *Nature* **227,** 680–685.

4. Graham, M. F., Willey, A., Adams, J., Yager, D., and Diegelmann, R. F. (1996) Interleukin 1 beta down-regulates collagen and augments collagenase expression in human intestinal smooth muscle cells. *Gastroenterology* **110,** 344–350.

5. Graham, M. F., Willey, A., Adams, J., and Diegelmann, R. F. (1995) Corticosteroids increase procollagen gene expression, synthesis, and secretion by human intestinal smooth muscle cells. *Gastroenterology* **1091,** 454–461.

6. Graham, M. F., Willey, A., Adams, J., Yager, D., and Diegelmann R. F. (1995) Role of ascorbic acid in procollagen expression and secretion by human intestinal smooth muscle cells. *J. Cell Physiol.* **162,** 225–233.

7. Rosenblat, G., Willey, A., Zhu, Y. N., Jonas, A., Diegelmann, R. F., Neeman, I., and Graham, M. F. (1999) Palmitoyl ascorbate: selective augmentation of procollagen mRNA expression compared with L-ascorbate in human intestinal smooth muscle cells. *J. Cell Biochem.* **73,** 312–320.

8. Graham, M. F., Gluck, U., Shah, M., and Ben-Ze'ev, A. (1994) β-tropomyosin and α-actin are phenotypic markers for human intestinal smooth muscle cells in vitro. *Mol. Cell. Diff.* **2(1),** 45–60.

9. Graham, M. F., Bryson, G. R., and Diegelmann, R. F. (1990) Transforming growth factor-β_1 selectively augments collagen synthesis by human intestinal smooth muscle cells. *Gastroenterology* **99,** 447–453.

33

Use of High-Throughput Microarray Membranes for cDNA Analysis of Cutaneous Wound Repair

Nicole S. Gibran and F. Frank Isik

1. Introduction

   Hypertrophic scar formation represents an abnormal wound-healing response following thermal injuries or partial-thickness wounds. Specific growth factors, cytokines, extracellular matrix molecules, and proteinases that are known to alter cell proliferation and migration have been implicated in the generation of hypertrophic scars. However, the etiology of hypertrophic scarring has not been identified. Given the complex molecular mechanisms of wound repair, differences in expression of isolated functional genes alone may not sufficiently explain clinical variations. Other genes, such as transcriptional regulators, control response to injury and may provide a more comprehensive explanation for the different responses to injury. Gene expression by Northern blot analysis or *in situ* hybridization (ISH) to determine levels of mRNA in tissue samples limits the study of tissues to a single gene and requires a large amount of sample. Reverse transcriptase polymerase chain reaction (PCR) and ribonuclease protection assays allow detection of smaller amounts of mRNA in less tissue but are still restricted by the limited number of genes that can be targeted per assay and by the time involved. With the advent of cDNA microarray technology, a broad-scale evaluation of differential gene expression in hypertrophic scar formation is attainable *(1–5)*. This technology permits simultaneous broad evaluation of previously unsuspected genes such as cell signaling and transcription genes.

   Because of the ability to store large data sets and compare different experiments, it is possible not only to compare hypertropic scar with normal scar or to normal skin, as we have previously reported, but also to compare the data from those arrays to other data sets—such as acute wounds. This allows a

From: *Methods in Molecular Medicine, vol. 78: Wound Healing: Methods and Protocols*
Edited by: Luisa A. DiPietro and Aime L. Burns © Humana Press Inc., Totowa, NJ

broad-scale evaluation of events that may be comparable in an early inflamed wound and a late inflamed hypertrophic scar. This versatility may elicit differences in the early wounds that define later events in wound repair.

High-throughput cDNA microarrays provide expression analysis of thousands of genes simultaneously. Most published microarray studies have focused on isolated cells in culture, rather than on human tissues. Whereas the multiple distinct cell types in skin magnify the complexity of interpreting cDNA microarray data, the most powerful applications of cDNA microarray technology will involve analysis of complex human tissues, such as skin, in normal and disease states *(6)*.

We describe one approach to cDNA microarray analysis using a commercially available microarray system (www.resgen.com/resources/apps/genefilters; Research Genetics, Huntsville, AL) to evaluate differences in expression of 4000 known human genes in hypertrophic scar *(7)*.

2. Materials

2.1. Equipment

1. Dewar flask.
2. Mortar and pestle capable of holding liquid nitrogen (*see* **Notes 1** and **2**).
3. Hybridization oven with roller tubes (Techne, Cambridge, UK).
4. Microcentrifuge tubes.
5. Cryovials.
6. PCR tubes.
7. Phosphor screens (Super resolution; Packard, Meridian, CT).
8. Phosphorimager (Cyclone; Packard).
9. DNA spin column filters (QIAspin; Qiagen, Valencia, CA).
10. Research Genetics microarrays (GF211 Human "Named Genes" GeneFilters). http://www.resgen.com/resources/apps/genefilters
11. Horizontal gel apparatus for RNA evaluation.
12. UV spectrophotometer for determining $A_{260/280}$ ratio of the extracted RNA.
13. Water bath at 37°C, for reverse transcription of RNA to cDNA.
14. Pentium III PC or higher.
15. Pathways® software (http://www.resgen.com/resources/apps/genefilters; Research Genetics).
16. Graphics and spreadsheet software (e.g., Adobe Photoshop® or Microsoft Excel®).
17. Zip drives or recordable CDs for data storage.

2.2. Reagents

1. Liquid nitrogen, to fast freeze the tissue sample and for homogenization.
2. Neutral buffered formalin, to fix a sample of the tissue for later correlation of array results with histology.

3. Tri-Reagent, for RNA extraction (5 cc/g of tissue) (Sigma, St. Louis, MO).
4. Alcohol.
5. Radioactive isotope (for labeling cDNA) [^{33}P]-dCTP (10 mCi/mL, 3000 Ci/mmol) (ICN, Costa Mesa, CA).
6. Oligo dT (1 µg/µL) (Research Genetics).
7. Superscript-II reverse transcriptase (Gibco Life Technologies, Rockville, MD).
8. 5X First-strand buffer (Gibco).
9. 0.1 *M* dithiothreitol (DTT) (Gibco).
10. 20 m*M* dNTP (minus dCTP) (Pharmacia, Arlington Heights, IL).
11. Agarose.
12. Formaldehyde.
13. 10X 3-(*N*-Morpholino)propanesulfonic acid (MOPS)
14. Ethidium bromide solution.
15. Diethylpyrocarbonate (DEPC) treated water.
16. Hybridization solution containing oligo dA (1 µg/µL) (Research Genetics); Cot-1 DNA (1 µg/µL) (Gibco Life Technologies), boiled at 100°C for 3 min prior to adding to buffer; MicroHyb (Research Genetics).

2.3. Buffers

1. Posthybridization wash solution: 2X saline sodium citrate (SSC)/0.1% sodium dodecyl sulfate (SDS).
2. Posthybridization wash solution: 0.5X SSC/0.1% SDS.
3. Boiling stripping solution: 0.5% SDS.
4. MOPS buffer.

3. Methods
3.1. Tissue Selection

Wounds must be carefully chosen as representative samples of tissue of interest by a knowledgeable clinician. This is especially important for hypertrophic scars. For hypertrophic scars, the age of the wound is vital for data interpretation. Just as a 0.5-h wound differs from a 12-h wound, a 5-mo-old hypertrophic scar is likely to have very different gene activity from a 12-mo hypertrophic scar (*see* **Note 1**).

A database must be maintained to track wound age, site and type (etiology), patient age, and race. Ideally, a photograph of the wound should be included in the data collection.

3.2. Sample Collection

It is important to emphasize the necessity of institutional review board approval for collection of any human tissues. Furthermore, collection of study samples must not interfere with clinical pathological evaluation of tissue where neoplasia is suspected. Because of the ethical issues of identifying altered expression of marker genes that are included on the Research Genetics membranes, there should be no patient identifiers. Codes should be assigned to the samples such that the data can be maintained in a separate database from the subject information.

1. Once the surgical site has been identified and prepped and draped for surgery, excise the tissue as expeditiously as possible. Even if a small sample of the scar must be excised separately from the wound site for the purposes of tissue collection, the specimen should not be allowed to stay on the operative field for a prolonged time.
2. When the sample is passed off the operative field, remove a full-thickness piece and place in neutral buffered formalin for eventual histological ISH correlation of array results.
3. Quickly and efficiently complete dissection of the subcutaneous fat. In addition, exclude the edges of the hypertrophic scar and scar tissues from the samples to prevent nonscar contamination.
4. Mince the sample into 0.5×0.5 cm pieces and place in a cryovial in liquid nitrogen as soon as possible after removing the sample from the operative field. The longer the sample is allowed to sit at room temperature, the more likely RNA degradation will occur. The smaller pieces will facilitate RNA extraction (*see* **Notes 4** and **5**).

3.3. RNA Extraction

1. Homogenize frozen skin samples (5–10 g) without further dissection in liquid nitrogen using a mortar and pestle. It is essential to homogenize under liquid nitrogen until the sample resembles talcum powder. Homogenization on the day of tissue collection is ideal (*see* **Notes 1** and **2**).
2. Extract RNA using Tri-Reagent (5 cc/g of tissue) according to the manufacturer's protocol. Repeat the final wash in 70% EtOH twice to ensure that no salt remains in the sample.
3. Precipitate RNA in 75% ethanol and store at $-20°C$ until assayed. Reconstitute the sample in DEPC-treated water.
4. Run an aliquot of each sample on 1% agarose-formaldehyde gels to verify the integrity of the RNA by demonstrating discrete 18S and 28S RNA bands prior to use for the microarray analysis. If the bands are not sharp, the microarray data will not be accurate.
5. Evaluate the samples by spectrophotometry to determine RNA concentration and purity with readings at 260 and 280 nm. Only samples with an $A_{260/280}$ spectrophotometric ratio of ≥ 1.8 should be included. Marginal samples with even minimal degradation evident on gel electrophoresis or $A_{260/280}$ ratios of <1.8 should not be further analyzed (*see* **Note 6**).

3.4. Reverse Transcription of RNA-Probe Generation

1. Reconstitute RNA in DEPC H_2O to a final concentration of 0.2–1.0 µg/µL.
2. Heat a sample comprising of 1 µg of sample RNA (volume depends on concentration of sample), 2 µL of oligo dT, and DEPC H_2O to total 10 µL at 70°C for 10 min.
3. Add to the sample (to total volume of 31.5 µL) 6 µL of 5X first-strand buffer, 1 µL of 0.1 M DTT, 3 µL of dNTP mix (20 mM), 1.5 µL of Superscript-II reverse transcriptase, and 10 µL [^{33}P]-dCTP.
4. Incubate the sample at 37°C for 90 min.
5. Purify with a QIASpin nucleotide removal kit.

3.5. Microarray Methodology

1. Prescan DNA microarray membranes from the same lot (GF211; Research Genetics) to ensure that all cDNA data points are present to exclude false positives and negatives.
2. Boil the membrane in 0.5% SDS in DEPC H_2O with for 5 min.
3. Incubate the membrane for 2 h at 42°C in a hybridization oven in a roller bottle containing 5 mL of microhybridization solution (1 µg/µL), 5 µL of Cot-1 DNA (1 µg/µL), and 5 µL of poly dA.
4. Add the entire purified sample of [^{33}P]-labeled probe to the prehybridization solution in the roller bottle.
5. Incubate the membrane in the hybridization oven at 42°C for 12–18 h.
6. Wash the membrane twice in 2X SSC with 0.1% SDS at 50°C for 20 min each in the roller bottle.
7. Wash the membrane once in 0.5X SSC with 0.1% SDS at room temperature for 15 min in the roller bottle.
8. Wrap the membrane in plastic wrap and seal. Expose to a superresolution phosphor screen.
9. Take multiple exposures until 60–90% of maximal detectable intensity is reached (usually 24–96 h).
10. If desired, RNA samples can be run on different membranes to ensure reproducibility and to verify results.
11. Detect hybridization signals by phosphorimager utilizing the maximum image resolution (600 dpi).

3.6. Image Analysis

Two independent observers should perform the image analysis using the Pathways software. It is imperative to save the native raw files as original data prior to manipulation in image-editing programs such as Adobe Photoshop. The Pathways program generates a quantitative value for the intensity detected at each spot on the membrane representing each gene analyzed. Care must be taken to ensure that the background is low and that screens are not overexposed.

The raw signal intensities for each cDNA spot are normalized against the 400 housekeeping genes spotted on the membrane as internal controls. The normalized signal intensity values of the 4000 known human genes can subsequently be compared among multiple samples. Data are exported into a Microsoft Excel for further analysis.

3.7. Data Analysis (see Note 7)

Mean intensities are calculated for each gene in each group (e.g., hypertrophic scar, scar, and skin). Ratios of the mean intensities of hypertrophic scar to scar, hypertrophic scar to skin, and scar to skin can be generated such that a ratio >1 indicates upregulation and a ratio <1 indicates downregulation of any particular gene, respectively. Since the distribution of ratios is positively skewed, ratios can be log transformed to generate a Gaussian distribution. Determination of differential expression depends on investigator preference for sensitivity. We have considered genes with log ratios >2 SDs from the mean to be differentially expressed in the affected tissue compared with control tissue.

4. Notes

1. The mortar and pestle should be washed with DEPC water and maintained RNase free. They should also be stored at $-70°C$ prior to use to prevent cracking when the liquid nitrogen and tissue are added for homogenization.

2. Comparison of homogenization with mortar and pestle, a motorized homogenizer, and ultrasonic disruption demonstrated that manual homogenization with the mortar and pestle resulted in samples with the highest $A_{260/280}$ ratios and best integrity of the RNA bands using horizontal gel electrophoresis. Each of these pieces of motorized equipment generated too much heat.

3. The results of cDNA analysis of wounds and hypertrophic scars can only be as good as the tissues chosen for analysis. Therefore, it is crucial that the samples accurately represent the process. Unless a temporal course of gene expression in maturing hypertrophic scars is the goal of the study, the samples must be as similar in age as possible. Likewise, body site may be an important factor in hypertrophic scar formation. It is known that certain parts of the body are more likely to develop hypertrophic scar than other sites. Therefore, consistency in body anatomical site is crucial—unless, of course, that is the aim of the study.

4. Based on our previous studies of cDNA array analysis of hypertrophic scars and normal scars, it may be important to perform an epidermal split of the samples prior to freezing. Weight for weight, hypertrophic scar has fewer basal epidermal cells compared to uninjured skin or normal scar. Therefore, equal weights of epidermal RNA extracts should be compared, and equal weights of dermal RNA can be compared separately.

5. Handling of the skin may be the most challenging aspect of these studies. The RNase in the skin very rapidly degrades any RNA in the samples. Tissue must be in liquid nitrogen <60 s after its removal from the subject. Rapid dissection of subcutaneous adipose tissue and transfer into liquid nitrogen is essential for intact RNA.

6. Integrity of the RNA is of the utmost importance for generation of valuable reproducible cDNA microarray data. RNA that is adequate for PCR or Northern blot analysis may not be suitable for microarray analysis. Therefore, using RNase-free methods and double-checking the purity and integrity of the RNA are crucial.

7. Although we have performed much of our initial data interpretation using Microsoft Excel 98 for statistical analysis, it is clearly not robust enough to seriously evaluate gene expression. Bioinformatics, defined as the application of computers, databases, and computational models to the management of biological information, has emerged as a crucial aspect of data management in modern biology *(8–10)*. Microarray techniques generate large volumes of data that require combined bioinformatics approaches and very advanced tools for analysis. In general, these tools use computational methods to group (cluster) the genes that have similar changes in expression levels. The assumption is that by distinguishing genes that behave similarly, it is possible to identify profiles of groups of genes that share regulatory functions or roles. Hierarchical clustering constitutes the most commonly used tool in gene expression analysis. In one such method, all values are paired and for each possible pairwise combination, modified Pearson correlations are calculated and used in distance matrices. Two integrated programs developed by Eisen et al. *(11)* are the most common applications used for the analysis and visualization of the data generated by microarray techniques. Cluster v 2.11 (http://rana.lbl.gov for Windows 95/98/NT only), a hierarchical clustering-based algorithm, performs a variety of types of cluster analysis on large microarray data sets *(11)*. The resulting clusters can be visualized using Treeview v1.50 (http://rana.lbl.gov for Windows 95/98/NT only), a simple visualization software package for displaying phylogenies generated by Cluster *(12)*. This method allows recognition of distinct groups of genes that behave similarly, such as functionally related genes, and identification of unique transcriptional features of a clinical condition (clustering of groups). The newest version of Cluster has several approaches to microarray data set analysis including self-organizing maps (SOMs), which are especially suited for exploratory data analysis *(13)*. They are considered superior to hierarchical clustering when analyzing data that include outliers, irrelevant variables, and nonuniform densities. The basic concept is that you impose a partial organizational structure on the data and then iteratively adjust the structure according to the data. The input data are the raw expression values (not ratios) obtained from the array experiments. The output is a series of SOMs represented

by their similar patterns. GeneCluster http://www-genome.wi.mit.edu/cancer/ software/software.html (for Apple Computer® or Windows PC) developed at the Whitehead Institute also produces and displays SOMs *(14)*.

References

1. Schena, M. (1996) Genome analysis with gene expression microarrays. *Bioessays* **18,** 427–431.
2. Kurian, K. M., Watson, C. J., and Wyllie, A. H. (1999) DNA chip technology [editorial]. *J. Pathol.* **187,** 267–271.
3. Ramsay, G. (1998) DNA chips: state-of-the art. *Nat. Biotechnol.* **16,** 40–44.
4. Schena, M., Heller, R. A., Theriault, T. P., Konrad, K., Lachenmeier, E., and Davis, R. W. (1998) Microarrays: biotechnology's discovery platform for functional genomics [see comments]. *Trends Biotechnol.* **16,** 301–306.
5. Bowtell, D. D. (1999) Options available—from start to finish—for obtaining expression data by microarray [published erratum appears in *Nat. Genet.* 1999 21(2):241]. *Nat. Genet.* **21,** 25–32.
6. Nelson, P. S., Hawkins, V., Schummer, M., Bumgarner, R., Ng, W. L., Ideker, T., Ferguson, C., and Hood, L. (1999) Negative selection: a method for obtaining low-abundance cDNAs using high-density cDNA clone arrays. *Genet. Anal.* **15,** 209–215.
7. Tsou, R., Cole, J. K., Nathens, A. B., Isik, F. F., Heimbach, D. M., Engrav, L. H., and Gibran, N. S. (2000) Analysis of hypertrophic and normal scar gene expression with cDNA microarrays. *J. Burn Care Rehabil.* **21,** 541–550.
8. Claverie, J. M. (1999) Computational methods for the identification of differential and coordinated gene expression [in process citation]. *Hum. Mol. Genet.* **8,** 1821–1832.
9. Zhang, M. Q. (1999) Large-scale gene expression data analysis: a new challenge to computational biologists. *Genome Res.* **9,** 681–688.
10. Ermolaeva, O., Rastogi, M., Pruitt, K. D., Schuler, G. D., Bittner, M. L., Chen, Y., Simon, R., Meltzer, P., Trent, J. M., and Boguski, M. S. (1998) Data management and analysis for gene expression arrays. *Nat. Genet.* **20,** 19–23.
11. Eisen, M. B., Spellman, P. T., Brown, P. O., and Botstein, D. (1998) Cluster analysis and display of genome-wide expression patterns. *Proc. Natl. Acad. Sci. USA* **95,** 14,863–14,868.
12. Page, R. D. (1996) TreeView: an application to display phylogenetic trees on personal computers. *Comput. Appl. Biosci.* **12,** 357–358.
13. Toronen, P., Kolehmainen, M., Wong, G., and Castren, E. (1999) Analysis of gene expression data using self-organizing maps. *FEBS Lett.* **451,** 142–146.
14. Tamayo, P., Slonim, D., Mesirov, J., Zhu, Q., Kitareewan, S., Dmitrovsky, E., Lander, E. S., and Golub, T. R. (1999) Interpreting patterns of gene expression with self-organizing maps: methods and application to hematopoietic differentiation. *Proc. Natl. Acad. Sci. USA* **96,** 2907–2912.

34

Particle-Mediated Gene Therapy of Wounds

Jeffrey M. Davidson, Sabine A. Eming, and Jayasri Dasgupta

1. Introduction

Advances in molecular biology and the understanding of the molecular basis of many diseases have provided tools necessary for a new approach to the treatment of both inherited and acquired diseases. This approach, called gene therapy, was initially focused on the correction of inherited diseases for which no therapeutic approaches were available *(1,2)*. However, it is now clear that the technique of gene therapy can potentially be applied to the local, temporary treatment of acquired diseases, including impaired wound healing and tissue repair *(3)*. Gene therapy is becoming a reality, and it is a particularly attractive approach for wound healing, since the wound site is often exposed, the treatment and condition should be transient, and gene products such as growth factors and cytokines suffer from problems with bioavailability and stability. Such approaches are often innovative and provide solutions to the problems inherent in cell-based drug delivery methods.

Wound healing is an organized response to tissue injury that involves a complex interaction and crosstalk of various cell types, extracellular matrix molecules, soluble mediators, and cytokines *(4–6)*. Knowledge of the signals temporally triggering and controlling wound healing is fundamental to our understanding of skin regeneration. Recently, it has become clear that various systemic (e.g., underlying internal disease, malnutrition, or therapeutic interventions) and local (e.g., bacterial infection, growth factor deficiency, or increased proteolytic activity) *(7)* factors can critically impair the wound-healing process. Therefore, an effective therapeutic regime for chronic wounds comprises both a systemic and a local approach.

From: *Methods in Molecular Medicine, vol. 78: Wound Healing: Methods and Protocols*
Edited by: Luisa A. DiPietro and Aime L. Burns © Humana Press Inc., Totowa, NJ

Many of the therapeutic strategies currently available for the local treatment of chronic wounds are based on the delivery of a drug or protein that promotes healing of the injured tissue. Growth factors have been the most important group of these molecules to be investigated during the last decade *(3,8–10)*. In numerous animal studies and clinical trials, it has been demonstrated that the topical application of cytokines can improve the tissue repair response *(11)*. Cytokines that have been tested include transforming growth factor-β (TGF-β), platelet-derived growth factor (PDGF), epidermal growth factor (EGF), basic fibroblast growth factor (bFGF), and granulocyte macrophage colony-stimulating factor *(6)*. Studies of these cytokines demonstrated that an important aspect of the growth factor wound-healing paradigm is the effective delivery of these polypeptides to the wound site; however, the wound site is a hostile environment. Current drug delivery strategies suffer from the inherent loss of the drug's activity owing to the combined effects of physical inhibition and biological degradation *(12)*. The biological activity of growth factors at the chronic wound site is limited by several circumstances, such as their short half-life, their inactivation by wound proteases, their adherence to extracellular matrix components, their poor bioavailability from the delivery vehicles, and the consequent need for high initial doses and frequent applications. Hence, a critical issue to address is the development of a strategy aimed at optimizing the delivery of growth factors to maximize their therapeutic efficacy. A molecular genetic approach in which genetically modified cells synthesize and deliver the desired growth factor in a time-regulated manner is a powerful means to overcome the limitations associated with the (topical) application of recombinant growth factor proteins.

1.1. Gene Transfer in Tissue Repair

Gene transfer techniques may aid in the sustained expression and release of proteins into surrounding tissues. By inserting a gene into those cells involved in the healing process, it would be possible to engineer the synthesis and delivery of a specific therapeutic protein into the wound site using a permanent or transient gene expression system. This process could enhance the therapeutic benefit of the wound-healing agent and might create an environment that promotes tissue repair, rather than destruction *(3,13)*.

Different delivery technologies for gene transfer applied in tissue repair have been investigated and successfully applied to ex vivo and in vivo gene therapy. The ex vivo approach permits the introduction of genetic material directly into a particular cell type by isolating the involved cells from the patient, genetically manipulating these cells in culture, and then transplanting them back into the donor. Although ex vivo gene therapy is limited to those tissues for which culture conditions and transplantation techniques are well defined, this strategy allows better control over the genetic modification of the target cell, and modified cells can be combined with biomaterials prior to transplantation. In vivo gene therapy obviates the need for proper cell culture and transplantation, since the genes are delivered directly into the target tissue. This method simply requires that the DNA vector harboring the encoding sequence be inserted into host cells in vivo. This straightforward approach, besides being simple, is especially relevant to tissues whose cells are difficult or impossible to culture and/or transplant, such as in the nervous system. Although there are clear advantages to this in vivo approach, it is sometimes difficult to target genes to specific cells of a particular tissue in vivo.

Viruses are natural vehicles for gene delivery and were the first obvious choice *(14)*. Recombinant viruses have had the sequences required for their self-replication removed and replaced with the foreign DNA sequences. The viral proteins necessary for efficient cell entry and gene delivery are supplied by packaging cell lines. Viruses, in general, efficiently transduce cells, and in some cases they permanently integrate the transgene into the host cell's genome. Retroviruses, adenoviruses, and adenoassociated viruses are the most widely tested viral gene delivery systems, and retroviruses and adenoviruses have been used in tissue repair gene therapy *(15–17)*. Distinct advantages and disadvantages govern the applicability of each viral system in gene therapy. These restrictions are based on the size of the insert, the characteristics of the target cells (dividing vs nondividing), the potential for long-term expression, immunogenicity, and the capacity for genomic integration.

Effective nonviral gene transfer systems (**Table 1**) have been developed that deliver genes to target cells without the inherent disadvantages of viral-based systems such as antigenicity, potential for recombination with wild-type viruses, and possible cellular damage owing to persistent or repeated exposure to the viral vectors *(18)*. These synthetic systems are also easier to manufacture on a large scale because they typically use plasmid constructs, which can be grown using existing fermentation technology. In addition, tedious measurements of viral titers and tests for replication-competent virus are avoided. Direct plasmid application, lipofection, and receptor-mediated delivery vectors are the most promising nonviral systems. There are many other nonviral transfection techniques that are too inefficient for clinical use (e.g., coprecipitation of DNA with calcium phosphate *[19]*, DNA complexed with DEAE-dextran *[20]*, electroporation *[21]*, or laborious microinjection of DNA *[22]*). Puncture techniques may also be a practical approach *(23,24)*. Recently, it has been demonstrated that naked DNA can be delivered to the epidermis by a physical means of gene delivery called particle bombardment. The application of this technique in tissue repair is outlined next.

Table 1
Nonviral Methods for Introduction of DNA into Cells and Tissues

Chemical
    Liposomes
    Nanoparticles
    Calcium phosphate precipitation
    DEAE-dextran
    Polybrene/DMSO
Physical
    Irradiation
    Microinjection
    Microseeding
    Muscle injection
    Electroporation
    Biolistics/particle-mediated bombardment

1.2. The Particle-Mediated Gene Transfer Approach

A novel approach for gene transfer is a physical means of gene delivery by the bombardment of cells/tissues with DNA-coated particles or microprojectiles *(25–28)*. Originally, particle-mediated gene transfer was developed by Sanford and colleagues in 1987 to deliver genes to plant cells using gunpowder acceleration *(28)*. Advancing the technique, an electrical discharge and then high-pressure helium replaced gunpowder as the particle propellant for most particle-mediated devices *(27,29)*. Currently, handheld instruments have been developed to utilize the biolistic, particle-mediated delivery system to deliver genes into skin in vivo (**Fig. 1A**).

Microparticles (e.g., gold, tungsten) coated with plasmid DNA are accelerated by a force (e.g., helium pressure) to penetrate the cells and to deliver the DNA (**Fig. 1B**). The gold particles are typically 1–3 μm in diameter, and plasmid DNA is attached to the gold particles by precipitation in the presence of polyvinylpyrrolidone (PVP), the polycation spermidine, and $CaCl_2$ (**Fig. 1C**). We have found that other charged polymers can give better performance. In particular, the Tetronic T704 compound (BASF) and other similar polymers gave severalfold higher transfection efficiency than spermidine formulations *(30)*. Because they are small, the DNA-loaded particles can penetrate through the cell membrane and carry the bound DNA into the cell. At this point the DNA disassociates from the gold particles and can be expressed. The effects of particle-mediated bombardment of skin can be easily visualized when plasmid DNA encoding the firefly luciferase gene is utilized (**Fig. 2**). Gene delivery

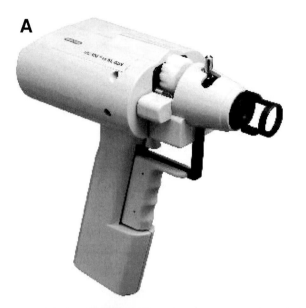

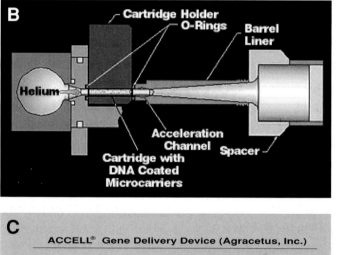

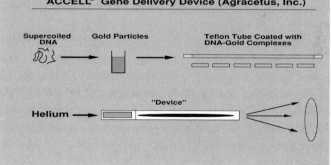

Fig. 1. Particle bombardment instrument for introduction of cDNA into skin. (A) Commercially available Helios gene gun; (B) design features of Helios device; (C) principles of particle-mediated gene transfer.

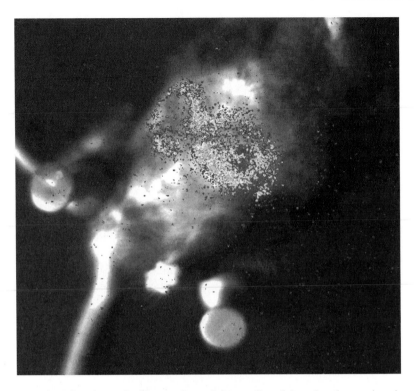

Fig. 2. Visualization of effects of particle-mediated bombardment in vivo. The ventral skin of a mouse was transfected at two adjacent sites by particle bombardment with 0.5 mg of plasmid DNA encoding the firefly luciferase gene under control of the cytomegalovirus promoter (pCMV-luc). Luciferase activity was visualized *in situ* *(51,52)* 1 d later by applying luciferin dissolved in dimethylsufloxide (DMSO) to the target sites of the anesthetized animal and performing a double exposure of the mouse and the photon emission from the hydrolysis of luciferin with an intensified charge-coupled device (CCD) camera. By 5 d after transfection, no further emission could be detected.

can be controlled by the degree of penetration into the tissue, which is directed by the size of the particles and the helium pressure (**Fig. 3**). Previous transfection experiments in different animal models using particle bombardment demonstrated high levels of local transgene expression in the epidermal and dermal compartments of the skin *(31,32)*.

When using different mammalian cell culture lines, 3–15% of bombarded cells in monolayer culture expressed high levels of the transgene. However, similar to the other nonviral transfection methods, the transferred genes are expressed transiently, and stable gene transfer occurred at a frequency of only

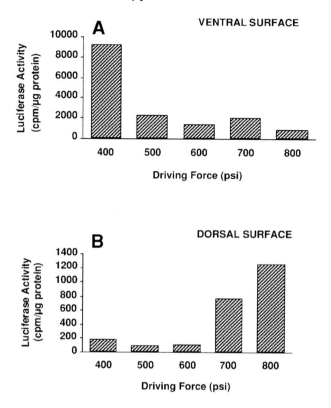

Fig. 3. Efficiency of transgene expression as function of pressure and site. (**A**) The ventral skin of rats was transfected with pCMV-luc at the pressures indicated. The animals were sacrificed at 24 h posttransfection, and luciferase activity was determined in homogenized skin extracts. (**B**) Pressure-dependent response in dorsal skin of rat. Efficiency of transfection is dependent on the thickness of the epidermis, which varies at different body sites. (Reprinted from **ref.** *32* with permission.)

10^{-3}–10^{-4} *(29,31–33)*. In skin, transient gene expression peaked between 1 and 3 d after bombardment and was minimal after 1 wk *(32,33)*.

Advantages of this technology include applicability to different cell types and tissues, the possibility of delivering large DNA molecules, and the ability to deliver multiple genes to the cells owing to the high loading capacity of the microprojectiles. This could facilitate the evaluation of the coordinate expression of multiple genes in a tissue. Another significant advantage is the applicability of this technology to in vivo gene transfer. Bombardment of many tissues including the skin, liver, pancreas, kidney, and muscle resulted in readily detectable transgene activities *(32–38)*. Current limitations of this technique are comparable to those of other nonviral transfection methods in that gene expression is transient, cellular uptake is moderate, and the frequency of stable gene integration is low.

1.3. Applications of Particle Bombardment in Tissue Repair

As a surface tissue, the skin makes an amenable organ for gene therapy and in particular for in vivo transfection by particle bombardment. Recently, particle-mediated DNA vaccination in mice has been successful in the immunization against a series of pathogens *(39–42)*. Additionally, this technique has been applied to the field of immunomodulation. Particle-mediated introduction of interferon-α *(43)*, interleukin-2 (IL-2), or IL-6 cDNA has been shown to produce local antitumor immunity in established tumor models *(44)*. Alternatively, gene gun delivery of IL-12 cDNA in a murine model showed that local expression of this cytokine in epidermal cells adjacent to tumor cells resulted in regression of underlying tumors, inhibition of systemic metastasis, and prolonged survival of test mice *(44–46)*. This study suggests that immune stimulation by particle bombardment can result in local as well as systemic anticancer effects.

A promising application of the gene gun technique relates to its use in tissue repair. We and others have investigated this approach to deliver DNA encoding therapeutically beneficial genes to wounds. Initially, Andree et al. *(36)* demonstrated that the in vivo transfection of porcine partial-thickness wounds with a vector expressing EGF increased the rate of reepithelization and shortened the time of wound closure by 20%. Recently, Nanney et al. *(31)* showed that the beneficial effect of topically applied EGF protein could be significantly increased by overexpression of the EGF–tyrosine kinase receptor. Increased epidermal EGF receptor expression had an integral impact on cell proliferation, rates of resurfacing, and dermal components.

We recently used this technique to evaluate the expression of different PDGF isoforms on wound healing in a rat incisional wound-healing model *(34)*. Using reverse transcriptase polymerase chain reaction analysis, transgene expression was readily detected up to d 3 after transfection, but expression of the transgene fell to detection limits by d 5. To examine the biological effect of transient local PDGF expression, we determined the wound breaking strength 7 and 14 d after a single administration of recombinant DNA to the skin. On average, we obtained a 75–100% increase in mechanical strength of incisions for up to 2 wk after transfection. Although we did not directly measure PDGF protein in this study, previous estimates of luciferase expression in this model showed a steady-state level of about 15 ng of gene product in tissue homogenates *(32)*. Previously, topical application of rPDGF-BB had been shown to enhance wound strength in incisional wounds in a rat model *(47)*.

A single application of 20 µg of rPDGF-BB in a collagen mixture resulted in a 1.3-fold increase in breaking strength at d 7, when compared with control animals. As shown here, in vivo transfection can result in a biological response that appears comparable with that obtained with the applications of the corresponding recombinant growth factor. These findings are supported by other studies using this technique. Benn et al. *(32)* demonstrated that overexpression of TGF-β also resulted in the significant increase in tensile strength of healing rat tissue. A single application of 2 µg of rTGF-β1 resulted in a 1.4-fold increase in breaking strength, whereas transfection with the TGF-β1 plasmid resulted in a 1.8-fold increase in breaking strength when compared with controls *(32)*. Overall, these studies demonstrate that particle-mediated transfection using appropriate expression vectors can be a simple and effective means of enhancing the rate of wound repair in an animal model.

Since the efficiency of cellular targeting with gene gun technology is about 10%, and the primary target is the basal cells of the epidermis, the principal application of gene gun therapy in the wound-healing arena has been to utilize targeted cells for production of secreted factors that can act in *trans*. Recently, one group has shown that transfection with the transcription factor Egr-1 also has a positive effect on wound repair *(48)*. This appears to be owing to the ability of this intracellular protein to stimulate the expression of several growth factors. Similarly, we have observed significant effects in two wound-healing models with a gene product involved in growth factor signal transduction (unpublished observations).

Because of the ease of generating the DNA/gold particles, the gene gun is an excellent experimental tool for developing DNA-based therapeutics and gene discovery. In recent studies, particle-mediated bombardment has been successfully used to show wound-healing effects with connective-tissue growth factor, activin βA, vascular endothelial growth factor, and a number of other novel cDNAs. The technology has been productively coupled with a gene discovery strategy that identifies novel genes involved in wound repair. New genes can be rapidly engineered into expression vectors and introduced into standardized wound-healing models such as incisional and excisional wounds in a variety of species. To date, collaborative efforts have validated at least four different genes with this method *(49)*.

Some growth factors have not exhibited biological activity when expressed by the epidermis. In particular, the heparin-binding growth factor FGF-2 has shown little activity by direct skin application of gold particles. Even when the coding sequence was fused with a secretory signal peptide *(50)*, no wound-healing or angiogenic activity was observed. We hypothesize that this may be owing to sequestration of secreted FGF at the epithelial surface or basal lamina, which is enriched in heparan sulfate proteoglycan. Indeed, when the gene gun is used to transfect soft connective tissue directly, one can obtain a spectacular, transient, angiogenic response (**Fig. 4**).

1.4. Future Developments

Molecular medicine holds considerable therapeutic promise and the potential range and versatility of gene therapy in tissue repair, particularly the use of particle bombardment outlined herein. The particle-mediated acceleration strategy in tissue repair offers several advantages over other in vivo transfection methods including adenoviral vectors or liposomal delivery. First, the transfection system is a simple, standardized, and reproducible technology for cutaneous applications. Second, the DNA/gold preparation is extremely stable, with a shelf life of at least 6 mo. Third, the preparation of the delivery system (once the expression vector has been designed, cloned, and purified) requires only a few hours. Fourth, no foreign protein is involved. The technique offers the possibility of beginning to build growth factor combinations; of incorporating into one chimeric molecule more than one growth factor activity; of facilitating diffusion of the molecules to their target sites; or protecting them from degradation by proteinases present in the wound environment. Another distinct advantage of the particle-mediated bombardment technology is the ability to coformulate several growth factor cDNAs into the same particle or to mix different populations of particles before loading them into the cartridge system. This enormous flexibility will allow researchers to explore much more rapidly the range and potential of applications of this novel DNA-mediated wound therapy.

Although the particle bombardment technique has proven to be useful in several experimental conditions of cutaneous gene transfer, the technique in its actual form is not suitable for clinical use yet. Current, practical limitations include the high helium pressure, which is needed to accelerate microparticles into the tissue. A helium pressure of 400–700 psi, which is needed to drive the particles into the epidermis, might damage underlying granulation tissue. Another issue to be addressed when applying this technology is that the currently available handheld device transfects approx 1 cm^2 per application, so that, depending on the wound size, multiple transfections are required. The transfection efficiency is on a par with other physical delivery systems, but an order of magnitude lower than viral transfection.

Overall, from an experimentalist's point of view, this system has remarkable advantages to screen for the effectiveness of DNA encoding therapeutically beneficial genes to the wound (**Fig. 5**). However, it appears that the current

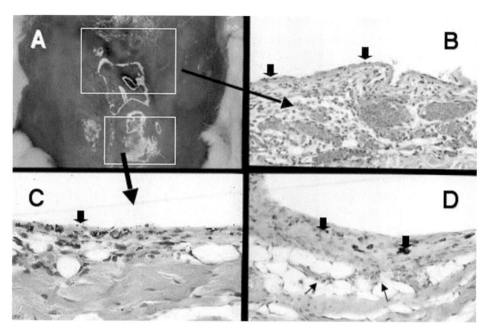

Fig. 4. Particle-mediated transfection of an angiogenic factor, FGF-2, produces transient neovascularization. Gold particles loaded with an expression vector that is a fusion between the signal peptide sequence of bovine IgG and human FGF-2 cDNA (IgbFGF) were targeted to the exposed abdominal fascia of adult Sprague-Dawley rats. In addition, a comparable site was targeted with particles containing a control plasmid expressing β-galactosidase. After particle bombardment at these two sites, the surgical wound was closed. Three days later, the targeted regions were exposed to observe the effect of transfection. (**A**) The upper outlined area indicates the site of IgbFGF transfection, which demonstrated an intense angiogenic response with a dense capillary plexus. (**B**) A histological cross section of this region after staining with hematoxylin and eosin is shown. A large number of dilated capillaries is seen immediately below the fascial surface. Thick arrows indicate sites on the surface that show embedded gold particles. (**C**) The histological response of adjacent fascial tissue targeted with gold containing the control vector is shown. Although many gold particles are plainly visible (thick arrow), the histological organization is identical to untreated regions. (**D**) The appearance of an IgbFGF-targeted area in another rat 3 d later, 6 d after transfection is shown. Most of the gold particles have been swept up by tissue phagocytes (thick arrows), and the capillary structures have collapsed and/or undergone marked regression (thin arrows).

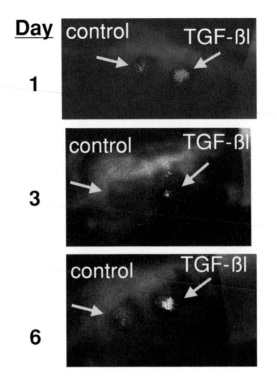

Fig. 5. Use of gene gun to validate growth factor action. The gene gun was used to propel 0.5 mg of plasmid DNA from an expression vector for β-galactosidase (control) or a constitutively active form of TGF-β1 *(32)* into separate sites on the ventral surface of a transgenic mouse bearing the firefly luciferase gene under control of the COL1A2 enhancer/promoter *(53,54)*. At the indicated time points, transgene activity was visualized as described in the legend to **Fig. 2**. The images confirm that local transfection of the fibrogenic cytokine TGF-β1 induces collagen expression. Similar strategies can be used to screen for many biological properties of genes thought to participate in wound repair.

technique does not yet provide the therapeutic solution for the gene transfer system in the clinical setting.

2. Materials

2.1. Sample Preparation

1. Supercoiled plasmid DNA.
2. 0.1 *M* Spermidine.
3. 2.5 *M* CaCl$_2$.
4. Absolute ethanol, dehydrated.
5. Gold particles, 1.6 µm diameter (Bio-Rad, Richmond, CA; www.biorad.com).

6. Ultrasonic water bath.
7. PVP/ethanol stock (20 mg/mL).

2.2. Cartridge Preparation

1. Helios Tubing Prep Station and Tubing Cutter (Bio-Rad).
2. Tefzel™ tubing, 1/8 in. od (McMaster-Carr, Atlanta, GA; www.mcmaster.com).
3. Nitrogen, extra dry, and regulator.
4. Syringe (5 mL).

2.3. Target Preparation

1. Hair clippers.
2. Commercial depilatory cream.
3. Gauze pads.
4. Isopropanol.
5. Stamp pad.
6. Biopsy punch (4 mm).
7. Lidocaine.
8. Semiocclusive dressing.

2.4. Loading Gene Gun

1. Cartridge holder.

2.5. Firing Gene Gun

1. Helios gene gun and helium regulator.
2. Helium, extra dry, 3000 psi.

3. Methods

The manufacturer provides a detailed user's guide with animation at its Web site (www.bio-rad.com/GeneTransfer/genegun/ggnsfrmst.htm).

3.1. Sample Preparation

1. Weigh ~50 mg of gold microcarriers into a 1.5-mL microcentrifuge tube.
2. Add 100–200 µL of 0.1 M spermidine to suspend the particles.
3. Briefly vortex and sonicate the mixture at room temperature to break up any gold clumps.
4. Add the required volume of plasmid DNA to produce a loading ratio of 2:1 (e.g., 100 mg DNA/50 mg of gold).
5. Mix the DNA (2 µg/mg of gold), spermidine, and gold by vortexing for 5 s.
6. While vortexing, add 2.5 M $CaCl_2$ dropwise to the mixture to equal two times the volume of the spermidine solution; continue vortexing for 5–10 s.
7. Allow the mixture to settle at room temperature for 5 min.
8. Microfuge for 30 s at low speed to pellet the gold.
9. Remove and discard the supernatant.

10. Resuspend and wash the pellet three times with fresh 100% ethanol. Spin briefly and discard the supernatant between each wash (*see* **Note 1**).
11. After the final ethanol wash, resuspend the pellet in 200 mL of ethanol solution containing 0.1 mg/mL of PVP from the stock solution.
12. Transfer the gold-ethanol slurry into a 15-mL tube with a screw cap.
13. Rinse the microfuge tube once with the same ethanol/PVP solution to collect any remaining sample.
14. Add the required volume of ethanol/PVP solution to the centrifuge tube to bring the DNA/microcarrier solution to the desired microcarrier loading ratio. The suspension is now ready for tube preparation.

3.2. Cartridge Preparation

1. Flush the tubing with absolute EtOH.
2. Load the appropriate length of Tefzel tubing into the Tubing Prep Station and flush with N_2 for 3 min to dry the tubing thoroughly.
3. Using a 5-mL syringe, draw the gold suspension into the tubing.
4. Leave the apparatus undisturbed for 3 min to allow the gold particles to settle.
5. Remove the excess ethanol.
6. Turn on the rotator for 20 s to distribute the slurry on the walls of the tube.
7. Flush the tubing for 5 min to dry the tubing thoroughly.
8. Cut the tubing into correct lengths with the tubing cutter. Store the cut lengths in a capped vial with a dessicant at –20°C.

3.3. Target Preparation

3.3.1. Rat Incision

1. Anesthetize the rats.
2. Shave the incisional site(s), and treat with a depilatory cream.
3. Wait 7 min and remove residual hair and dead skin with a gauze pad.
4. Clean and prep the site(s) with isopropanol and sterile gauze.
5. Use stamp pad ink to mark the targeting sites.
6. An adult rat is conveniently targeted at two sites on either side of the dorsal midline (*see* **Note 2**). Evaluate the response of the anterior and posterior sites independently, since the thickness of the skin varies considerably along the longitudinal axis. For each pair of treatment sites, include a microcarrier control loaded with an inert/reporter plasmid to correct for nonspecific responses to transfection of foreign DNA.
7. Maintain anesthesia until the firing step is complete.

3.3.2. Mouse Excision

1. Anesthetize the mouse.
2. Carefully shave the incisional site(s), and treat with a depilatory cream.
3. Wait 2 min and remove residual hair and dead skin with a gauze pad.
4. Clean and prep the site(s) with isopropanol and sterile gauze.

5. Use stamp pad ink to mark the targeting sites.
6. A mouse can be targeted at two sites on either side of the dorsal midline. Although in mice the thickness of the skin varies less along the longitudinal axis, for each pair of treatment sites include a microcarrier control loaded with an inert/reporter plasmid to correct for nonspecific responses to transfection of foreign DNA.
7. Carry out excisional surgery with a sterile biopsy punch (4 mm).

3.3.3. Rabbit Excision

1. Anesthetize the rabbits.
2. Depilate the inner aspect of each ear.
3. After 5 min clean the surface with isopropanol and gauze.
4. Carry out excisional surgery after lidocaine infusion with a sterile biopsy punch, taking great care not to let the blade penetrate or damage the auricular cartilage.
5. Remove the skin and scrape off the perichondrium to leave an avascular wound base of naked cartilage.
6. Center the gene gun on the target site. Multiple firings may be used to obtain greater coverage.
7. Cover each wound with an adherent semiocclusive dressing.

3.4. Loading Gene Gun

1. Arrange the cartridges in the cylinder.
2. Place the cylinder in the Helios gene gun.

3.5. Firing Gene Gun

1. Set the regulator to 400 psi.
2. If control and experimental particles are being fired in the same series, shoot the control cartridges first (*see* **Note 3**).
3. Place the gene gun against the skin, centered over the target area, and fire.

4. Notes

1. This step is critical in the procedure—it is important that the ethanol does not absorb any water. The bottle should be kept closed between uses, or use a fresh bottle each time.
2. Our experimentation with the gene gun has used a wound design that accommodates the skin field that is targeted for transfection. This occupies a circular area (if the gun is perpendicular to the target) of about 2 cm in diameter. There is a reasonably uniform distribution of particles within this field, with some diminution at the target margins. Experimental wounds are designed to fit within the target area (i.e., <1 cm in greatest dimension), whether they are incisions or excisions. On the other hand, it is certainly possible to apply multiple doses to cover a larger area. This can be accomplished by a series of overlapping shots or by using a moveable mask that divides the target area into contiguous,

nonoverlapping sectors. Some investigators may wish to exclude certain regions of the wound from biolistic targeting. For example, the central region of an immature excisional wound contains largely granulation tissue, which may not be an efficient target for biolistic therapy. The epithelialized wound margins can be selectively targeted by overlaying the exposed granulation tissue with a mask consisting of plastic or metal foil sheeting.

3. The gene gun is a gun. As with any mechanical means of introducing material into tissue, the gene gun produces a certain amount of tissue damage on discharge. There are two separate effects to consider: the impact of the gold projectiles on living cells and the influence of the pressure wave. The projectile impact can produce a mild inflammatory response, consistent with that elicited by abrasion of the epidermis. Since the keratinocyte is replete with inflammatory cytokines, only slight physical disturbance is needed to cause the release of paracrine signals. A slight, transient edema can ensue, with accompanying infiltration of leukocytes. In our experience, this reaction subsides within a few hours to days. There is no question that each treatment site needs to have its response normalized to a comparable site treated with either uncoated gold particles or those coated with a control plasmid at the same loading. The second potential artifact is the ability of the helium pulse to cause dehiscence of fresh wounds. If the user is contemplating multiple, postsurgical applications of a test gene by the biolistic method to an incision, the integrity needs to be secured by sufficient sutures or wound clips. The helium pulse is not strong enough to displace material from open, excisional wounds.

Acknowledgments

This work was supported by National Institute of Health grant AG06528; the Department of Veterans Affairs; the German Research Society; and, in part, the Research Program Köln Fortune and the Nolting Foundation.

References

1. Anderson, W. F. (1984) Prospects for human gene therapy. *Science* **226,** 401–409.
2. Anderson, W. F. (1992) Human gene therapy. *Science* **256,** 808–813.
3. Davidson, J. M., Whitsitt, J. S., Pennington, B., Ballas, C. B., Eming, S. and Benn, S. I. (1999) Gene therapy of wounds with growth factors. *Curr. Top. Pathol.* **93,** 111–121.
4. Martin, P. (1997) Wound healing—aiming for perfect skin regeneration. *Science* **276,** 75–81.
5. Hoff, C. R. and Davidson, J. M. (1996) Cellular and biochemical mechanisms of wound repair, in *Cellular and Biochemical Mechanisms of Wound Repair* (Lonai, P., ed.), Harwood, London, pp. 293–320.
6. Singer, A. J. and Clark, R. A. (1999) Cutaneous wound healing. *N. Engl. J. Med.* **341,** 738–746.

7. Falanga, V. (1993) Chronic wounds: pathophysiologic and experimental considerations. *J. Invest. Dermatol.* **100,** 721–725.
8. Falanga, V. (1992) Growth factors and chronic wounds: the need to understand the microenvironment. *J. Dermatol.* **19,** 667–672.
9. Bennett, N. T. and Schultz, G. S. (1993) Growth factors and wound healing: biochemical properties of growth factors and their receptors. *Am. J. Surg.* **165,** 728–737.
10. Bennett, N. T. and Schultz, G. S. (1993) Growth factors and wound healing: part II. Role in normal and chronic wound healing. *Am. J. Surg.* **166,** 74–81.
11. Pierce, G. F. and Mustoe, T. A. (1995) Pharmacologic enhancement of wound healing. *Annu. Rev. Med.* **46,** 467–481.
12. Lauer, G., Sollberg, S., Cole, M., Flamme, I., Sturzebecher, J., Mann, K., Krieg, T., and Eming, S. A. (2000) Expression and proteolysis of vascular endothelial growth factor is increased in chronic wounds. *J. Invest. Dermatol.* **115,** 12–18.
13. Eming, S. A., Morgan, J. R., and Berger, A. (1997) Gene therapy for tissue repair: approaches and prospects. *Br. J. Plast. Surg.* **50,** 491–500.
14. Friedmann, T. (1992) A brief history of gene therapy. *Nat. Genet.* **2,** 93–98.
15. Chandler, L. A., Doukas, J., Gonzalez, A. M., et al. (2000) FGF2-Targeted adenovirus encoding platelet-derived growth factor-B enhances de novo tissue formation. *Mol. Ther.* **2,** 153–160.
16. Spector, J. A., Mehrara, B. J., Luchs, J. S., Greenwald, J. A., Fagenholz, P. J., Saadeh, P. B., Steinbrech, D. S., and Longaker, M. T. (2000) Expression of adenovirally delivered gene products in healing osseous tissues. *Ann. Plast. Surg.* **44,** 522–528.
17. Liechty, K. W., Nesbit, M., Herlyn, M., Radu, A., Adzick, N. S., and Crombleholme, T. M. (1999) Adenoviral-mediated overexpression of platelet-derived growth factor-B corrects ischemic impaired wound healing. *J. Invest. Dermatol.* **113,** 375–383.
18. Felgner, P. L. and Rhodes, G. (1991) Gene therapeutics. *Nature* **349,** 351,352.
19. Chen, C. and Okayama, H. (1987) High-efficiency transformation of mammalian cells by plasmid DNA. *Mol. Cell. Biol.* **7,** 2745–2752.
20. Pagano, J. S., McCutchan, J. H., and Vaheri, A. (1967) Factors influencing the enhancement of the infectivity of poliovirus ribonucleic acid by diethylaminoethyl-dextran. *J. Virol.* **1,** 891–897.
21. Neumann, E., Schaefer-Ridder, M., Wang, Y., and Hofschneider, P. H. (1982) Gene transfer into mouse lyoma cells by electroporation in high electric fields. *EMBO J.* **1,** 841–845.
22. Capecchi, M. R. (1980) High efficiency transformation by direct microinjection of DNA into cultured mammalian cells. *Cell* **22,** 479–488.
23. Eriksson, E., Yao, F., Svensjo, T., Winkler, T., Slama, J., Macklin, M. D., Andree, C., McGregor, M., Hinshaw, V., and Swain, W. F. (1998) In vivo gene transfer to skin and wound by microseeding. *J. Surg. Res.* **78,** 85–91.
24. Ciernik, I. F., Krayenbuhl, B. H., and Carbone, D. P. (1996). Puncture-mediated gene transfer to the skin. *Hum. Gene Ther.* **7,** 893–899.

25. Yang, N. S. (1992) Gene transfer into mammalian somatic cells in vivo. *Crit. Rev. Biotechnol.* **12,** 335–356.

26. Yang, N. S. and Sun, W. H. (1995) Gene gun and other non-viral approaches for cancer gene therapy. *Nat. Med.* **1,** 481–483.

27. Yang, N. S., McCabe, D. E., and Swain, W. F. (1997) Methods for particle-mediated gene transfer into skin, in *Gene Therapy Protocols* (Robinson, P. D., ed.), Humana, Totowa, NJ, pp. 281–296.

28. Klein, R. M., Wolf, E. D., Wu, R., and Sanford, J. C. (1992) High-velocity microprojectiles for delivering nucleic acids into living cells. 1987. *Biotechnology* **24,** 384–386.

29. Yang, N.-S., Burkholder, J., Roberts, B., Martinelli, B., and McCabe, D. (1990) In vivo and in vitro gene transfer to mammalian somatic cells by particle bombardment. *Proc. Natl. Acad. Sci. USA* **87,** 9568–9572.

30. Prokop, A., Kozlov, E., Carlesso, G., and Davidson, J. M. (2001) Hydrogel-based colloidal polymeric systems for protein and drug delivery: physical and chemical characterization, permeability control and applications. *Adv. Polymer Sci.* **160,** 119–173.

31. Nanney, L. B., Paulsen, S., Davidson, M. K., Cardwell, N. L., Whitsitt, J. S., and Davidson, J. M. (2000) Boosting epidermal growth factor receptor expression by gene gun transfection stimulates epidermal growth in vivo. *Wound Rep. Reg.* **8,** 117–127.

32. Benn, S. I., Whitsitt, J. S., Broadley, K. N., Nanney, L. B., Perkins, D., He, L., Patel, M., Morgan, J. R., Swain, W. F., and Davidson, J. M. (1996) Particle-mediated gene transfer with transforming growth factor-beta1 cDNAs enhances wound repair in rat skin. *J. Clin. Invest.* **98,** 2894–2902.

33. Cheng, L., Ziegelhoffer, P. R., and Yang, N.-S. (1993) In vivo promoter activity and transgene expression in mammalian somatic tissues evaluated by using particle bombardment. *Proc. Natl. Acad. Sci. USA* **90,** 4455–4459.

34. Eming, S. A., Whitsitt, J. S., He, L., Krieg, T., Morgan, J. R., and Davidson, J. M. (1999) Particle-mediated gene transfer of PDGF isoforms promotes wound repair. *J. Invest. Dermatol.* **112,** 297–302.

35. Lu, B., Scott, G., and Goldsmith, L. A. (1996) A model for keratinocyte gene therapy: preclinical and therapeutic considerations. *Proc. Assoc. Am. Physician* **108,** 165–172.

36. Andree, C., Swain, W. F., Page, C. P., Macklin, M. D., Slama, J., Hatzis, D., and Eriksson, E. (1994) In vivo transfer and expression of a human epidermal growth factor gene accelerates wound repair. *Proc. Natl. Acad. Sci. USA* **91,** 12,188–12,192.

37. Sun, L., Xu, L., Chang, H., Henry, F. A., Miller, R. M., Harmon, J. M., and Nielsen, T. B. (1997) Transfection with aFGF cDNA improves wound healing. *J. Invest. Dermatol.* **108,** 313–318.

38. Mahvi, D. M., Burkholder, J. K., Turner, J., Culp, J., Malter, J. S., Sondel, P. M., and Yang, N. S. (1996) Particle-mediated gene transfer of granulocyte-macrophage

colony-stimulating factor cDNA to tumor cells: implications for a clinically relevant tumor vaccine. *Hum. Gene Ther.* **7,** 1535–1543.

39. Haynes, J. R. (1999) Genetic vaccines. *Infect. Dis. Clin. North Am.* **13,** 11–26.
40. Olsen, C. W. (2000) DNA vaccination against influenza viruses: a review with emphasis on equine and swine influenza. *Vet. Microbiol.* **74,** 149–164.
41. Johnston, S. A. and Tang, D. C. (1993) The use of microparticle injection to introduce genes into animal cells in vitro and in vivo. *Genet. Eng.* **15,** 225–236.
42. Fynan, E. F., Webster, R. G., Fuller, D. H., Haynes, J. R., Santoro, J. C., and Robinson, H. L. (1995) DNA vaccines: a novel approach to immunization. *Int. J. Immunopharmacol.* **17,** 79–83.
43. Tuting, T., Gambotto, A., Baar, J., Davis, I. D., Storkus, W. J., Zavodny, P. J., Narula, S., Tahara, H., Robbins, P. D., and Lotze, M. T. (1997) Interferon-alpha gene therapy for cancer: retroviral transduction of fibroblasts and particle-mediated transfection of tumor cells are both effective strategies for gene delivery in murine tumor models. *Gene Ther.* **4,** 1053–1060.
44. Tuting, T., Storkus, W. J., and Falo, L. D. Jr. (1998) DNA immunization targeting the skin: molecular control of adaptive immunity. *J. Invest. Dermatol.* **111,** 183–188.
45. Elder, E. M., Lotze, M. T., and Whiteside, T. L. (1996) Successful culture and selection of cytokine gene-modified human dermal fibroblasts for the biologic therapy of patients with cancer. *Hum. Gene Ther.* **7,** 479–487.
46. Rakhmilevich, A. L., Turner, J., Ford, M. J., McCabe, D., Sun, W. H., Sondel, P. M., Grota, K., and Yang, N. S. (1996) Gene gun-mediated skin transfection with interleukin 12 gene results in regression of established primary and metastatic murine tumors. *Proc. Natl. Acad. Sci. USA* **93,** 6291–6296.
47. Pierce, G. F., Mustoe, T. A., Senior, R. M., Reed, J., Griffin, G. C., Thomason, A., and Deuel, T. F. (1988) In vivo incisional wound healing augmented by platelet-derived growth factor and recombinant c-sis gene homodimeric proteins. *J. Exp. Med.* **167,** 974–987.
48. Bryant, M., Drew, G. M., Houston, P., Hissey, P., Campbell, C. J., and Braddock, M. (2000) Tissue repair with a therapeutic transcription factor. *Hum. Gene Ther.* **11,** 2143–2158.
49. Bittner, M., Halle, J.-P., Regenbogen, J., Hof, P., Dopazo, A., Reitmaier, B., Werner, S., DasGupta, J., Davidson, J., and Goppelt, A. (2001) Identification of target genes for the development of innovative drugs to heal chronic wounds. *Wound Rep. Reg.* **9,** 146.
50. Yayon, A. and Klagsbrun, M. (1990) Autocrine transformation by chimeric signal peptide-basic fibroblast growth factor: reversal by suramin. *Proc. Natl. Acad. Sci. USA* **87,** 5346–5350.
51. Contag, C. H., Contag, P. R., Mullins, J. I., Spilman, S. D., Stevenson, D. K., and Benaron, D. A. (1995) Photonic detection of bacterial pathogens in living hosts. *Mol. Microbiol.* **18,** 593–603.
52. Contag, P. R., Olomu, I. N., Stevenson, D. K., and Contag, C. H. (1998) Bioluminescent indicators in living mammals. *Nat. Med.* **4,** 245–247.

53. Bou-Gharios, G., Garrett, L. A., Rossert, J., Niederreither, K., Eberspaecher, H., Smith, C., Black, C., and Crombrugghe, B. (1996) A potent far-upstream enhancer in the mouse pro alpha 2(I) collagen gene regulates expression of reporter genes in transgenic mice. *J. Cell. Biol.* **134,** 1333–1344.
54. Chatziantoniou, C., Boffa, J. J., Ardaillou, R., and Dussaule, J. C. (1998) Nitric oxide inhibition induces early activation of type I collagen gene in renal resistance vessels and glomeruli in transgenic mice: role of endothelin. *J. Clin. Invest.* **101,** 2780–2789.

Index

A

Actin,
  immunostaining of α-smooth
    muscle actin in angiogenesis
    model, 170, 172
  intestinal smooth muscle cell
    Western blot analysis, 421
Activin A, overexpression effects on
    wound healing in mice,
    200–202
Aging,
  animal models, 220
  clinical aspects of wound healing,
    227
  medication impairment of wound
    healing, 219, 220
  prospects for wound healing
    research, 227–230
  skin alterations, 217–219
  ultraviolet irradiation exposure
    effects in skin, 219
  wound healing alterations,
    extracellular matrix deposition,
      221
    fibronectin expression, 221
    growth factors, 222, 223
    history of study, 220, 221
    inflammatory phase of wound
      healing, 223–225
    matrix metalloproteinase
      expression, 222, 223
    proliferative phase of wound
      healing, 225, 226
    remodeling phase of wound
      healing, 226

Airway wound, *see* Tracheal injury
Alkaline phosphatase,
  immunostaining in
    angiogenesis model, 170,
    172
Alloxan, diabetes induction,
    182, 183
Angiogenesis,
  blood vessel density
    quantification in wound
    repair,
    anesthesia and euthanasia, 321,
      322, 325
    full-thickness excisional
      wound model, 322, 326
    image analysis, 323, 324
    immunohistochemistry, 322,
      323, 326
    markers, 319
    materials, 320, 321, 324
    rationale, 320
    sectioning of tissue, 322, 326
    software, 319, 320
  developmental angiogenesis, 319
  endothelial cell assays,
    see Endothelial cell
  Matrigel models,
    in vitro,
      angiogenic assay, 313, 3140
      cell culture, 312, 314
      conditioned medium
        preparation, 312–314
      imaging, 313, 314
      materials, 312–314
      Matrigel preparation, 313

overview, 311, 312
in vivo,
    angiogenic compound
        testing, 332–334
    antiangiogenic compound
        testing, 330, 333, 334
    materials, 331, 332
    microscopy, 333, 334
    mouse selection
        considerations, 330, 331
    overview of plug assay,
        329, 330
overview of in vivo models,
    161, 162
pathology, 337
severe combined
        immunodeficient mouse
        model,
    advantages, 168, 169
    biodegradable polymer
        matrices,
        fabrication, 169, 171
        types, 162
    human dermal microvascular
        endothelial cell
        transplantation, 162, 169,
        171, 173, 174
    immunostaining of
        microvessels,
        alkaline phosphatase,
            170, 172
        apoptosis, 170–174
        CD31, 170–174
        CD34, 170–172
        Flag, 170–172
        intracellular adhesion
            molecule-1, 166, 167,
            170–172
        overview, 166, 167
        α-smooth muscle actin,
            170, 172

vascular cell adhesion
            molecule-1, 166, 167,
            170–172
        von Willebrand factor,
            170–172
    materials, 169–171
    organizational stages of
        microvessel formation,
        167, 168
    principles, 162, 166
    steps, 337, 338
Antisense, *see* Plasminogen
        activator inhibitor type-1
Apoptosis,
    immunostaining in angiogenesis
        model, 170–174
    TUNEL assay of corneal injury
        samples, 78, 80, 81

B

BMP-6, *see* Bone morphogeneic
        protein-6
Bone morphogeneic protein-6
        (BMP-6), overexpression
        effects on wound healing in
        mice, 202
Boyden chamber migration assay,
        see Endothelial cell
Breaking strength, incisional
        wound,
    definition, 41
    determination, 39, 40
Burn injury, *see also* Partial-
        thickness injury,
    degree classification, 242
    histology of partial thickness
        burn, 243
    ideal criteria, 107
    mortality, 241
    porcine models, *see also*
            Partial-thickness injury,

advantages, 108, 109
contact burn induction, 113, 116
disadvantages, 109
dressing application, 113, 116, 118
hair removal, 112
healing outcome measurements,
  overview, 113
  reepithelialization, 114, 115, 118
  scarring, 115, 116
macroscopic description of
  burns, 113
materials, 110–112
preconditioning and
  anesthesia, 112, 116
scald versus contact burn
  induction, 110
site selection for wounding,
  109, 110
sepsis models in mice,
  anesthesia, 96–98, 104
  burn wound induction, 96, 98
  cecal ligation and puncture,
    controls, 103
    overview, 95
    technique, 101, 103–105
  materials, 96, 97
  Pseudomonas aeruginosa
    seeding of burn wounds,
    bacteria preparation,
      98–100, 104
    seeding, 100, 101
  resuscitation, 103
specimen collection and analysis
  from humans,
  burn wound specimens, 246
  controls, 248, 252
  immunohistochemical
    processing,

automation, 248, 253
cellular infiltrate evaluation,
  250, 251
controls, 249
overview, 248, 252, 253
staining, 249, 250
standards, 249
infected wound specimens,
  246, 247
institutional review board
  approval, 247, 251, 252
materials, 243, 245, 246
transport and storage of tissue,
  247, 248, 252
water scald model, 22

C

CD31, immunostaining in
  angiogenesis model,
  170–174
CD34, immunostaining in angiogenesis model, 170–172
Chemokines,
  amino-terminal processing,
    379–381
  classification, 378, 379
  CXCR2, knockout effects on
    wound healing in mice,
    204, 205
  domains, 381
  enzyme-linked immunosorbent
    assay,
    advantages, 382, 383
    incubation conditions, 383
    lung allograft rejection, 385
    materials, 383, 384
    pneumonia, 384, 385
    sample preparation, 383
  longevity and stability, 379–381
  receptors, 378, 379, 382
  specificity of action, 377, 378

Collagen, *see also* Fibroblast-
    populated collagen lattice,
    expanded polytetrafluoroethylene
    model,
    deposition of collagen, 266,
        267
    hydrolysis and amino acid
        determination, 270–272
    functions, 349
    polyvinyl alcohol sponge model
        analysis, 88, 92
    procollagen secretion assay in
        intestinal smooth muscle
        cells,
        cell culture and radiolabeling,
            419, 421, 422
        gel electrophoresis, 420
        materials, 418, 421
    synthesis assays,
        materials, 350–352, 355, 356
        overview, 349, 350
        quantitative analysis, 354–357
        radiolabeling tissue
            biopsies, 352
        sample preparation and
            hydrolysis, 353, 355, 356
        scintillation counting, 353,
            354, 356
Complementary DNA microarray,
    data analysis, 430–432
    hypertrophic scar formation study
        rationale, 425
    image analysis, 429, 430
    materials, 426, 427
    membrane hybridization, 429
    overview, 425, 426
    reverse transcription for RNA
        probe generation, 429
    RNA extraction, 428, 430, 431
    sample collection, 427, 428,
        430, 431

tissue selection, 427, 430
Corneal injury,
    advantages of models, 67, 68
    anatomy, 67
    mouse and rabbit models,
        anesthesia and euthanasia, 69,
            70, 78
        animals, 68, 70
        hemotoxylin and eosin
            staining, 78
        microinjection into stroma, 69,
            75, 76
        propidium iodide staining, 78
        sectioning of tissue, 70, 77, 78,
            80
        tissue procurement and
            fixation, 69, 76, 77
        TUNEL assay, 78, 80, 81
        wounding,
            lamellar flap formation,
                73–75, 78, 80
            laser injury, 71–73, 78, 80
            scrape injury, 71, 78, 80
CXCR2, knockout effects on
        wound healing in mice,
        204, 205

D

Diabetes mellitus models,
    chemical induction, 182, 183
    genetic models,
        insulin-dependent diabetes
            mellitus, 184
        insulin-resistant obese models,
            184–187
        overview, 183
    surgical induction, 182
    ulcer,
        pathogenesis, 181, 182
        platelet-derived growth factor
            treatment, 187

wound healing impairment, 181
DNA microarray, *see* Complementary
    DNA microarray

E

EGF, *see* Epidermal growth factor
ELISA, *see* Enzyme-linked
    immunosorbent assay
Endothelial cell,
    angiogenesis assays in vitro,
        capillary formation assay,
            338, 339
        chemokinesis assay, 339
        endothelial cell proliferation,
            338
        migration assay in Boyden
            chamber,
            chamber cleaning and
                sterilization, 343
            chamber setup and assay,
                341, 342, 344
            endothelial cell propagation
                and freezing, 341, 344
            materials, 340, 344
            membrane preparation,
                341, 344
            principles, 339, 340
            quantitative analysis, 342–345
        overview, 338, 343, 344
        wound model, 338
    severe combined
        immunodeficient mouse
        model of angiogenesis,
        advantages, 168, 169
        biodegradable polymer
            matrices,
            fabrication, 169, 171
            types, 162
        human dermal microvascular
            endothelial cell transplanta-
            tion, 162, 169, 171, 173, 174

immunostaining of micro-
    vessels, 166, 167, 170–174
materials, 169–171
organizational stages of
    microvessel formation,
    167, 168
principles, 162, 166
Enzyme-linked immunosorbent
    assay (ELISA), chemokines,
    advantages, 382, 383
    incubation conditions, 383
    lung allograft rejection, 385
    materials, 383, 384
    pneumonia, 384, 385
    sample preparation, 383
Epidermal growth factor (EGF),
    particle-mediated gene
    transfer, 440
Evaporimetry, epidermal healing
    assay, 29, 30
Excisional wound healing model,
    advantages, 5
    embedding tissue for histology,
        7, 12, 14
    excisional wounding, 5, 7–9, 12, 13
    materials, 5–7, 12
    overview, 3, 4
    protein preparation, 7, 12–14
    RNA preparation, 5, 6, 10, 12
    wound biopsy specimen isolation,
        5, 9, 10, 13
Expanded polytetrafluoroethylene
    model,
    collagen,
        deposition, 266, 267
        hydrolysis and amino acid
            determination, 270–272
    materials, 267, 268
    polymer tubes,
        delipidization and drying,
            269–271

implantation and removal, 268, 269, 271
measurement of dried tubes, 270, 272
preparation and sterilization, 268, 271
principles, 266, 267

F

Fetal wound,
cytokine modulation of repair, 149
fibroblast explantation,
explanting of skin, 156, 158
materials, 150, 151
preparation, 154, 158
skin harvesting, 154–156
rat model,
anesthesia, 151, 156, 157
harvesting of wounds, 154
materials, 150, 151
overview, 149
wound creation, 151–154, 157, 158
FGF, *see* Fibroblast growth factor
Fibroblast,
aging effects on wound healing response, 225
explantation from fetal wound,
explanting of skin, 156, 158
materials, 150, 151
preparation, 154, 158
skin harvesting, 154–156
isolation from polyvinyl alcohol sponge model, 89, 92
Fibroblast growth factor (FGF),
fibroblast growth factor-2 knockout mouse and delayed reepithialization, 196, 197
receptors, 192

types, 192
Fibroblast-populated collagen lattice (FPCL),
casting of free-floating lattice, 284, 289
cell morphology, 282, 283
cell sources, 286–288
collagen,
concentration, 284, 285
isolation and purification, 283, 284
limited proteolysis, 286
types, 285, 286
contraction mechanism,
fibroblasts and tractional forces, 280–282
myofibroblast role, 280
overview, 279, 280
fatty acid enrichment of membranes, 288, 289
fibroblast density effects, 289
materials, 283–289
modifications,
attached model, 278, 279
stress-relaxed model, 279
principles, 277, 278
Flag, immunostaining in angiogenesis model, 170–172
FPCL, *see* Fibroblast-populated collagen lattice

G

Gene therapy,
delivery approaches, 434, 435
growth factors and cytokines, 434
particle-mediated gene transfer,
advantages and limitations, 439, 440
applications, 440–442, 444
cartridge preparation, 446

gene expression response, 438, 439

gene gun loading and firing, 447, 448

growth factor delivery, 440–442

materials, 444, 445

principles, 436, 438

prospects, 442, 444

sample preparation, 445–447

target preparation by incision, mouse, 446, 447

rabbit, 447

rat, 446–448

wound repair prospects, 229, 230, 433

Guinea pig models, *see* Tracheal injury

H

Hunt-Shilling wire mesh chamber model, features, 265

Hydrogen peroxide, macrophage assay, 371, 374

I

ICAM-1, *see* Intracellular adhesion molecule-1

IL-6, *see* Interleukin-6

IL-10, *see* Interleukin-10

Implantable wound healing models, *see also* Expanded polytetrafluoroethylene model; Polyvinyl alcohol sponge model,

Hunt-Shilling wire mesh chamber model, 265

microdialysis, 264, 265

overview, 263

viscose cellulose sponge model, 263, 264

Incisional wound healing, animal models, 40

breaking strength, definition, 41

determination, 39, 40

clinical significance, 37

formalin fixation of tissue, 42

impairing factors, 38, 39

limitations of models, 133, 134

mouse model, clip removal, 45, 51

materials, 42–44

wound disruption strength determination, 46, 47, 51, 52

wounding, 44, 45, 47–50

phases, 37, 38

tensile strength, 40, 41

Interferon-γ-inducible protein-10 (IP-10), overexpression effects on wound healing in mice, 203, 204

Interleukin-6 (IL-6), aging effects on wound healing response, 226

knockout effects on wound healing in mice, 202, 203

Interleukin-10 (IL-10), null graft scarring in mice, 205

Intestinal anastomosis models, mouse models, colon anastomosis, 136

euthanasia and anastomoses preparation, 136, 137

materials, 134, 135, 137

postoperative care, 136, 138

preoperative preparation, 135

small intestine anastomosis, 135–138

tensiometry, 137–139

overview, 133, 134

Intestinal smooth muscle cell,

immunoblotting of cytoskeletal
proteins,
materials, 418, 421
Western blot, 420, 421
isolation and culture,
culture, 419
dissection, 419
harvesting, 418
materials, 417, 418, 421
procollagen secretion assay,
cell culture and radiolabeling,
419, 421, 422
gel electrophoresis, 420
materials, 418, 421
Intracellular adhesion molecule-1
(ICAM-1), immunostaining
in angiogenesis model, 166,
167, 170–172
IP-10, *see* Interferon-γ-inducible
protein-10
Ischemic wound healing,
overview of models, 55, 56
rabbit model,
advantages, 56
animal preparation, 56, 57
materials, 56, 56, 62
microscopic analysis, 57, 61,
62, 64
pedicle dissection, 57, 58, 60,
62
principles, 56
treatment with healing
agents, 60
wound harvesting, 57, 60, 61, 64
wounding, 57, 60, 63
rat model, 56, 62

K

Keratinocyte,
plasminogen activator inhibitor
type-1 expression,

see Plasminogen activator
inhibitor type-1
skin organ culture, *see* Skin organ
culture
Keratinocyte growth factor (KGF),
dominant-negative mutant
impairment of
reepithialization, 192, 193
knockout mouse effects on
wound healing, 193, 195
KGF, *see* Keratinocyte growth
factor
Knockout mouse, *see* Transgenic/
knockout mouse, wound-
healing studies

L

Laser, corneal injury, 71–73, 78, 80
Leukocyte,
extravasation, 378
immunostaining at injury site,
analysis, 364, 366, 367
immunostaining of T-cells,
362–366
materials, 360–362, 364
overview, 360
sample collection and
sectioning, 360, 361, 365
mononuclear cell retrieval from
polyvinyl alcohol sponge
model, 90, 92
wound invasion and healing, 359
Lucigenin-dependent
chemiluminescence,
macrophage assay, 371, 374

M

Macrophage,
assays,
hydrogen peroxide release,
371, 374

lucigenin-dependent
chemiluminescence, 371, 374
materials, 370–372, 375
oxygen consumption, 371,
372, 375
superoxide formation in cell-
free lysates, 370, 373, 374
superoxide release, 370, 372,
373, 375
characteristics in wounds, 369
mononuclear cell retrieval from
polyvinyl alcohol sponge
model, 90, 92
Matrigel angiogenesis model, *see*
Angiogenesis
Microarray, *see* Complementary
DNA microarray
Microdialysis,
implantable wound healing
models, 264, 265
oxygen assay, 405–407
Mouse models, *see* Angiogenesis;
Burn injury; Corneal injury;
Excisional wound healing
model; Incisional wound
healing; Intestinal
anastomosis models;
Peritoneal adhesion
formation; Transgenic/
knockout mouse, wound-
healing studies

N

Neutrophil, *see* Leukocyte
Nitric oxide (NO), aging effects on
wound healing response, 224
NO, *see* Nitric oxide
Northern blot, plasminogen activator inhibitor type-1
expression analysis in wound
healing, 295, 298, 299

O

Oxygen,
cell culture measurement, 407–
409
historical perspective of
measurement in wounds,
389, 390
macrophage assay of
consumption, 371, 372, 375
microdialysis assay, 405–407
microelectrodes for measurement,
389, 400
rabbit ear chamber model for
measurement,
advantages, 394, 410, 411
materials, 390, 391, 409, 410
overview, 393, 394
technique, 394–396, 411
subcutaneous wound tissue
oximetry,
materials, 392, 393, 410
overview, 399–401
Psqo$_2$ measurement, 392, 393,
402–404, 412–414
tonometer,
placement, 392, 401, 402, 412
preparation, 392, 401, 412
removal, 404
transcutaneous measurement in
lower extremity ulcers,
materials, 393
overview, 404, 405
technique, 405, 414, 415
wire mesh cylinder model,
cylinder preparation,
rabbit, 398
rat, 397
implantation, 399, 411, 412
materials, 391, 392
overview, 396, 397
wound healing role, 389, 394

P

PAI-1, *see* Plasminogen activator
   inhibitor type-1
Partial-thickness injury,
  definition, 19
  epidermal regeneration
    mechanism, 19, 20
  excision models, 21
  porcine thermal injury model,
   advantages, 23, 24
   anesthesia, 26, 31
   burn injury, 26, 27, 31, 32
   data analysis, 30, 31, 33
   disadvantages, 24, 25
   dressing and treatment of
    injury, 27, 28, 32
   epidermal healing assays,
    evaporimetry, 29, 30
    planimetric analysis, 28,
     29, 33
    strip biopsy, 29, 33
    wound excision, 29
   materials, 25, 26, 31
   monitoring of wounds and
    anesthesia, 28
   overview, 22, 23
Particle-mediated gene transfer,
  see Gene therapy
PDGF, *see* Platelet-derived growth
  factor
Peritoneal adhesion formation,
  assessment, 141, 142
  clinical significance, 141
  mouse model,
   abdominal wall tissue
    harvesting, 144, 147
   data interpretation and
    statistical analysis, 147
   materials, 142, 143
   overview, 142
   talc injection, 143, 144, 147

tissue analysis,
    microscopy and histology,
     145–147
    processing, 144
    sectioning, 145
    staining, 145
Plasminogen activator inhibitor
  type-1 (PAI-1), expression
  in epithelial injury model,
  antisense vector transfection of
   keratinocytes,
   materials, 295, 296, 302
   plasmid preparation, 299
   transfection, 299, 300
   vector construction, 295, 302
  keratinocyte culture, 294
  materials, 294–296, 300–302
  microscopy of wound closure
   rate, 294, 296–298
  Northern blot analysis, 295,
   298, 299
  overview, 293, 294
  Western blot analysis, 296, 300
Platelet-derived growth factor
  (PDGF),
  diabetic ulcer treatment, 187
  particle-mediated gene transfer,
   440, 441
  wound healing in aging, 227, 228
Polyvinyl alcohol sponge model,
  animal species selection, 84
  cell retrieval from wounds,
   fibroblasts, 89, 92
   mononuclear cells, 90, 92
   overview, 89
   RNA preparation, 91
  collagen analysis, 88, 92
  fluid harvesting from wounds,
   88, 92
  human models, 92
  materials, 84–86

principles, 83, 265, 266
rationale, 84
sponge,
    preparation, 86, 87
    removal, 88, 92
wounding, 87
wound manipulation model, 91,
    92
Porcine models, *see* Burn injury;
    Partial-thickness injury
Propidium iodide, corneal injury
    sample staining, 78
Pseudomonas aeruginosa seeding of
    burn wounds,
    bacteria preparation, 98–100, 104
    seeding, 100, 101

R

Rabbit models, *see* Corneal injury;
    Ischemic wound healing
Rat models, *see* Fetal wound;
    Ischemic wound healing

S

Scarring,
    burn injury analysis, 115, 116
    complementary DNA microarray
        analysis, *see*
        Complementary DNA
        microarray
    interleukin-10 null graft scarring
        in mice, 205
Senescence, wound repair
    studies, 228
Sepsis, *see* Burn injury
Severe combined immunodeficient
    mouse, *see* Angiogenesis
Skin, function and anatomy, 242
Skin organ culture,
    advantages, 305, 306
    culture, 306

hemotoxylin and eosin staining,
    307, 309
immunohistochemical techniques,
    308
keratinocyte,
    preparation, 307
    transplantation, 306, 307, 309
materials, 306
punch biopsy, 306, 308, 309
reepithelialization studies, 305
Smad3, knockout effects on wound
    healing in mice, 199, 200
Smooth muscle cell, *see* Intestinal
    smooth muscle cell
Sponge model, *see* Implantable
    wound healing models
Sponge model, *see* Polyvinyl
    alcohol sponge model
Stat-3, knockout effects on wound
    healing in mice, 203
Streptozotocin, diabetes induction,
    182, 183
Strip biopsy, epidermal healing
    assay, 29, 33
Suction blister model,
    analysis,
        intact blisters, 259
        open blisters, 258, 259
    applications, 255
    blister induction, 257, 258, 260
    healing process, 255, 256
    materials, 256, 257, 259, 260
    principles, 21, 22
Superoxide, macrophage assay,
    formation in cell-free lysates,
        370, 373, 374
    release, 370, 372, 373, 375

T

Tape abrasion model, principles, 20
T-cell, *see* Leukocyte

Telomere, shortening in aging, 228, 229

Tensile strength,
incisional wound, 40, 41
intestinal anastomoses, 137–139
tensiometers, 134

TGF-α, *see* Transforming growth factor-α

TGF-β, *see* Transforming growth factor-β

TNF-α, *see* Tumor necrosis factor-α

Tracheal injury,
guinea pig model,
adaptation to other species, 130, 131
digital imaging of wounds, 125, 127, 128, 131
materials, 123–125
overview, 122, 123
tracheal injury, 123–125, 130
healing overview, 121, 122

Transforming growth factor-α (TGF-α), knockout effects on wound healing in mice, 195, 196

Transforming growth factor-β (TGF-β),
functions, 197
isoforms, 197
superfamily members, 197
transforming growth factor-β1
aging effects on wound healing response, 225, 226
knockout effects on wound healing in mice, 197–199, 207
overexpression effects on wound healing in mice, 199
particle-mediated gene transfer, 441

Transgenic/knockout mouse, wound-healing studies,
activin A overexpression effects, 200–202
bone morphogeneic protein-6 overexpression effects, 202
CXCR2 knockout effects, 204, 205
fibroblast growth factor-2 knockout and delayed reepithialization, 196, 197
inducible systems, 207, 208
interferon-γ-inducible protein-10 overexpression effects, 203, 204
interleukin-6 knockout effects, 202, 203
interleukin-10 null graft scarring, 205
keratinocyte growth factor,
dominant-negative mutant impairment of reepithialization, 192, 193
knockout mouse, 193, 195
overview, 191, 192, 194, 195
Smad3 knockout effects, 199, 200
Stat-3 knockout effects, 203
transforming growth factor-α knockout studies, 195, 196
transforming growth factor-β1 knockout effects, 197–199, 207
overexpression effects, 199
vimentin knockout studies in embryo wound repair, 205

Tumor necrosis factor-α (TNF-α), aging effects on wound healing response, 224

TUNEL assay, corneal injury samples, 78, 80, 81

V

Vascular cell adhesion molecule-1 (VCAM-1),
immunostaining in angiogenesis model, 166, 167, 170–172

Vascular endothelial growth factor (VEGF), aging effects on wound healing response, 225

VCAM-1, *see* Vascular cell adhesion molecule-1

VEGF, *see* Vascular endothelial growth factor

Vimentin, knockout studies in mouse embryo wound repair, 205

Viscose cellulose sponge model, features, 263, 264

von Willebrand factor, immunostaining in angiogenesis model, 170–172

W

Water scald model, principles, 22

Western blot,
cytoskeletal proteins in intestinal smooth muscle cells, 420, 421
plasminogen activator inhibitor type-1 expression analysis in wound healing, 296, 300

Wound healing, *see also* specific models and wound types,
growth factor enhancement, 17, 19, 20
phases, 17, 223–226
timeline for burn healing, 250, 251

Wound oximetry, *see* Oxygen

About the Editors

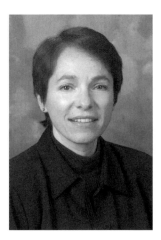

Luisa A. DiPietro received her DDS and PhD in Microbiology and Immunology from the University of Illinois at Chicago. Dr. DiPietro is currently an Associate Professor in the Department of Surgery at Loyola University Medical Center in Maywood, Illinois, where she is the Vice Chair for Research for the Department of Surgery and the Director of Research for the Burn and Shock Trauma Institute.

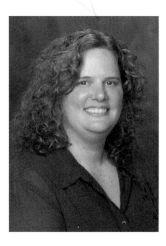

Aime L. Burns received her BS in Biology from Kalamazoo College and MS in Neuroscience from Yale University. She has held positions at Mt. Sinai Medical Center, New York, and Northwestern University, Chicago. She is currently a member of the Burn and Shock Trauma Institute at Loyola University Medical Center in Maywood, Illinois.